CHROMOSOMAL ABNORMALITIES - A HALLMARK MANIFESTATION OF GENOMIC INSTABILITY

Edited by **Marcelo L. Larramendy**
and **Sonia Soloneski**

Chromosomal Abnormalities - A Hallmark Manifestation of Genomic Instability
http://dx.doi.org/10.5772/65142
Edited by Marcelo L. Larramendy and Sonia Soloneski

Contributors

Ksenija Gersak, Ziva Miriam Gersak, Nevim Aygun, Tatiana Gindina, Nikolay Mamaev, Boris Afanasyev, Rasime Kalkan, Benjamín Rodríguez-Garay, Yoko Matsuda, Olga Simonova, Roman Cherezov, Julia Vorontsova, Pinar Tulay, Alicia Leonor Basso Abraham, Diana CJ Spierings, Hilda Van Den Bos, Floris Foijer, Peter M Lansdorp

Published by InTech

Janeza Trdine 9, 51000 Rijeka, Croatia

Publishing Process Manager Marijana Francetic
Technical Editor SPi Global
Cover InTech Design team

First published August, 2017
Printed in Croatia
Legal deposit, Croatia: National and University Library in Zagreb

Additional hard copies can be obtained from orders@intechopen.com

Chromosomal Abnormalities - A Hallmark Manifestation of Genomic Instability, Edited by Marcelo L. Larramendy and Sonia Soloneski
p. cm.
Print ISBN 978-953-51-3473-2
Online ISBN 978-953-51-3474-9

For EU product safety concerns:
IN TECH d.o.o., Prolaz Marije Krucifikse Kozulić 3, 51000 Rijeka, Croatia,
info@intechopen.com or visit our website at intechopen.com.

Meet the editors

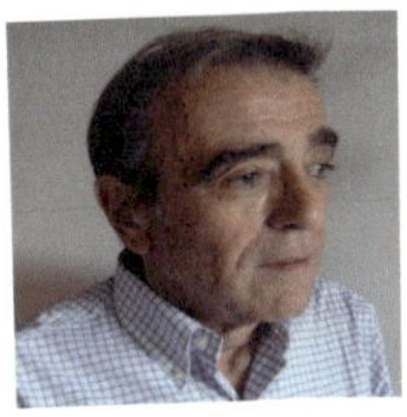

Marcelo L. Larramendy, Ph.D., serves as Professor of Molecular Cell Biology at the School of Natural Sciences and Museum (National University of La Plata, Argentina). Appointed Senior Researcher of the National Scientific and Technological Research Council of Argentina. Former Member of the Executive Committee of the Latin American Association of Environmental Mutagenesis, Teratogenesis and Carcinogenesis. Author of more than 470 contributions, including scientific publications, research communications and conferences worldwide. Recipient of several national and international awards. Prof. Larramendy is a regular Lecturer at the international A. Hollaender Courses organized by the IAEMS and former guest scientist at NIH (USA) and University of Helsinki, (Finland). He is expert in Genetic Toxicology and is, or has been, referee for more than 30 international scientific journals. Member of the International Panel of Experts at the International Agency for Research on Cancer (IARC, WHO, Lyon, France) in 2015 for the evaluation of DDT, 2,4-D and Lindane. Presently, Prof. Dr. Larramendy is Head of the Laboratory of Molecular Cytogenetics and Genotoxicology at the UNLP.

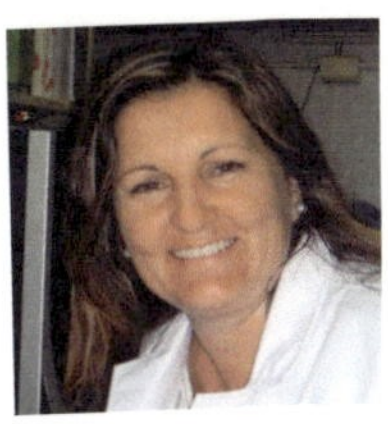

Sonia Soloneski is PhD in Natural Sciences and Professor Assistant of Molecular Cell Biology at the Faculty of Natural Sciences and Museum of La Plata, National University of La Plata, Argentina. She became a member of the National Scientific and Technological Research Council (CONICET) of Argentina in Genetic Toxicology field. Presently, she is member of the Latin American Association of Environmental Mutagenesis, Teratogenesis and Carcinogenesis (ALAMCTA), the Society of Environmental Toxicology and Chemistry, the Argentinean Society of Toxicology (ATA), and the Argentinean Society of Genetics (SAG). She is authored of more than 320 scientific publications on the field, including scientific publications in research papers, reviewed journals and conferences worldwide. She is a referent for on issues related to Genetic Toxicology, Mutagenesis and Ecotoxicology field.

Contents

Preface

Genome replication is a highly conserved, essential biological process to preserve genetic information across generations. Perturbations in genome replication represent significant challenges for cells from prokaryotic and eukaryotic organisms. Thus, this process needs to be highly regulated to occur only once per cell cycle in order to ensure the preservation of genome integrity and to promote faithful genome propagation from a parental cell to the two daughter cells. Living cells have developed several mechanisms to preserve genome stability. The genome replication process includes several aspects to ensure the fidelity of DNA replication, an efficient DNA repair system, if required, and an optimal mechanical mechanism for achieving a normal segregation of the genetic material into the daughter cells.

Genomic instability in the form of mutations and chromosomal abnormalities has a key role in pathological disorders as well as in the evolution process by generating genetic variation. Chromosomal instability is a process that leads to cells with unbalanced genomes, containing both numerical and/or structural abnormalities. For more than a century, the loss of stability of the genome has been and is still accepted as one of the most important aspects of carcinogenesis. In humans, it is often associated with premature aging and with inherited diseases. Chromosomal abnormalities have been recognized for a long time and have generally proven to be a highly specific biomarker of malignancy in the majority of, if not all, neoplastic processes. Furthermore, it is well known that chromosomal abnormalities represent one of the leading causes of pregnancy loss and developmental disabilities and are the highest risk factors that might contribute to the natural aging process. Understanding the structural and molecular bases of chromosomal abnormalities remains a basic challenge in cellular biology in general and in cytogenetics in particular.

Chromosomal abnormalities are mainly classified into two groups: structural aberrations and numerical alterations. Structural rearrangements encompass several different classes of events such as gene amplification or deletion, translocation, duplication, inversion, and ring formation, whereas numerical abnormalities include euploidy or aneuploidy. Structural chromosome abnormalities can originate from DNA breakage of the double helices in the genome at two different locations, followed by a rejoining of the broken ends to produce a new chromosomal rearrangement, whereas numerical abnormalities can form through various errors in the mitotic spindle checkpoint and some cellular processes during mitosis. Numerous genetic testing methodologies have been developed rapidly over the last decade, including cytogenetic, biochemical, and molecular approaches, to detect these different types of abnormalities. However, the causes and consequences of these aberrations still remain far from being fully understood. Thus, further investigations into the mechanisms of the origins of chromosomal instability would broaden insights regarding the structure and function of chromosomes.

This single volume comprises 10 high-quality chapters describing the implications of the generation of chromosomal abnormalities in genetic material. The first chapter comprises an excellent review about the general principles of chromosomal abnormalities and the molecular cytogenetic techniques that can help in the identification of the presence or absence of a particular DNA sequence or the evaluation of the number or organization of chromosomes or a chromosomal region, as well as the importance of employing these methodologies in diagnostic procedures in numerous areas of clinical medicine, including hematology, perinatology, and obstetrics. This is followed by the second chapter providing information from morphological markers of chromosomal instability employed for prognoses of cancers, with special emphasis on descriptions of atypical mitosis including multipolar, ring, dispersed, asymmetrical, and lag-type mitoses as well as nuclear atypia such as micronuclei formation. The third chapter presents an update in the field, describing the acquired structural and numerical chromosomal abnormalities in solid tumors and presents potential formation mechanisms. In this chapter, the relationship between long inverted repeat sequences and *MYCN* oncogene amplification in neuroblastoma is also discussed. The fourth chapter discusses specific treatment options, including allogeneic hematopoietic stem cell transplantation in both acute myeloid and acute lymphoblastic patients, with some prognostically proven cytogenetic variants such as the presence of hyperdiploid karyotypes, monosomies, and complex chromosomal rearrangements. The fifth chapter provides an overview about the occurrence of the aneuploidy process in brain cells from normal individuals and Alzheimer's patients as well as a discussion of the possible mechanisms to explain the origin of aneuploidy and the pros and cons of different techniques used to analyze aneuploidy in brain cells. The sixth chapter presents a contribution showing how X chromosome abnormalities as well as low-level mosaicism for this chromosome can be implicated in reproductive consequences in phenotypically normal women with recurrent pregnancy loss and/or fertility problems. The seventh chapter is a detailed overview about the applications of two genetic tests, preimplantation genetic diagnosis (also known as PGD) and preimplantation genetic screening (also known as PGS), for the estimation of translocations and detection of aneuploidy, respectively. The eighth chapter highlights how a decrease in expression of the basic transcription factor TRF2 can result in chromatin condensation abnormalities in a validated experimental organism model, *Drosophila* sp.. The ninth chapter presents a description of normal karyotypes and chromosomal abnormalities through comprehension of chromosomal variation within fruit fly populations as models for studying genetic polymorphisms. The book ends with a chapter describing a hypothesis showing how frying pan–shaped chromosomes are formed by sister chromatid exchanges and a premature kinetochore movement in prophase II in two agave plants, *Agave stricta* and *A. angustifolia*. Furthermore, the authors postulate the presence of genes that are prone to act under diverse kinds of environmental stress.

The editors of *Chromosomal Abnormalities - A Hallmark Manifestation of Genomic Instability* are enormously grateful to all the contributing authors for sharing their knowledge and insight in this book project. They have made an extensive effort to arrange the information included in every valuable chapter. This book is designed to provide an introduction and overview and could be consulted by scientific readers and readers not familiar with the field. The publication of this book is of high importance for those researchers, scientists, biologists, geneticists, and veterinarians, as well as teachers and advanced-level students, who make use of these different investigations to understand the origin and implications of chromosomal aberrations and to guide them in the future investigations.

Sonia Soloneski, PhD, and Marcelo L. Larramendy, PhD
School of Natural Sciences and Museum
National University of La Plata
La Plata, Argentina

Chapter 1

The Use of Molecular Cytogenetic Techniques for the Identification of Chromosomal Abnormalities

Rasime Kalkan

Additional information is available at the end of the chapter

http://dx.doi.org/10.5772/67415

Abstract

Chromosomal analysis is an increasingly important diagnostic procedure in numerous areas of clinical medicine that includes haematology, perinatology or obstetrics. Chromosomal disorders are viewed as a major category of genetic diseases, and sometimes the identification of abnormal chromosomes is not easily applicable. Just like the identification of the marker chromosome or the identification of the complex karyotypes is important in clinics for the evaluation of the patient prognosis as well as the treatment response, needless to say; fluorescence in situ hybridization (FISH) is the most suitable and rapid method in the above-mentioned situations. It gives chance to the rapid analysis of chromosomal aneuploidies in dividing and non-dividing cells. In this chapter, we will discuss the general principles of the chromosomal abnormalities and the molecular cytogenetic techniques that can help the identification of presence or absence of a particular DNA sequence or the evaluation of the number of organization of a chromosome or chromosomal region.

Keywords: FISH, chromosomal abnormalities, marker chromosome, molecular cytogenetics, cytogenetics

1. Introduction

A chromosome is the condensed version of the DNA, and it contains two sister chromatids. The critical parts are consisted of centromere, telomere and nucleolar organizing regions [1]. Depending on the mechanism, chromosomal abnormalities can be classified under two-major groups, numerical and structural abnormalities. The non-disjunction of chromosomes or anaphase lagging is the major cause of the numerical chromosome abnormalities. The structural abnormalities can be classified as balanced and unbalanced abnormalities. Balanced structural abnormalities include translocations, insertions and inversions. Unbalanced structural abnormalities include deletions, duplications, marker and ring chromosomes [2, 3]. The identification of these numerical and structural abnormalities has an impact on the diagnosis of the syndromes, understanding of the phenotypic effects of chromosomal abnormalities, identification of the diagnosis and prognosis of haematological malignancies or solid tumours [3]. From that perspective, one can say that the identification of chromosome abnormalities has an important role in several conditions.

The diagnosis of chromosomal abnormalities is the most important factor in haematology, prenatal genetics and postnatal diagnosis of genetic conditions [4–6]. The identification of the chromosomal abnormalities in foetus is one of the most important thing in modern perinatology, or the identification of the BCR/ABL translocation in CML (Chronic Myeloid Leukaemia) is the most important diagnostic and prognostic factor in haematology. Chromosomal abnormalities involve the pathogenesis of several clinical conditions like infertility or hematologic malignancies and are important indicators for their diagnosis and prognosis [4, 5, 7]. There are a several methods that can be used to detect the genetic changes in genetic clinics include:

(a) conventional cytogenetics (karyotyping on cells derived from cell cultures using banding analysis; G-banding);

(b) molecular cytogenetics, e.g., fluorescence in situ hybridization (FISH), multicolour FISH, locus-specific FISH;

(c) molecular techniques to analyse DNA, RNA or proteins directly, e.g. the polymerase chain reaction (PCR), reverse transcriptase PCR (RT-PCR), quantitative real-time RT-PCR (RQ-PCR; qRTPCR), array CGH (comparative genomic hybridization), NGS (next generation sequencing), and microarray analysis [8].

Conventional cytogenetics is the golden standard and most comprehensive method to assess chromosomal abnormalities, especially numerical and structural chromosome aberrations. Technical issues like the need for fresh sample, difficulties in identification of masked or cryptic aberrations due to limited resolution by classic banding techniques have resulted in an increased use of molecular cytogenetic techniques, such as FISH, to identify specific abnormalities that are useful in either the diagnosis or management of hematologic disorders and are important tools for the identification of the cryptic translocations and sub-telomeric deletions in dysmorphic or mentally/developmentally retarded patients [8–12].

This chapter summarizes the structural abnormalities and the use of molecular cytogenetics as well as the identification of the chromosomal abnormalities.

1.1. Indications of the chromosome analysis in prenatal, postnatal ctyogenetics and haematological malignancies

Chromosomal analysis can be used as a golden standard for pre-natal and post-natal genetic diagnostic testing.

- In prenatal diagnosis, prenatal chromosomal analysis is applied during the following conditions.
- Presence of structural chromosomal or genome abnormality in one of the parents.
- Previous child with de novo chromosomal aneuploidy or another genomic imbalance.
- Higher maternal ages.
- Positive family history.
- Abnormal findings during the maternal serum screening.
- Abnormal USG finding.
- Stillbirth or neonatal deaths [2].

Postnatally chromosome analysis is applied during the following conditions:

- Fertility problems.
- Suspected syndrome identification.
- Mentally or developmentally retarded patients.
- Problems of early growth and development.
- Family history.
- Neoplasm [2].

Prognostic and predictive chromosome analysis in haematological malignancies:

Chromosomal abnormalities are important for the chromosomal and molecular changes as well as the identification of specific hematologic malignancies and syndromes and have important therapeutic and prognostic impacts, which include [13]:

- t(15;17)PML/RARa is characteristic for acute promyelocytic leukaemia (APL), that is a unique variant of acute myeloid leukaemia (AML) treated with ATRA and arsenic dioxide.
- t(8;21) or inv(16) comprises the favourable risk group of AML.
- Deletions of 5q, monosomy 7, deletion of 7q, trisomy 8, deletion of 9q, trisomy 11, trisomy 13, and trisomy 1 are the unbalanced abnormalities in AML.
- Acute myeloid leukaemia with associated abnormalities of 11q23 has an intermediate survival. The *MLL* gene at 11q23 is involved in a number of translocations with different partner chromosomes. The more common translocations observed in childhood AML are t(9;11)(p21;q23) and t(11;19)(q23;p13).
- The complex karyotype in AML predicts a poor prognosis.

- t(9;22)BCR/ABL is typical for chronic myeloid leukaemia (CML), although it may be seen in AML, where it is associated with a poor prognosis.
- In MDS, the typical abnormalities are partial and complete chromosome loss, most commonly −5, 5q−, −7, 7q−, +8, 11q−, 13q−, 20q−, and −Y [6, 14, 15].

Understanding the role of chromosomal abnormalities in the pathogenesis of haematological malignancies led to the development of a selective treatment options and gives prognosis information [13, 16–20].

1.2. FISH development

The development fluorescence in situ hybridization (FISH) technique increased the resolution of visualization of the chromosome rearrangements which is at the submicroscopic level [12, 21]. The FISH is applied on metaphase chromosomes, interphase nuclei, fixed tissues or cells and solid tumour samples [22]. The procedure contains denaturation, hybridization, post hybridization washes, which removes unbound single-strand DNA and after washing, an anti-fade solution containing DAPI (4′,6-diamidino-2-phenylindole) is applied to the slide, and a coverslip must be added (**Figure 1**) [23]. For FISH analysis, epifluorescence microscopes with specific filters and for identifying fluorochromes, a charge-coupled device (CCD) camera that captures the images were needed. A huge range of probes can be used for the identification of the chromosome abnormalities, which includes whole-chromosome painting probes, chromosome-arm painting probes, repetitive centromeric, subtelomeric and locus-specific

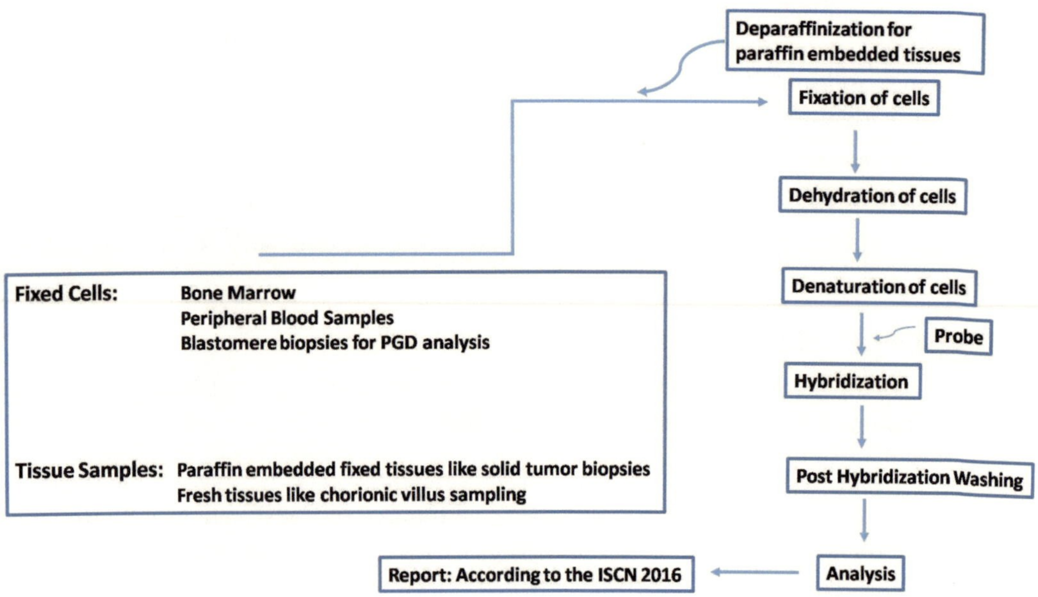

Figure 1. Algorithm for FISH analysis.

probes [24]. First, FISH probes obtained chromosome flow sorting [25] or microdissection [26] using universal degenerate oligonucleotide-primed PCR (DOP-PCR) [26].

There are different applications which used FISH-based methods like reverse-FISH [27], fibre-FISH [28, 29], M-FISH (multicolor FISH) [30], SKY (spectral karyotyping FISH) [31], flow-FISH [32], Q-FISH (quantitative FISH) [33], COBRA-FISH (combined binary ratio labelling FISH) [34], cenM-FISH (centromere-specific M-FISH) [35], podFISH (parental origin determination FISH) [36] and heterochromatin-M-FISH [37]. The most advanced FISH-based approaches included COBRA-FISH, M-FISH and SKY. These techniques give chance to the simultaneous visualization and the detection of all human chromosomes. These three FISH techniques use similar probes to be able to stain each of the 24 human chromosomes with a different colour [38].

Another high-resolution molecular cytogenetic technique for metaphase chromosomes, which gives chance to analyse chromosomes, is called multicolour banding (MCB). This technique involves the microdissection of chromosomal loci to obtain a set of probes that produce multi-colour pseudo-G-banding [39].

1.3. The use of FISH analysis in clinical diagnosis

Fluorescent in situ hybridization (FISH) was used for mapping human genes [40–43], and today, this technology is utilized for the characterization of chromosomal rearrangements and marker chromosomes [25, 44], the detection of microdeletions [45], and the prenatal diagnosis of common aneuploidies [46, 47], the detection of prognostic or predictive chromosomal abnormalities in haematological malignancies in clinical cytogenetic laboratories. At the same time, numerous DNA probes have been commercialized, further promoting the wide-spread clinical applications of molecular cytogenetic. Many new FISH techniques have been developed, including primed in situ labelling (PRINS [48]), fibre FISH [29, 49], comparative genomic hybridization (CGH) [50], chromosome microdissection [51, 52], spectral karyotyping (SKY [31]), multiple colour FISH (M-FISH [30, 53]), colour banding [54], FISH with multiple sub-telomeric probes [55], and array-based CGH [56, 57]. With the current FISH techniques, deletion or rearrangement of a single gene can be detected, cryptic chromosome translocations can be visualized, the copy number of oncogenes amplified in tumour cells can be assessed, and very complex rearrangements can be fully characterized. Using interphase FISH, genomic alterations can be studied in virtually all types of human tissues at any stage of cell division, without the need of cell culture and chromosome preparation. In that case, FISH is a unique technique that gives way to identification of numerical or structural chromosomal abnormalities in 1–3 days. The biggest advantage of the FISH technique is that it is more cost effective and labour intensive than the quantitative PCR (q-PCR) or other molecular genetics techniques.

Depending on the suspected genetic abnormalities type, the FISH probes can be generally subclassified into the following categories:

(a) Centromere-specific probes.

(b) Whole chromosome ('painting') probes.

(c) Single-copy (locus-specific) genomic probes.

(d) Spectral karyotyping (SKY; multiplex metaphase FISH; multi-colour FISH).

(e) Translocation fusion probes [58].

2. Identification of the translocations

Translocation involves the exchange of chromosome segments between two chromosomes [2]. The balanced reciprocal translocation carrier individuals are clinically normal; they do have an increased risk for having children with unbalanced karyotypes secondary to meiotic non-disjunction of their translocation [1]. In addition to being inherited, reciprocal translocations can also occur as new or de novo mutations and can be disrupt the proto-oncogenes and can cause uncontrolled cell division and cancer development.

The identification of translocations is mostly used for the evaluation of the haematopoietic malignancies. There are two types of probes, which are used to detect translocations: (single- or dual-) fusion probes and break-apart probes. A dual-fusion probe consists of a pair of probes labelled with two different colours (fluorochromes), green (e.g. FITC) and red (e.g. rhodamine), directed against translocation breakpoint regions in the two different genes involved in a reciprocal translocation. Variant and complex patterns may also be identified and provide additional clinical information on the underlying chromosomal changes. One locus is adjacent to another locus like in a normal cell, but the second pair is separated. This implies some type of rearrangement, which separated two loci that are usually found together, and this kind of probes was called break-apart. Commonly used BA probes in hematologic malignancies include MYC-BA (Burkitt lymphoma; BL), ALK-BA (anaplastic large cell lymphoma; ALCL) and IGH-BA (lymphoma/MM) [8].

Whole chromosome probes (WCPs; chromosome 'painting' probes) consist of numerous overlapping probes that recognize and bind to specific nonrepetitive DNA sequences along the entire length of targeted chromosomes. WCPs can be used to identify marker chromosomes (rearranged chromosomes of unidentified origin) or translocations that are otherwise not evident or difficult to interpret with routine banding cytogenetics. Whole chromosome probes do not give information about the deletion or inversions [8].

3. Duplications

The presence of an extra genomic copy of a chromosomal segment, which causes a partial trisomy, is called duplication. A duplication can be derived as a de novo duplication or as a consequence of the unbalanced chromosomal organizations like isochromosomes, dicentrics, derivatives, recombinants and markers [1, 3]. When the duplicated regions contain genes, genomic rearrangements involving the duplicated sequences can result in the deletion of the region between the copies and thus give rise to disease like 22q11.2 duplication or

http://dx.doi.org/10.5772/67415

the 15q11-q13 microduplication [3]. Most cytogenetically detectable tandem duplications in humans appear to be direct [59]. The phenotypes of the duplications are typically less severe than those associated with comparable deletions. Same as the deletions, the locus-specific FISH analysis should be applied when the duplication is suspected.

4. Deletions

The autosomal chromosome deletions can be detected by conventional, high-resolution or molecular cytogenetic methods and produce monosomies that are generally associated with significant disorders [1]. Deletions are classified into two groups: interstitial and terminal deletions. Due to the haploinsufficiency of the regions or the continuous gene deletions, the phenotypes of these patients are highly variable [2].

The deletions, which have a pathological significance, can be detected by routine methodology. Larger deletions have a more severe phenotype and associated with the major malformation than smaller ones. The gene continent of the deleted material is also important for the phenotypic severity of the patients and an important point in determining whether a specific deletion is viable [1]. The deletion of the chromosome segment can cause complex birth defects like Cri du chat syndrome, Wolf-Hirschhorn syndrome and DiGeorge Syndrome [2]. The locus-specific FISH analysis should be applied when the deletion is suspected. All stable chromosomes have telomeres at the end of the chromosomes. The sub-telomeric deletions were associated with the severe problems, which include mental retardation, developmental delay, and this terminal deletions cannot detect with the conventional cytogenetic techniques. The sub-telomeric FISH analysis is the appropriate technique to evaluate the abnormalities [10, 11, 21]. Some exceptions occur like loss of the short arm material from acrocentric chromosomes during the formation of Robertsonian translocations has no impact on phenotype [1].

5. Inversions

An inversion is an intrachromosomal rearrangement, which occurs when a single chromosome undergoes two breaks and is reconstituted with the segment between the breaks inverted. Two types of inversions occur: a paracentric inversion which both breaks occur in one arm and pericentric inversion which there is a break in each arm of the chromosomes [1]. The pericentric inversions can be easier to identify cytogenetically when they change the proportion of the chromosome arms as well as the banding pattern. The inversion does not usually cause an abnormal phenotype in carriers because it is a balanced rearrangement. The major problem of these patients is at risk for producing abnormal gametes that may lead to unbalanced offspring [2]. The breakpoints could be identified by visual inspection of the GTG image. However, further molecular cytogenetic analysis would be required to define the exact breakpoints. The locus-specific FISH is a suitable method, and also the break-apart FISH probes or m-banding is the useful molecular cytogenetics techniques for determining the inversions [60].

6. Complex chromosomal abnormalities

The complex chromosomal rearrangements (CCRs) involve two or more chromosomes, and at least three breakpoints are generally considered to be complex [61]. The greater the number of chromosome breaks and the higher the probability that an essential gene has been interrupted or that genetic material has been lost or gained during its formation. This CCRs are rarely seen in constitutional karyotypes and mostly seen in hematologic malignancies, and the identification of the structurally abnormal chromosomes is more important to be evaluated for the prognosis of haematological malignancies and important for the treatment response [62].

7. Identification of the marker chromosome

A marker chromosome is the extra structurally abnormal chromosomes in cytogenetics [2]. The precise characterization of marker chromosomes is important for prenatal and postnatal diagnosis and proper genetic counselling [63].

Mostly, the banding pattern of this abnormal chromosome does not permit for identification of the marker chromosome [62]. The chromosomal origin of marker chromosomes can be identified by using a combination of banding cytogenetics and molecular cytogenetic techniques including diverse fluorescence in situ hybridization (FISH) and array comparative genomic hybridization (array CGH) (**Figure 2**) [63].

The small structurally abnormal chromosomes, which are called as supernumerary marker chromosomes (sSMCs), are generally equal or smaller in size than a chromosome 20 of the

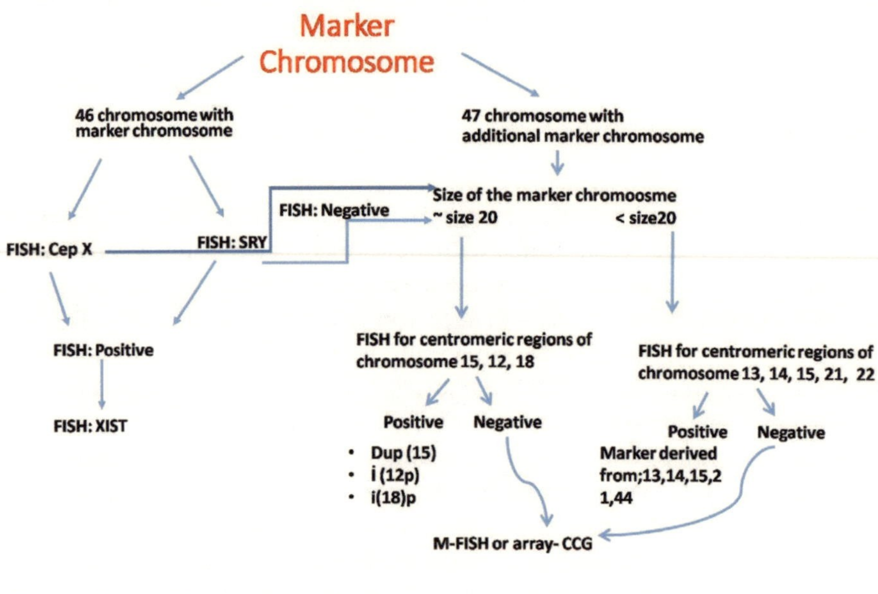

Figure 2. The possible algorithm chart for the identification of the marker chromosome.

same metaphase spread [64], and the chromosomal origin can be identified by conventional banding techniques, and molecular cytogenetic techniques are necessary for their characterization. **Figure 2** could be used for the identification of the marker chromosome.

Due to the effect of two or more chromosomal abnormalities, the conventional cytogenetics is limited to the identification. The m-FISH or the SKY is the best molecular cytogenetics choice to identify these CCRs.

8. Oncogenic amplifications

Amplification refers to the increasing copy number of a gene. Amplification causes gene upregulation of gene expression. The oncogenic amplification has described several solid tumours, which are often associated with progression, therapeutic response and prognostic markers of the cancer [65].

The oncogenes coded proteins, which have a role on control cell proliferation and programmed cell death. These oncogenes are activated by mutation, gene amplification and translocation. The oncogenic amplification mostly occurs in metastatic and low-differentiated tumours and reflects the genetic instability of solid tumour cell [66]. MYC, EGFR and RAS gene families are frequently amplified oncogenes in solid tumours. MYCN amplification in neuroblastoma or Her-2 amplification has been demonstrated, and the locus-specific probes allow accurate enumeration of each locus within individual nuclei [65]. Also, dual colour break apart rearrangement probes were used for the identification of these gene rearrangements [67].

9. Final remarks and conclusion

FISH techniques do not require mitotically active cells for evaluation of the chromosomal abnormalities, do not require culturing and allow disease monitoring in haematological malignancies. FISH can be applied on fixed, fresh tissue and on paraffin-embedded materials like paraffin-embedded solid tumours. It allows the analysis of a large number of cells. The SKY, M-FISH or COBRA-FISH techniques provide an overall evaluation of the whole genome. On the other hand, FISH analysis is not a screening test and cannot detect small intragenic mutations, deletions or insertions. Because it requires chromosome-specific FISH probes and generally less sensitive than the molecular genetics techniques.

Instead of array-CGH technology, in developed countries, the cytogenetic testing is the first line test in the diagnostic investigation detection of novel or rare chromosomal abnormalities like microdeletions, microduplications or trisomies. With the increased technology, array-based analysis like array comparative genome hybridization can help easily assess the relative copy number of genomic DNA sequences in a comprehensive, genome-wide manner, but the main disadvantage in aCGH is that it cannot detect translocation or balanced abnormalities, and in these conditions, FISH is important to determine the nature of the abnormality and its risk of recurrence.

Author details

Rasime Kalkan

Address all correspondence to: kalkanr@yahoo.com

Department of Medical Genetics, Faculty of Medicine, Near East University, Nicosia, TRNC

References

[1] Gersen SL, Keagle BM: The Principles of Clinical Cytogenetics. 2nd edition. Humana Press Inc., Totowa, New Jersey, 2005, pp. 1-113.

[2] Nussbaum RL, McInnes RR, Willard HF: Thompson & Thompson Genetics in Medicine. 8th edition. Elsevier Inc, 2016, pp. 57-102.

[3] Gardner RJM, Sutherland GR, Shaffer LG: Chromosome Abnormalities and Genetic Counseling. 4th edition. Oxford University Press, 2011. pp. 27-53. doi: 10.1093/ med/ 9780195375336.001.0001

[4] Wieacker P, Steinhard J: The prenatal diagnosis of genetic diseases. Dtsch Arztebl Int. 2010; 107(48): 857-862. doi: 10.3238/arztebl.2010.0857.

[5] Vundinti BR, Ghosh K: Chromosomal aberrations in hematological malignancies: a guide to the identification of novel oncogenes. Indian J Hum Genet. 2011: 17(2): 43-44. doi: 10.4103/0971-6866.86168.

[6] Provan D, Gribben JG: Molecular Hematology. 3rd edition. Wiley-Blackwell, 2010, p. 318. John Wiley & Sons Ltd, The Atrium, Southern Gate, Chichester, West Sussex

[7] Baccarani M, Saglio G, Goldman J, Hochhaus A, Simonsson B, Appelbaum F, Apperley J, Cervantes F, Cortes J, Deininger M, Gratwohl A, Guilhot F, Horowitz M, Hughes T, Kantarjian H, Larson R, Niederwieser D, Silver R, Hehlmann R, European LeukemiaNet: Evolving concepts in the management of chronic myeloid leukemia: recommendations from an expert panel on behalf of the European LeukemiaNet. Blood. 2006;108:1809-20. doi: 10.1182/blood-2006-02-005686.

[8] Gorczyca W: Cytogenetics, FISH and Molecular Testing in Hematologic Malignancies. 1st edition. Informa UK Ltd, 2008, pp. 31-108.

[9] Czepulkowski B: Analyzing Chromosomes. 1st edition. Bios Scientific Publishers Limited. 2001, pp. 1-106. Springer-Verlag New York Inc. 175 Fifth Avenue, New York.

[10] Mohan S, Koshy T, Vekatachalam P, Nampoothiri S, Yesodharan D, Gowrishankar K, Kumar J, Ravichandran L, Joseph S, Chandrasekaran A, Paul SF: Subtelomeric rearrangements in

Indian children with idiopathic intellectual disability/developmental delay: frequency estimation & clinical correlation using fluorescence in situ hybridization (FISH). Indian J Med Res. 2016 Aug;144(2):206-214. doi: 10.4103/0971-5916.195031.

[11] Charalsawadi C, Khayman J, Praphanphoj V, Limprasert P: Screening for subtelomeric rearrangements in Thai patients with intellectual disabilities using FISH and review of literature on subtelomeric FISH in 15,591 cases with intellectual disabilities. Genet Res Int. 2016;2016:9153740.

[12] Henegariu O, Artan S, John GM, Xiao-Ning C, Julie RK, Gail VH, Lisa S, Bray-Ward P, David WC: Cryptic translocation identification in human and mouse using several telomeric multiplex FISH (TM-FISH) strategies. Lab Investig (00236837) 2001;81(4):483.

[13] Ren R: Mechanisms of BCR-ABL in the pathogenesis of chronic myelogenous leukaemia. Nat Rev Cancer. 2005; 5:172-83.

[14] Durak BA, Akay OM, Sungar G, Bademci G, Aslan V, Caferler J, Ozdemir M, Cilingir O, Artan S, Gülbaş Z: Conventional and molecular cytogenetic analyses in Turkish patients with multiple myeloma. Turk J Haematol. 2012 Jun;29(2):135-42. doi: 10.5152/tjh.2011.42.

[15] Sahin DG, Durak B, Gündüz E, Artan S, Akay OM: A new case of dic(1;15)(p11;p11) in AML M1: apropos of a case and a review of the literature. Case Rep Genet. 2013;2013:462896. doi: 10.1155/2013/462896.

[16] Kantarjian H, Sawyers C, Hochhaus A, Guilhot F, Schiffer C, Gambacorti-Passerini C, Niederwieser D, Resta D, Capdeville R, Zoellner U, Talpaz M, Druker B, Goldman J, O'Brien SG, Russell N, Fischer T, Ottmann O, Cony-Makhoul P, Facon T, Stone R, Miller C, Tallman M, Brown R, Schuster M, Loughran T, Gratwohl A, Mandelli F, Saglio G, Lazzarino M, Russo D, Baccarani M, Morra E: Hematologic and cytogenetic responses to imatinib mesylate in chronic myelogenous leukemia. N Engl J Med. 2002;346:645-52.

[17] O'Brien SG, Guilhot F, Larson RA, Gathmann I, Baccarani M, Cervantes F, Cornelissen JJ, Fischer T, Hochhaus A, Hughes T, Lechner K, Nielsen JL, Rousselot P, Reiffers J, Saglio G, Shepherd J, Simonsson B, Gratwohl A, Goldman JM, Kantarjian H, Taylor K, Verhoef G, Bolton AE, Capdeville R, Druker BJ, IRIS Investigators: Imatinib compared with interferon and low-dose cytarabine for newly diagnosed chronic-phase chronic myeloid leukemia. N Engl J Med. 2003; 348:994-1004.

[18] Faderl S, Talpaz M, Estrov Z, O'Brien S, Kurzrock R, Kantarjian HM: The biology of chronic myeloid leukemia. N Engl J Med. 1999;341:164-72.

[19] Goldman JM, Melo JV: Chronic myeloid leukemia – advances in biology and new approaches to treatment. N Engl J Med. 2003;349:1451-64.

[20] Jones RJ: Biology and treatment of chronic myeloid leukemia. Curr Opin Oncol. 1997;9:3-7.

[21] Hélias-Rodzewicz Z, Bocian E, Stankiewicz P, Obersztyn E, Kostyk E, Jakubów-Durska K, Kutkowska-Kaźmierczak A, Mazurczak T: Subtelomeric rearrangements detected by FISH in three of 33 families with idiopathic mental retardation and minor physical anomalies. J Med Genet 2002;39:e53. doi: 10.1136/jmg.39.9.e53

[22] Bishop R: Applications of fluorescence *in situ* hybridization (FISH) in detecting genetic aberrations of medical significance. Biosci Horiz. 2010;3:85-95. doi: 10.1093/biohorizons/hzq009 first published online February 27, 2010.

[23] Shah P, Vedarethinam I, Kwasny D, Andresen L, Skov S, Silahtaroglu A, Tümer Z, Dimaki M, Svendsen WE: FISH prep: a novel integrated device for metaphase FISH sample preparation. Micromachines. 2011;2:116-128. doi:10.3390/mi2020116.

[24] Riegel M: Human molecular cytogenetics: from cells to nucleotides. Genet Mol Biol. 2014 Mar;37(1 Suppl):194-209.

[25] Pinkel D, Landegent J, Collins C, Fuscoe J, Segraves R, Lucas J, Gray JW: Fluorescence in situ hybridization with human chromosome-specific libraries: detection of trisomy 21 and translocations of chromosome 4. Proc Natl Acad Sci USA. 1988;85:9138-9142.

[26] Telenius H, Carter NP, Bebb CE, Nordenskjöld M, Ponder BA, Tunnacliffe A: Degenerate oligonucleotide-primed PCR: general amplification of target DNA by a single degenerate primer. Genomics. 1992;13:718-725.

[27] Carter NP, Ferguson-Smith MA, Perryman MT, Telenius H, Pelmear AH, Leversha MA, Glancy MT, Wood SL, Cook K, Dyson HM, *et al.*: Reverse chromosome painting: a method for the rapid analysis of aberrant chromosomes in clinical cytogenetics. J Med Genet. 1992; 29:299-307.

[28] Florijn RJ, Bonden LA, Vrolijk H, Wiegant J, Vaandrager JW, Baas F, den Dunnen JT, Tanke HJ, van Ommen GJ, Raap AK: High-resolution DNA Fiber-FISH for genomic DNA mapping and colour bar-coding of large genes. Hum Mol Genet. 1995 May;4(5):831-6.

[29] Heiskanen M, Hellsten E, Kallioniemi OP, Mäkelä TP, Alitalo K, Peltonen L and Palotie A: Visual mapping by fiber-FISH. Genomics. 1995;30:31-36.

[30] Speicher MR, Ballard SG, Ward DC: Karyotyping human chromosomes by combinatorial multifluor FISH. Nat Genet. 1996;12:368-375.

[31] Schröck E, du Manoir S, Veldman T, Schoell B, Wienberg J, Ferguson-Smith MA, Ning Y, Ledbetter DH, Bar-Am I, Soenksen D, *et al.*: Multicolor spectral karyotyping of human chromosomes. Science. 1996;273:494-497.

[32] Rufer N, Dragowska W, Thornbury G, Roosnek E, Lansdorp PM: Telomere length dynamics in human lymphocyte subpopulations measured by flow cytometry. Nat Biotechnol. 1998;16:743-747.

[33] Martens UM, Zijlmans JM, Poon SS, Dragowska W, Yui J, Chavez EA, Ward RK, Lansdorp PM: Short telomeres on human chromosome 17p. Nat Genet. 1998;18:76-80.

[34] Tanke HJ, Wiegant J, van Gijlswijk RP, Bezrookove V, Pattenier H, Heetebrij RJ, Talman EG, Raap AK, Vrolijk J: New strategy for multi-colour fluorescence in situ hybridisation: COBRA: COmbined Binary RAtio labelling. Eur J Hum Genet. 1999;7:2-11.

[35] Nietzel A, Rocchi M, Starke H, Heller A, Fiedler W, Wlodarska I, Loncarevic IF, Beensen V, Claussen U, Liehr T: A new multicolor-FISH approach for the characterization of marker chromosomes: centromere-specific multicolor- FISH (cenM-FISH). Hum Genet. 2001;108:199-204.

[36] Weise A, Gross M, Mrasek K, Mkrtchyan H, Horsthemke B, Jonsrud C, Von Eggeling F, Hinreiner S, Witthuhn V, Claussen U, *et al.*: Parental-origin-determination fluorescence in situ hybridization distinguishes homologous human chromosomes on a single-cell level. Int J Mol Med. 2008; 21:189-200.

[37] Bucksch M, Ziegler M, Kosayakova N, Mulatinho MV, Llerena Jr JC, Morlot S, Fischer W, Polityko AD, Kulpanovich AI, Petersen MB, *et al.*: A new multicolor fluorescence in situ hybridization probe set directed against human heterochromatin: HCM-FISH. J Histochem Cytochem. 2012;60:530-536.

[38] Schröck E, Zschieschang P, O'Brien P, Helmrich A, Hardt T, Matthaei A, Stout Weider K: Spectral karyotyping of human, mouse, rat and ape chromosomes—applications for genetic diagnostics and research. Cytogenet Genome Res. 2006;114:199-221.

[39] Liehr T, Heller A, Starke H, Rubtsov N, Trifonov V, Mrasek K, Weise A, Kuechler A, Claussen U: Microdissection based high resolution multicolor banding for all 24 human chromosomes. Int J Mol Med. 2002;9:335-339.

[40] Pinkel D, Straumer T, Gray IW: Cytogenetic analysis using quantitative, high-sensitivity, fluorescence in situ hybridization. Proc Natl Acad Sci USA. 1986;83:2934-2938.

[41] Lawrence JB, Villnave CA, Singer RH: Sensitive, high-resolution chromatin and chromosome mapping in situ: presence and orientation of two closely integrated copies of EBV in a lymphoma line. Cell. 1988;52:51-61.

[42] Fan YS, Davis LM, Shows TB: Mapping small DNA sequences by fluorescence in situ hybridization directly on banded metaphase chromosomes. Proc Natl Acad Sci USA. 1990;87:6223-6227.

[43] Lichter P, Ward DC: High resolution mapping of human chromosome 11 by in situ hybridization with cosmid clones. Science.1990; 247:64-69.

[44] Blennow E, Anneren G, Bui T-H, Berggren E, Asadi E, Nordenskjold M: Characterization of supernumerary ring marker chromosomes by fluorescence in situ hybridization. Am J Hum Genet. 1993; 53:433-442.

[45] Ledbetter DH, Ballabio A: Molecular cytogenetics of continuous gene syndromes: mechanisms and consequences of gene dosage imbalances, in Scriver CR, Beaudet A, Sly W, Valle D, eds., The Metabolic and Molecular Bases of Inherited Diseases, 7th edition, McGraw Hill, New York. 1995, pp. 811-839.

[46] Klinger K, Landes G, Shook, D., Harvey R, Lopez L, Locke P, Lerner T, Osathanondh R, Leverone B, Houseal T: Rapid detection of chromosome aneuploidies in uncultured amniocytes by using fluorescence in situ hybridization (FISH). Am J Hum Genet. 1992;51, 55-65.

[47] Ward BE, Gersen SL, Carelli MP, McGuire NM, Dackowski WR, Weinstein M, Sandlin C, Warren R, Klinger KW: Rapid prenatal diagnosis of chromosomal aneuploidies by fluorescence in situ hybridization: clinical experience with 4,500 specimens. Am J Hum Genet. 1993;52:954-865.

[48] Koch J, Kovarra S, Gregersen N, Petersen KB, Bolund L: Oligonucleotide-priming methods for the chromosome-specific labeling of alpha satellite DNA in situ. Chromosoma. 1989; 98:259-262.

[49] Heng HHQ, Squire J, Tsui L-C: High resolution mapping of mammaliangenes by in situ hybridization to free chromatin. Proc Natl Acad Sci USA. 1992; 89:9509-9513.

[50] Kallioniemi A, Kallioniemi OP, Suder D, Rutovitz D, Gray JW, Waldman F, Pinkel D: Comparative genomic hybridization for molecular cytogenetic analysis of solid tumors. Science. 1992;258:818-821.

[51] Su Y, Trent J, Guan XY, Meltzer P: Direct isolation of genes encoded within a homogeneously staining region by chromosome microdissection. Proc Natl Acad Sci USA. 1994; 91:9121-9125.

[52] Guan XY, Meltzer P, Dalton W, Trent J: Identification of cryptic sites of DNA sequence amplification in human breast cancer by chromosome microdissection. Nat Genet. 1994;8:155-160.

[53] Eils R, Uhring S, Saracoglu, Sätzler K, Bolzer A, Petersen I, Chassery J, Ganser M, Speicher MR: An optimized, fully automated system for fast and accurate identification of chromosome rearrangements by multiplex-FISH (M-FISH). Cytogenet Cell Genet. 1998; 82:160-171.

[54] Müller S, Rocchi M, Ferguson-Smith MA, Wienberg J: Toward a multicolor chromosome bar code for the entire human karyotype by fluorescence in situ hybridization. Hum Genet. 1997; 100:271-278.

[55] Knight SJL, Horsley SW, Regan R, Lawrie NM, Maher EJ, Cardy DL, Flint J, Kearney L: Development and clinical application of an innovative fluorescence in situ hybridization technique which detects submicroscopic rearrangements involving telomeres. Eur J Hum Genet. 1997;5:1-8.

[56] Pinkel D, Segraves R, Sudar D, *et al.*: High resolution analysis of DNA copy number variation using comparative genomic hybridization to microarrays. Nat Genet. 1998;20: 207-211.

[57] Pollack JR, Perou CM, Alizadeh AA, Eisen MB, Pergamenschikov A, Williams CF, Jeffrey SS, Botstein D, Brown PO: Genome-wide analysis of DNA copy-number changes using cDNA microarrays. Nat Genet. 1999; 23:41-46.

[58] Weise A, Liehr T: In Thomas L. ed., Fluorescence In Situ Hybridization (FISH)—Application Guide. 2009 Springer-Verlag Berlin Heidelberg, pp. 113-143

[59] Van Dyke DL: Isochromosomes and interstitial tandem direct and inverted duplications. In Daniel A, ed., The Cytogenetics of Mammalian Autosomal Rearrangements, Alan R. Liss, New York. 1988, pp. 635-666.

[60] Schmidt S, Claussen U, Liehr T, Weise A: Evolution versus constitution: differences in chromosomal inversion. Hum Genet. 2005;117:213-219.

[61] Pai GS, Thomas GH, Mahoney W, Migeon BR: Complex chromosome rearrangements; report of a new case and literature review. Clin Genet. 1980;18:436-444.

[62] Kalkan R, Özdağ N, Bundak R, Serakıncı N: A unique mosaic Turner syndrome patient with Androgen Receptor gene derived marker chromosome. Syst Biol Reprod Med. 2016;62(1):77-83. 10.3109/19396368.2015.1109007.

[63] Jang W, Chae H, Kim J, Son JO, Kim SC, Koo BK, Kim M, Kim Y, Park IY, Sung IK: Identification of small marker chromosomes using microarray comparative genomic hybridization and multicolor fluorescent in situ hybridization. Mol Cytogenet. 2016 Aug 8;9:61. doi: 10.1186/s13039-016-0273-5. eCollection 2016.

[64] Liehr T, Claussen U, Starke H: Small supernumerary marker chromosomes (sSMC) in humans. Cytogenet Genome Res. 2004;107:55-67.

[65] Bagci O, Kurtgöz S: Amplification of Cellular Oncogenes in Solid Tumors. N Am J Med Sci. 2015 Aug;7(8):341-6. doi: 10.4103/1947-2714.163641.

[66] Fan Y-S: In Yao-Shan ed. Molecular Cytogenetics. Humana Press. 2003, pp. 11-12.

[67] Yoon JH, Baek YS, Jeon J, Oh CH, Song HJ: Dual-color, break-apart fluorescence in situ hybridization probe for distinguishing clear cell sarcoma of soft tissue from malignant melanoma. Int J Dermatol. 2014 Dec;53(12):1464-7. doi: 10.1111/j.1365-4632.2011.05009.x.

Chapter 2

Morphological Markers of Chromosomal Instability

Yoko Matsuda, Junko Aida, Naoshi Ishikawa,

Kaiyo Takubo, Toshiyuki Ishiwata and Tomio Arai

Additional information is available at the end of the chapter

http://dx.doi.org/10.5772/67416

Abstract

Cancer is characterized by genomic complexity and chromosomal instability (CIN). Atypical mitosis and nuclear atypia such as micronuclei have been reported as morphological characteristics of chromosomal instability. An atypical mitotic figure is defined as anything other than the typical form of normal mitosis, including multipolar, ring, dispersed, asymmetrical, and lag-type mitoses. A micronucleus is defined as the small nucleus that forms whenever a chromosome or its fragment is not incorporated into one of the daughter nuclei during cell division. A telomere plays a key role in chromosomal instability. Telomere dysfunction induces fusion of chromatids and chromosome missegregation and this phenomenon can be observed as abnormal mitotic figures and micronuclei. Detection of morphological markers of chromosomal instability using pathological specimens, even small biopsy or cytological specimens, may provide valuable information concerning the prognosis of cancers. Here, we discuss morphological assessment of chromosomal instability using routine pathological specimens.

Keywords: chromosomal instability, cancer, pathology, mitosis, atypical mitosis

1. Introduction

Cancer is characterized by genomic complexity and chromosomal instability (CIN); mutations of cancer-related genes, telomere dysfunction, aneuploidy, polyploidy, nuclear atypia, and abnormal mitosis are all contributors to this phenotype [1–4]. The greatest risk factor for cancer is considered to be aging, via telomere shortening, accumulation of mutations, and perturbations in the microenvironment [5, 6]. Previously, we showed that age-related shortening of telomere length in various tissues is correlated to aging-related diseases, such as cancers, diabetes mellitus, and cognitive disorders [7]. Telomere shortening often occurs in cancers, as well as in precancerous lesions [8–10]. Telomere shortening induces fusion of chromatids and chromosome missegregation and this phenomenon can be observed as abnormal mitotic figures and micronuclei. In this article, we discuss the morphological markers to determine chromosomal instability in cancer tissues.

2. Chromosomal instability

CIN is defined as a persistently high rate of loss or gain of full or partial chromosomes induced by defects in cohesion, the spindle assembly checkpoint, centrosomes, kinetochore-microtubule attachment dynamics, or cell cycle regulation [11, 12]. Cells with CIN make errors in chromosome segregation in approximately 20% of cell divisions and the unequal distribution of DNA to daughter cells upon mitosis induces a failure to maintain euploidy leading to aneuploidy. Most solid tumors and hematological cancers are aneuploidy and many missegregate chromosomes at very high rates [11]. However, the presence of aneuploidy in cells does not necessarily mean CIN is present; a high rate of errors is definitive of CIN. Detection of CIN requires the determination of chromosome missegregation rates, however the ability to detect CIN from fixed tumor tissues is limited [13]. Therefore, when we need to determine CIN using fixed tumor samples in the clinical setting, we usually perform indirect methods such as karyotype analysis, fluorescent *in situ* hybridization, or array-based comparative genomic hybridization analyses. Analysis of atypical mitotic figures and nuclear atypia is considered a useful method to distinguish chromosomally unstable from chromosomally stable malignancies [14–18].

3. Mitotic figures

Mitosis is divided into five stages: prophase, prometaphase, metaphase, anaphase, and telophase. During mitosis, chromosomes thicken and condense, allowing them to be visualized by light microscopy. Most malignant tumors show a high mitotic index and for some tumors, a diagnosis of malignancy is based on mitotic index. A higher mitotic index is correlated with malignancy grade and prognosis [19, 20]. Structural chromosomal abnormalities may arise during somatic cell divisions. Cells with CIN have a higher probability of causing chromosome missegregation during mitosis as compared to normal cells, suggesting a close relationship between high mitotic index and CIN in malignancies, possibly as a result of mitotic arrest as opposed to high frequency of mitoses.

Cytological smears and formalin-fixed paraffin-embedded tissue samples are useful materials for evaluating mitotic figures because they are routinely performed in laboratories around the world. Metaphase figures can be evaluated using hematoxylin and eosin (H&E), Giemsa, or Papanicolaou-stained slides examined at high power magnification. The mitotic index value is assessed by counting the number of mitoses per 1000 or 2000 nuclei or per 50 high power fields.

http://dx.doi.org/10.5772/67416

Mitotic figures are defined as figures without a nuclear membrane, which indicates that the cell has passed prophase and in which clear hairy extensions of nuclear material are present. Pyknotic nuclei or nuclei with basophilic cytoplasm are not thought to distinguish mitosis from apoptosis or degenerative cells [21]. Recently, immunohistochemical determination of proliferating cells using primary antibodies for Ki67, PCNA, or phosphohistone H3 has become popular; however, sometimes there is a discrepancy between mitotic index and Ki67 index [22–24]. We believe that this phenomenon represents the frequent mitotic arrest mentioned above.

4. Atypical mitosis

Mitosis is classified into normal and atypical mitosis [25]. An atypical mitotic figure is defined as anything other than the typical form of normal mitosis, including an anaphase bridge, multipolar, ring, dispersed, asymmetrical, and lag-type mitoses [25, 26] (**Figure 1**). Cells in mitosis are often seen in normal tissues exhibiting rapid turnover, such as the epithelium of the gut, but the most important morphologic features of malignancy are atypical and bizarre mitotic figures. In our analysis, 30% of mitosis in pancreatic cancer cells was atypical mitosis, while normal epithelium did not show atypical mitosis and precancerous lesions showed only a few instances of atypical mitosis [9, 18].

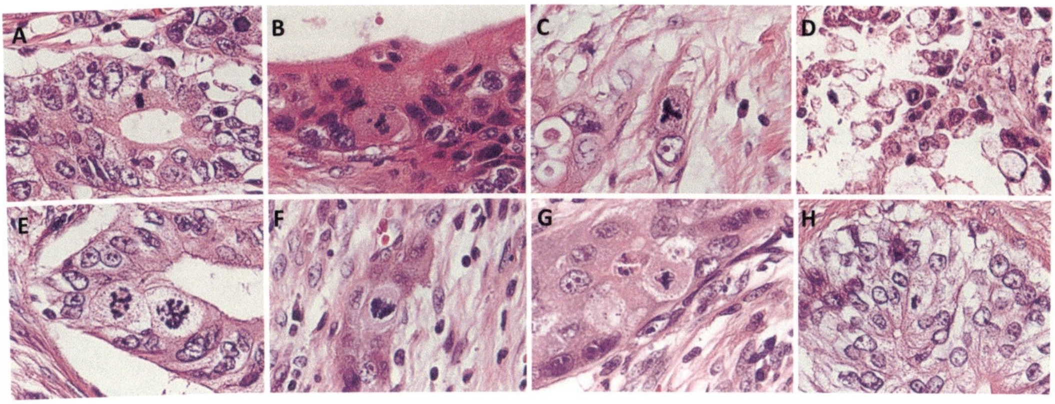

Figure 1. Normal and atypical mitosis in cancer cells. A, normal mitosis; B, anaphase bridge; C, multipolar mitosis; D, ring mitosis; E, dispersed mitosis; F, asymmetrical mitosis; G, lag-type mitosis; and H, micronuclei. H&E stain. Original magnification 400×.

An anaphase bridge is defined as a filamentous connection linking two well-separated and parallel-aligned groups of anaphase chromosomes [14, 15]. Telomeres protect each end of the chromosome from fusion; therefore, telomere dysfunction can be observed as an anaphase bridge [15, 17]. A lot of evidence has shown that telomere dysfunction plays a key role in carcinogenesis via induction of CIN [9, 27]; thus, detection of an anaphase bridge has been considered a useful method of indirectly evaluating telomere dysfunction and CIN.

Multipolar mitosis is metaphase with an abnormal configuration of the equatorial plate and the chromosomes are located along several radial axes. These figures are subdivided into tripolar mitoses, quadripolar mitoses, and others. Multipolar mitosis might be associated with multipolar spindles and numerical and functional abnormalities of centrosomes [28, 29]. It has been reported that multipolar mitosis determined by cytologic smears is useful to distinguish malignancies from benign tissue [30, 31]. Recently, we have reported that the existence of multipolar mitosis, but not other atypical mitotic figures, was an independent prognostic factor for in pancreatic cancers [18]. Multipolar mitosis-positive pancreatic cancer cases may have high invasiveness into surrounding tissue and arteries, in part, because of chromosomal instability and abnormality of the centrosome.

Lag-type mitoses are figures with nonattached condensed chromatin in the area of the mitotic figure. These are subdivided into metaphases with nonattached condensed chromatin at one polar side, metaphases with nonattached condensed chromatin at equidistant positions at the two polar sides and others. Furuta et al. has reported lag-type mitosis as a marker of high-risk human papilloma virus associated cervical cancers [32].

Medication-induced atypical mitoses have been reported. Docetaxel, paclitaxel, and colchicine can cause mitotic arrest, ring mitoses, and epithelial atypia mimicking dysplasia [33, 34]. They bind to the β-tubulin subunit of the microtubules of the mitotic spindle apparatus and therefore prevent mitotic spindle formation.

The interrelationship of each atypical mitotic figure has not been well clarified; however, each type of atypical mitosis is a morphologically important marker of CIN.

5. Telomere dysfunction

Aging drives telomere dysfunction. Inflammation, alcohol drinking, and diabetes mellitus also accelerate telomere attrition [35–37]. Furthermore, telomere shortening initiates the early phase of carcinogenesis even when there are no histopathological changes [9, 17]. Telomere dysfunction can be seen as nuclear atypia including the presence of micronuclei, nuclear buds, and anaphase bridges [38]. In our analysis, telomere length in the normal pancreatic duct was negatively correlated with mitotic index [9], which is consistent with telomere shortening of 100 base pairs in each mitosis. Normal epithelial cells in pancreatic cancer patients showed shorter telomeres than those in patients without cancers. Furthermore, telomere shortening was correlated to *KRAS* mutation in pancreatic cancer. These data indicate that telomere shortening occurs prior to CIN and drives CIN [39]. As a result, CIN drives gene mutation, deletion, or amplification.

In addition to this pathway, microsatellite instability also induces genetic abnormality and there seems to be organ specificity. Some colon and uterine cancers are caused by microsatellite instability [40], but most pancreatic cancers are microsatellite stable. All of the conventional pancreatic ductal adenocarcinomas showed telomere dysfunction and it progressed according to malignancy grade of pancreatic carcinogenesis steps [9]. Organ specificity as well as the difference of carcinogens might influence such difference of carcinogenesis steps. In CIN cancers, mitosis and atypical mitosis might have a predictive value of malignancy grade and prognosis [18].

6. Morphological markers of chromosomal instability

The usefulness of micronuclei in distinguishing malignant lesions from benign lesions using cytological specimens has been well clarified [41–43]. A micronucleus is the small nucleus that forms whenever a chromosome or its fragment is not incorporated into one of the daughter nuclei during cell division and it serves as an indicator of CIN. Samanta et al. reported that in the evaluation of the number of micronuclei in 1000 cells from fine needle aspiration samples of the breast, cancer cells showed a higher number of micronuclei than benign lesions [44]. Tyagi et al. assessed the number of anaphase bridges, multipolar mitoses, micronuclei, and nuclear budding in 1000 cells in Giemsa stained smears of ascitic fluid and found that these markers were correlated with the cytological diagnosis [30]. Moreover, Verma and Dey counted anaphase bridges, multipolar mitoses per smear, micronuclei and nuclear budding per 1000 carcinoma cells using fine needle aspiration samples of breast cancer and these markers were correlated with cytological grades [31]. We also counted normal and atypical mitoses in 1000 cells using surgically resected pancreatic cancer tissues and they were correlated with tumor stage and prognosis [18]. The number of mitotic figures is sometimes very low even in cancer tissues. For example, the mitotic index of pancreatic cancers was only 0.4%, suggesting the potential need to analyze more than 1000 cells [45].

Micronuclei, nuclear budding, anaphase bridging, and multipolar mitoses have been well evaluated among various morphological markers of CIN. The molecular methods to determine CIN are costly, require expertise, and may not be available in many laboratories. In the future, these aforementioned markers can be applied to diagnose malignancy in difficult cases of suspected malignancy.

Author details

Yoko Matsuda[1]*, Junko Aida[2], Naoshi Ishikawa[2], Kaiyo Takubo[2], Toshiyuki Ishiwata[2] and Tomio Arai[1]

*Address all correspondence to: yoko_matsuda@tmghig.jp

1 Department of Pathology, Tokyo Metropolitan Geriatric Hospital, Tokyo, Japan

2 Research Team for Geriatric Pathology, Tokyo Metropolitan Institute of Gerontology, Tokyo, Japan

References

[1] Weyrer, K, et al.: p53, Ki-ras, and DNA ploidy in human pancreatic ductal adenocarcinomas. Lab Invest, 1996. **74**: 279-89.

[2] Korc, M: Driver mutations: A roadmap for getting close and personal in pancreatic cancer. Cancer Biol Ther, 2010. **10**: 588-91. DOI: 13128 [pii]

[3] Bardeesy, N and DePinho, RA: Pancreatic cancer biology and genetics. Nat Rev Cancer, 2002. **2**: 897-909. DOI: 10.1038/nrc949 [pii]

[4] Hezel, AF, et al.: Genetics and biology of pancreatic ductal adenocarcinoma. Genes Dev, 2006. **20**: 1218-49. DOI: 20/10/1218 [pii] 10.1101/gad.1415606

[5] Pandol, S, et al.: Epidemiology, risk factors, and the promotion of pancreatic cancer: role of the stellate cell. J Gastroenterol Hepatol, 2012. **27** Suppl 2: 127-34. DOI: 10.1111/j.1440-1746.2011.07013.x

[6] Lillemoe, KD, Yeo, CJ, and Cameron, JL: Pancreatic cancer: State-of-the-art care. CA Cancer J Clin, 2000. **50**: 241-68.

[7] Ishikawa, N, et al.: Changes of telomere status with aging: An update. Geriatr Gerontol Int, 2016. **16** Suppl 1: 30-42. DOI: 10.1111/ggi.12772

[8] Aida, J, et al.: Short telomeres in an oral precancerous lesion: Q-FISH analysis of leukoplakia. J Oral Pathol Med, 2011. **41**: 372-8. DOI: 10.1111/j.1600-0714.2011.01120.x

[9] Matsuda, Y, et al.: Gradual telomere shortening and increasing chromosomal instability among PanIN grades and normal ductal epithelia with and without cancer in the pancreas. PLoS One, 2015. **10**: e0117575. DOI: 10.1371/journal.pone.0117575

[10] Ikeda, H, et al.: Quantitative fluorescence in situ hybridization measurement of telomere length in skin with/without sun exposure or actinic keratosis. Hum Pathol, 2014. **45**: 473-80. DOI: S0046-8177(13)00424-3 [pii] 10.1016/j.humpath.2013.10.009

[11] Thompson, SL, Bakhoum, SF, and Compton, DA: Mechanisms of chromosomal instability. Curr Biol, 2010. **20**: R285-95. DOI: 10.1016/j.cub.2010.01.034

[12] Negrini, S, Gorgoulis, VG, and Halazonetis, TD: Genomic instability—An evolving hallmark of cancer. Nat Rev Mol Cell Biol, 2010. **11**: 220-8. DOI: 10.1038/nrm2858

[13] McGranahan, N, et al.: Cancer chromosomal instability: Therapeutic and diagnostic challenges. EMBO Rep, 2012. **13**: 528-38. DOI: 10.1038/embor.2012.61

[14] Montgomery, E, et al.: Analysis of anaphase figures in routine histologic sections distinguishes chromosomally unstable from chromosomally stable malignancies. Cancer Biol Ther, 2003. **2**: 248-52.

[15] Takubo, K, et al.: Q-FISH analysis of telomere and chromosome instability in the esophagus with and without squamous cell carcinoma in situ. J Pathol, 2010. **221**: 201-9. DOI: 10.1002/path.2704

[16] Izumiyama-Shimomura, N, et al.: Short telomeres and chromosome instability prior to histologic malignant progression and cytogenetic aneuploidy in papillary urothelial neoplasms. Urol Oncol, 2014. **32**: 135-45. DOI: 10.1016/j.urolonc.2012.12.005

[17] Aida, J, et al.: Telomere lengths in the oral epithelia with and without carcinoma. Eur J Cancer, 2010. **46**: 430-8. DOI: 10.1016/j.ejca.2009.10.018

[18] Matsuda, Y, et al.: Mitotic index and multipolar mitosis in routine histologic sections as prognostic markers of pancreatic cancers: A clinicopathological study. Pancreatology, 2016. **16**: 127-32. DOI: S1424-3903(15)00675-4 [pii] 10.1016/j.pan.2015.10.005

[19] Valente, K, et al.: A histomorphologic grading system that predicts overall survival in diffuse malignant peritoneal mesothelioma with epithelioid subtype. Am J Surg Pathol, 2016. **40**: 1243-8. DOI: 10.1097/PAS.0000000000000696

[20] Weidner, N, et al.: Correlation of bromodeoxyuridine (BRDU) labeling of breast carcinoma cells with mitotic figure content and tumor grade. Am J Surg Pathol, 1993. **17**: 987-94.

[21] van Diest, PJ, et al.: Reproducibility of mitosis counting in 2,469 breast cancer specimens: results from the Multicenter Morphometric Mammary Carcinoma Project. Hum Pathol, 1992. **23**: 603-7.

[22] Jalava, P, et al.: Ki67 immunohistochemistry: A valuable marker in prognostication but with a risk of misclassification: Proliferation subgroups formed based on Ki67 immunoreactivity and standardized mitotic index. Histopathology, 2006. **48**: 674-82. DOI: 10.1111/j.1365-2559.2006.02402.x

[23] Tetzlaff, MT, et al.: Immunodetection of phosphohistone H3 as a surrogate of mitotic figure count and clinical outcome in cutaneous melanoma. Mod Pathol, 2013. **26**: 1153-60. DOI: 10.1038/modpathol.2013.59

[24] Kure, S, et al.: Expression of cancer stem cell markers in pancreatic intraepithelial neoplasias and pancreatic ductal adenocarcinomas. Int J Oncol, 2012. **41**: 1314-24. DOI: 10.3892/ijo.2012.1565

[25] Rubio, CA: Atypical mitoses in colorectal adenomas. Pathol Res Pract, 1991. **187**: 508-13. DOI: 10.1016/S0344-0338(11)80015-4

[26] Van Leeuwen, AM, et al.: Atypical mitotic figures and the mitotic index in cervical intraepithelial neoplasia. Virchows Arch, 1995. **427**: 139-44.

[27] Takubo, K, et al.: Changes of telomere length with aging. Geriatr Gerontol Int, 2010. **10** Suppl 1: S197-206. DOI: 10.1111/j.1447-0594.2010.00605.x

[28] Kalatova, B, et al.: Tripolar mitosis in human cells and embryos: Occurrence, pathophysiology and medical implications. Acta Histochem, 2015. **117**: 111-25. DOI: S0065-1281(14)00285-2 [pii] 10.1016/j.acthis.2014.11.009

[29] Sato, N, et al.: Correlation between centrosome abnormalities and chromosomal instability in human pancreatic cancer cells. Cancer Genet Cytogenet, 2001. **126**: 13-9. DOI: S0165-4608(00)00384-8 [pii]

[30] Tyagi, R, et al.: Analysis of morphological markers of chromosomal instability in ascitic fluid. Diagn Cytopathol, 2015. **43**: 855-8. DOI: 10.1002/dc.23249

[31] Verma, S and Dey, P: Correlation of morphological markers of chromosomal instability in fine needle aspiration cytology with grade of breast cancer. Cytopathology, 2014. **25**: 259-63. DOI: 10.1111/cyt.12096

[32] Furuta, R, et al.: Ectopic chromosome around centrosome in metaphase cells as a marker of high-risk human papillomavirus-associated cervical intraepithelial neoplasias. Int J Cancer, 2003. **106**: 167-71. DOI: 10.1002/ijc.11216

[33] Martinez-Lopez, JI: ECG of the month. Hammer and nails. Atrial fibrillation. J La State Med Soc, 1992. **144**: 437-40.

[34] Mackler, NJ and Pienta, KJ: Drug insight: Use of docetaxel in prostate and urothelial cancers. Nat Clin Pract Urol, 2005. **2**: 92-100; quiz 1 p following 112. DOI: 10.1038/ncpuro0099

[35] Tamura, Y, et al.: beta-cell telomere attrition in diabetes: Inverse correlation between HbA1c and telomere length. J Clin Endocrinol Metab, 2014. **99**: 2771-7. DOI: 10.1210/jc.2014-1222

[36] Aida, J, et al.: Alcoholics show reduced telomere length in the oesophagus. J Pathol, 2011. **223**: 410-6. DOI: 10.1002/path.2817

[37] Ishii, A, et al.: Telomere shortening with aging in the human pancreas. Exp Gerontol, 2006. **41**: 882-6. DOI: 10.1016/j.exger.2006.06.036

[38] Pampalona, J, et al.: Telomere dysfunction and chromosome structure modulate the contribution of individual chromosomes in abnormal nuclear morphologies. Mutat Res, 2010. **683**: 16-22. DOI: 10.1016/j.mrfmmm.2009.10.001

[39] Soler, D, et al.: Telomere dysfunction drives chromosomal instability in human mammary epithelial cells. Genes Chromosomes Cancer, 2005. **44**: 339-50. DOI: 10.1002/gcc.20244

[40] Arai, T, et al.: Hypermethylation of the hMLH1 promoter with absent hMLH1 expression in medullary-type poorly differentiated colorectal adenocarcinoma in the elderly. Mod Pathol, 2004. **17**: 172-9. DOI: 10.1038/modpathol.3800018 [pii]

[41] Hemalatha, A, Suresh, TN, and HarendraKumar, ML: Micronuclei in breast aspirates. Is scoring them helpful? J Cancer Res Ther, 2014. **10**: 309-11. DOI: 10.4103/0973-1482.136588

[42] Goel, S, Bhatia, A, and Dey, P: Spontaneously occurring micronuclei in infiltrating ductal carcinoma of breast: A potential biomarker for aggressive phenotype detection? Diagn Cytopathol, 2013. **41**: 296-302. DOI: 10.1002/dc.21836

[43] Bhatia, A and Kumar, Y: Cancer cell micronucleus: An update on clinical and diagnostic applications. APMIS, 2013. **121**: 569-81. DOI: 10.1111/apm.12033

[44] Samanta, S, Dey, P, and Nijhawan, R: The role of micronucleus scoring in fine needle aspirates of ductal carcinoma of the breast. Cytopathology, 2011. **22**: 111-4. DOI: 10.1111/j.1365-2303.2010.00773.x

[45] Baak, JP: Mitosis counting in tumors. Hum Pathol, 1990. **21**: 683-5.

Chapter 3

Acquired Chromosomal Abnormalities and Their Potential Formation Mechanisms in Solid Tumours

Nevim Aygun

Additional information is available at the end of the chapter

http://dx.doi.org/10.5772/67733

Abstract

Solid tumours include numerous malign or relatively less benign types of carcinomas and sarcomas. Acquired chromosomal abnormalities in solid tumours are hallmarks of gene deregulation and genome instability. Chromosomal abnormalities are mainly classified into two groups: structural and numerical alterations. Structural rearrangements involve chromosomal aberrations such as deletion, translocation, duplication, inversion and gene amplification, whereas numerical abnormalities result in aneuploidy or polyploidy. Structural chromosome abnormalities can arise from non-allelic homologous recombination (NAHR), non-homologous end joining (NHEJ) and fork stalling and template switching (FoSTeS). Numerical abnormalities can form through various errors in the mitotic spindle checkpoint and some cellular processes during mitosis. This chapter reviews acquired structural and numerical chromosomal abnormalities in solid tumours and presents potential formation mechanisms. In this chapter, the relationship between long inverted repeats (LIRs) and *MYCN* amplification in neuroblastoma was also investigated. The distribution of LIRs was determined at chromosome 2p25.3–2p24.3, using inverted repeat finder (IRF) software. LIRs were also identified at boundaries of amplicons in 14 neuroblastoma cell lines and 42 solid tumours, involving *MYCN* amplification. Statistical analysis showed a significant association between LIRs and *MYCN* amplification loci. Present data provide important insights into *MYCN* amplification mechanism. Therefore, a new model mechanism for formation of the *MYCN* amplification is proposed at the end of the chapter.

Keywords: solid tumour, chromosomal abnormalities, model mechanisms, long inverted repeats (LIRs), neuroblastoma, *MYCN* amplification mechanism

1. Introduction

Acquired chromosomal abnormalities during clonal evolution of tumour cells, which can influence biological or clinical behaviour in a solid neoplasm, are hallmarks of gene deregulation and genome instability [1, 2]. Acquired clonal cytogenetic abnormalities have been reported in more than 50,000 cases (current total number of the cases: 66,675, updated in 2016) in all main cancer types [3, 4]. Secondary chromosomal aberrations that are considered important unbalanced changes acquired during tumour progression usually result in large-scale genomic imbalances, whereas primary balanced abnormalities can cause a disease-specific gene rearrangement in cancer initiation [3, 5].

Chromosomal abnormalities are mainly classified into two groups: structural and numerical alterations [6]. Gross structural rearrangements involve the chromosomal changes including deletion, translocation, duplication, inversion, and gene amplification, whereas numerical abnormalities lead to abnormal number of a whole chromosome or entire chromosome set, resulting in aneuploidy and polyploidy, respectively.

Solid tumours include various malign or relatively less benign cancer types observed in multiple solid organs, systems and tissues, involving many carcinomas and sarcomas such as thyroid adenocarcinoma and Ewing sarcoma or adenomas such as salivary gland adenoma, respectively, as summarised in **Table 1** [7]. The Atlas of Genetics and Cytogenetics in Oncology and Haematology represents a large number of chromosomal abnormalities including translocation, deletion and inversion reported in solid tumours [7]. Together, the Mitelman Database of Chromosome Aberrations and Gene Fusions in Cancer presents the recurrent structural and numerical chromosome abnormalities reported in at least two cases with the same morphology at any topography of the body in solid tumours (**Table 1**) [4].

Recurrent aberrations share a common size and consistently recur in different individuals, leading to clustering of the breakpoints, whereas the nonrecurrent rearrangements formed within a region are in different size in each patient, but these rearrangements may share a smallest region of overlap (SRO), which may cause similar clinical phenotypes [8]. Recurrent abnormalities mostly occur via non-allelic homologous recombination (NAHR) between low copy repeats (LCRs) [9]. Nonrecurrent rearrangements are usually explained by non-homologous end joining (NHEJ) and the fork stalling and template switching (FoSTeS) models [8].

The recurrent structural rearrangements and chromosomal gains that are present in at least two cells in a neoplasia are accepted as clonal; however, according to the International System for Human Cytogenetic Nomenclature (ISCN), missing chromosomes that are observed in at least three cells are accepted as clonal [10]. The chromosome abnormalities detected at a frequency of less than 5% in an examined cell population are considered non-recurrent or non-clonal [11].

The balanced structural chromosomal rearrangements involving mostly translocations and some inversions, such as t(12;16)(q13;p11) in myxoid liposarcoma and t(X;1)(p11;q21) in papillary renal cell carcinoma, are decidedly more disease specific than the unbalanced changes [12]. However, unbalanced structural alterations are more frequently observed than the balanced aberrations in solid tumours, see **Table 1** in Ref. [12].

http://dx.doi.org/10.5772/67733

		Chromosomal abnormalities[b]				
		Structural				Numeric.
Site[a]	Solid tumour[a]	Trans.	Del	Dup	Inv	Aneup.
Bones	Ewing sarc. malign	t(11;22) (q24;q12)	del(22)(q12)	—	—	+8, +2 +12, −10
	Osteoblast. benign	—	—	—	—	+16, −13 −22
	Osteosarc. malign	der(1)t(1;3) (p36;p21)	del(1)(q11)	—	—	+7, +20 −13, −10
Digestive organs	Hepatoblast. malign	der(4)t(1;4) (q12;q34)	del(1)(p22) del(1)(q12)	—	—	+20, +2 +8, −18
Female organs	Ovary AC malign/benign	t(6;14) (q21;q24)	del(6)(q21) del(3)(q21) del(1)(q21)	dup(1) (q21q32)	inv(3) (p13p25)	+12, +3 −15, −X
	Breast AC malign	t(14;15) (p11;q11)	del(1)(p13) del(1)(p22)	dup(1) (q21;q44)	inv(1) (p22p36)	+1, +7 −X, −22
Head and neck	Larynx SCC malign	t(1;2) (p22;q21)	del(22)(q13) del(3)(p11) del(8)(p21)	—	—	+7, +20 −21, −Y
	Salivary gland Ad. benign	t(3;8) (p21;q12)	del(3)(p21) del(8)(p12)	—	inv(12) (q15q24)	+7, +8 −19, −Y
Lung heart skin	Myxoma benign	—	—	—	—	+7, −X −Y
	Malignant Melanoma Malign	t(1;14) (q21;q32)	del(9)(p21) del(6)(q13)	—	—	+7, +20 −10, −21
Male organs	Prostate AC malign	t(8;21) (q24;q22)	del(7)(q22) del(10)(q24)	dup(7) (q22q32)	—	+7, +Y −8, −Y
	Testis teratoma benign	der(1)t(1;14) (p11;q11)	del(6)(q21) del(1)(p35)	—	—	+8, +21 −13, −18
Nervous system	Glioblast. malign	der(1)t(1;12) (p36;q13)	del(9)(p21) del(9)(p13)	dup(1) (p11p36)	inv(19) (p13q13)	+7, +20 −10, −Y
Neuro-endoc./ endoc. system	Thyroid AC malign	t(2;3) (q13;p25)	del(12)(p11)	—	inv(10) (q11q21)	+7, +20 −22, −Y
	Pituitary AD.	—	—	—	—	+7, +12 −21, −22
	Benign neuroblast. malign	der(1)t(1;17) (p32;q21)	del(1)(p22)	—	inv(2) (p13p23)	+7, +17 −19, −X
Soft tissues	Alveolar rhabdo-myosarc. malign	t(2;13) (q35;q14)	del(13)(q14) del(16)(q22)	—	—	+2, +20 −3, −10
	Synovial Sarc. Malign	t(X;18) (p11;q11)	del(3)(p21) del(11) (q13q21)	—	—	+8, +12 −3, −14

		Chromosomal abnormalities[b]				
		Structural				Numeric.
Site[a]	Solid tumour[a]	Trans.	Del	Dup	Inv	Aneup.
Urinary system	Kidney AC malign	der(3)t(3;5) (p13;q22) t(X;1) (p11;q21)	del(3)(p14) del(3)(p13)	–	inv(1) (p36q21)	+7, +16 −14, −Y
	Wilms tumour malign	t(2;14) (q21;q24)	del(1)(p13) del(11) (p13p14)	–	–	+8, +12 −16, −22

[a]Information regarding solid tumours and their sites was obtained from database: 'Atlas of Genetics and Cytogenetics in Oncology and Haematology' [7].

[b]Chromosomal abnormalities were selected among the recurrent aberrations that are reported at most cases in the 'Mitelman Database of Chromosome Aberrations and Gene Fusions in Cancer' [4].

Abbreviations: AC, adenocarcinoma; AD, adenoma; Aneup., aneuploidy; Endoc., endocrine; Glioblast., glioblastoma; Hepatoblast., hepatoblastoma; Neuroblast., neuroblastoma; Numeric., numerical; Osteoblast., osteoblastoma; Sarc., sarcoma; SCC, squamous cell carcinoma; Trans., translocation.

Table 1. Common chromosomal abnormalities in solid tumours.

Aneuploidy (91.1%), an abnormal chromosome number deviated from euploid, is a very common feature in solid tumours, see **Table 1** in Ref. [13]. Aneuploidy is one of the main resultants of chromosomal instability and probably contributes to tumourigenesis through genomic variation and gene/protein dosage changes [14].

Gene amplifications are predominantly observed in solid tumours, as compared with haematological malignancies and lymphomas; see **Table 1** in Ref. [15]. Oncogene amplification can play an important role in the progression of solid tumours. Genomic DNA amplifications lead to a selective increase in the dosage of cellular oncogenes, usually resulting in overexpression of those genes and thus may provide contribution to the tumourigenesis [16]. *MYCN* amplification is a poor prognostic factor in neuroblastoma [17]. In addition, gene amplification, which involves multiple genes such as *MDM2, EGFR, MYCN, CCND1* and *CDK4*, is associated with poor prognosis in anaplastic grade III oligodendrogliomas, regardless of the gene involved [18].

Cytogenetic analysis in solid tumours is performed in a limited number of mitoses due to low mitotic index of tumour tissues, problems in disaggregation of sample, and intense necrosis in the periphery. Moreover, most of metaphases obtained from tissue culture have insufficient quality for karyotype analysis [19]. The technological developments in conventional cytogenetic, molecular cytogenetic, and molecular biological methods increased the quality and number of mitoses, which enhance efficiency and accuracy of karyotype analysis in solid tumours [20–22], while in vivo experimental models provided important insights into the mechanisms of chromosomal abnormalities [23, 24]. However, the mechanisms of chromosome abnormalities remain to be completely clarified.

Primary model mechanisms proposed for formation of structural chromosome abnormalities in genomic disorders and cancer are NAHR, NHEJ, and FoSTeS [8]. NAHR events are mostly associated with LCRs, but any evidence for such a direct association of NHEJ and FoSTeS with a specific DNA element was not yet provided. However, it was proposed that FoSTeS may be stimulated by a palindrome or cruciform structure [8]. In addition, the location of multiple DNA elements showed significant associations with the breakpoint regions of in particular non-recurrent rearrangements. This subject was argued in non-recurrent rearrangements section of this chapter. The numerical chromosome abnormalities can arise from various errors in the mitotic spindle checkpoint and cellular processes such as kinetochore assembly, chromatid cohesion and centrosome replication, leading to missegregation of chromosomes during mitosis [25].

On the other side, multiple models involving replication and/or breakage-fusion-bridge (BFB) cycles for formation mechanism of gene amplification have been proposed. These mechanisms are clearly described in Section 3.1.7. *MYCN* amplicon units within amplification locus are often arranged as clustered head-to-tail tandem repeats in direct orientation, suggesting that *MYCN* amplification may be formed via a mechanism different than those involving BFB cycles that produce inverted arrangements [26]. Some replication-based mechanisms for *MYCN* amplification were proposed, see Section 3.1.7. This chapter reviews acquired structural and numerical chromosomal abnormalities and their potential formation mechanisms in solid tumours. Furthermore, in light of present data, the chapter proposes a new model mechanism for formation of *MYCN* amplification that is a poor prognostic factor in neuroblastoma.

2. Cancer and chromosomal abnormalities: past to present

The earliest known malignant neoplasm was diagnosed in skeleton of a resident lived in Mauer (Vienna, Austria) in the Neolithic period, around 4000 BC [27]. It was reported that this example exhibited the signs of multiple myeloma rather than a metastatic carcinoma. The word cancer comes from term karkinos, which was first used to describe a non-healing swelling or ulceration in a medical text, 'Hippocratic corpus', written in about fifth century BC [28]. Hippocrates also used the terms karkinoma and scirrhus to describe malignant nonhealing tumours and hard tumours, respectively. In addition, he recognised and described the nasal carcinoma, later proposed a treatment for this cancer.

Claudius Galenus, known as Galen of Pergamum, classified the tumours into three categories as onkoi (lumps or masses in general), karkinos (malignant ulcers), and karkinomas (nonulcerating cancers) in the second century AD [29]. He also distinguished the lumps and growths as benign and malignant types. Ibn Sina, known as Avicenna, addressed the esophagus cancer in Iran of the eleventh century [30]. He was the first physician to refer to this disease as cancer of the esophagus. A century after the cancer studies of Avicenna, the physician Ibn Zuhr or Avenzoar made the first clinical description of the polyploid colorectal tumour, uterine cancer, and basal cell carcinoma in his monumental treatise Al Taysir during the twelfth century [31]. In the sixteenth century, Gabriele Fallopius accurately described the clinical differences between benign and malignant tumours [29].

Gregor Mendel examined the offspring of hybrids after hybridization of pea plants and discovered the fundamental laws of inheritance in 1865 [32]. Charles Darwin developed the first comprehensive theory of heredity, based on the transmission of physical entities that are the basis of development through inheritance in 1868 [33]. Between 1874 and 1876, Walther Flemming described the stages of cell division in more detail and showed the transformation of fibrous scaffold and network within the nucleus into 'threads', resulting in two daughter cells [34]. Fleming decided that this fibrous scaffold and arrangement of nuclear threads were termed chromatin (stainable material) and mitosen in 1879 and 1882, respectively. Heinrich Wilhelm Waldeyer coined the term chromosomen (chromosome) for stainable bodies in 1888, after he observed the stainability of the nuclear 'threads' during division [34].

David von Hansemann was first person to describe aneuploidy in 1890 [35]. He observed abnormal mitotic figures in several carcinoma samples. These findings were later developed by Theodor Boveri. Boveri showed the unequal distribution of chromosomes to the daughter cells after the fertilization of sea-urchin eggs by two sperms between 1902 and 1914 [36]. He revealed that the chromosome is a unit of heredity and proposed that chromosomal aberrations caused the cancer. At the same time, Walter Sutton showed that chromosomes occurred in distinct pairs and segregated at meiosis in his study with grasshopper chromosomes [37]. Sutton was the first to point out that the chromosomes conformed to Mendel's heredity rules. In other words, Sutton and Bovery developed the first clear chromosome theory of heredity.

Nowell and Hungerford first showed that the chromosomal abnormality was associated with a specific cancer [38]. They discovered a minute chromosome known as Philadelphia (Ph) chromosome today in the neoplastic cells of cases with chronic granulocytic leukaemia in 1960.

Spriggs *et al.* reported that many solid tumours included the aneuploid cell clones, which are hiperdiploid and/or relatively less hipodiploid, harbouring chromosomes in varying numbers detectable even in same case in 1962 [39]. They suggested that the biological success of these aneuploid clones is due presumably to the natural selection of successful variants. Rowley detected the Philadelphia (Ph) chromosome in the bone marrow and a few blood samples from the patients with chronic myelogenous leukaemia (CML), using the quinacrine fluorescence and Giemsa staining techniques in 1973 [40]. Author also observed the second Ph chromosome in a case and trisomy 8 in two patients in blast crisis.

The homogeneously staining region (hsr) was first detected in drug-resistant Chinese hamster sublines and two neuroblastoma cell lines, SK-N-BE(2) and IMR-32, using the trypsin-Giemsa banding methods in 1976 [41]. The authors also showed that the hsr replicated relatively, rapidly and synchronously before the midpoint of the S phase. In addition, two identical giant marker chromosomes 1 (bearing der(1)t(1;17) translocation containing 2p24 hsr) including 1p deletion, in addition to intact 1, were identified in IMR-32 neuroblastoma cell line in 1977 [42].

Atkin and Baker revealed that the pericentric inversions involving the heterochromatic regions of the chromosomes 1 are relatively common in cancer patients including solid tumours in 1977 [43].

http://dx.doi.org/10.5772/67733

The fluorescence *in situ* hybridization (FISH) method was developed by Bauman *et al.* in 1980 [44]. By *in situ* hybridization and Southern blotting methods, N-myc oncogene and its amplification in the hsrs were discovered in numerous neuroblastoma cell lines and a neuroblastoma tumour tissue by Schwab *et al.* in 1983 [45].

Comparative genomic hybridization (CGH) method was developed for detecting and mapping the relative DNA sequence copy number between genomes by Kallioniemi *et al.* in 1992 [46]. Multicolor spectral karyotyping (SKY), a molecular cytogenetic technique, for detecting and analyzing the chromosomal aberrations in clinical samples was developed by Schröck *et al.* in 1996 [47].

3. Chromosomal abnormalities

3.1. Structural chromosomal abnormalities

3.1.1. Recurrent genomic rearrangements

Recurrent structural genomic rearrangements often result from NAHR between LCRs in direct or inverted orientation [48]. NAHR involving nonallelic crossover is one of the homologous recombination mechanisms of two-ended double-strand break (DSB) repair and occurs in both meiotic and mitotic cells in human [49].

LCRs, also called segmental duplications (SDs), are region-specific DNA blocks of 10–400 kb in length with ≥97% identity between repeat copies [50]. SDs define hotspot of the chromosomal rearrangements and hence can act as mediator of normal variation or recurrent chromosomal aberrations associated with a genomic disease [51]. LCR-mediated NAHR mechanism occurs preferentially at the hotspots inside low copy repeats and yields the recurrent rearrangements with common size and clustered (fixed) breakpoints in unrelated individuals (**Figure 1a**) [8].

Ectopic interchromosomal and interchromatidal (intrachromosomal) recombination (NAHR) between directly oriented LCRs *in trans* can produce both deletion and duplication (**Figure 1b**), whereas intrachromatidal crossover *in cis* can result in only deletion [52]. Inversion can occur through ectopic crossing-over between inversely oriented LCRs *in cis* (**Figure 1c**). In addition, NAHR between inversely oriented LCRs on sister chromatids can cause an isochromosome formation [52]. NAHR between interchromosomal LCRs on nonhomologous chromosomes can lead to recurrent translocations [53]. Besides the segmental duplications, NAHR between interspersed repeats such as LINEs and Alus can result in de novo unbalanced translocation and interstitial deletion, respectively [54, 55].

NAHR hotspots, specific to meiosis, can cause *de novo* alterations in copy number of dosage-sensitive genes associated with some genomic disorders in germ line cells, resulting in structural rearrangements such as deletion and duplication [56]. NAHR also mediates the recurrent genomic rearrangements occurring at relatively high frequency in particular adults in human somatic cells, suggesting the accumulation of *de novo* variations after birth [57].

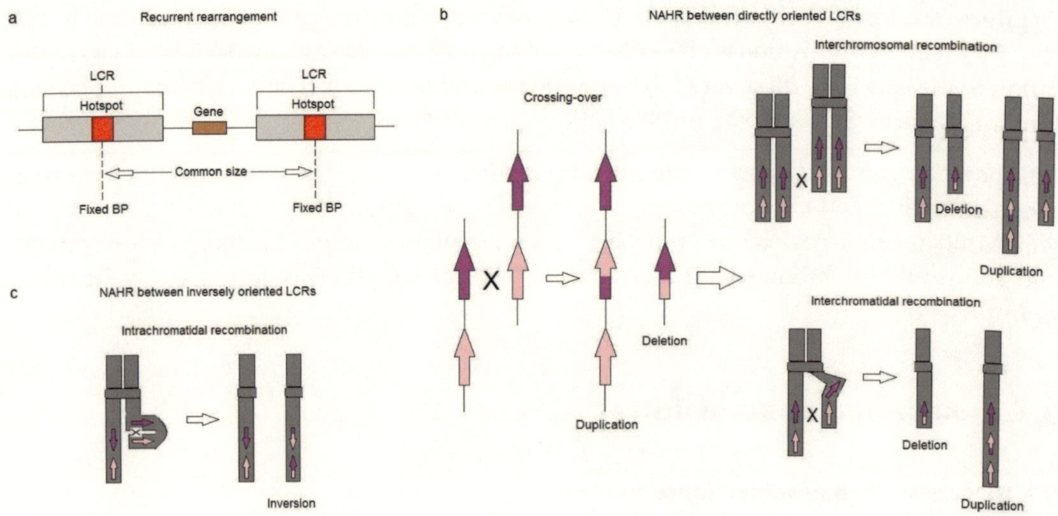

Figure 1. LCR-mediated nonallelic homologous recombination (NAHR). (**a**) Recurrent rearrangement with common size and clustered (fixed) breakpoints (BPs) resulting from NAHR between LCRs. (**b**) NAHR between directly oriented LCRs can yield both deletion and duplication through interchromosomal and interchromatidal (intrachromosomal) recombination. (**c**) NAHR between inversely oriented LCRs can result in an inversion through intrachromatidal recombination.

In addition, segmental duplications are markedly enriched at the multi-allelic CNVs, complex CNVs and loci including both deletion and duplication in human genome [58]. Carcinoma-associated breakpoint regions in human genome frequently contain SDs [59]. However, literature includes a limited number of the chromosomal abnormalities caused by NAHR mechanism in solid tumours. Of these studies, four reported that NAHR involved in large deletion of EXT1 and EXT2 genes in multiple osteochondromas and large deletion and duplication of NF1 gene in neurofibromatosis type 1 (NF1) [60–63].

3.1.2. Non-recurrent genomic rearrangements

Non-recurrent rearrangements are characterized by unique breakpoint junction in each individual but share an overlapped genomic region between the scattered breakpoints [8]. This SRO may encompass one or more genes (**Figure 2**), which are associated with a genetic disease or neoplasm. Due to the SRO region, the patients are likely to display similar clinical phenotypes. Like LCR in the recurrent rearrangement, any specific repeat causing a nonrecurrent rearrangement was not reported. However, one of the breakpoint locations of a nonrecurrent rearrangement in the genomic region can include relatively less scattered breakpoints in a smaller defined area, termed breakpoint grouping (**Figure 2**), suggesting that a genomic architecture such as palindrome or cruciform was extruded near this defined area [8].

The repetitive DNA sequence elements, such as inverted repeats, direct repeats, long inverted repeats (LIRs), *Alu* repeats, G-guadruplex-forming G-rich repeats and palindromic AT-rich repeats (PATRRs) were often detected in the breakpoint regions of many non-recurrent chromosomal abnormalities associated with genomic disorder, inherited disease or cancer in human [64–73].

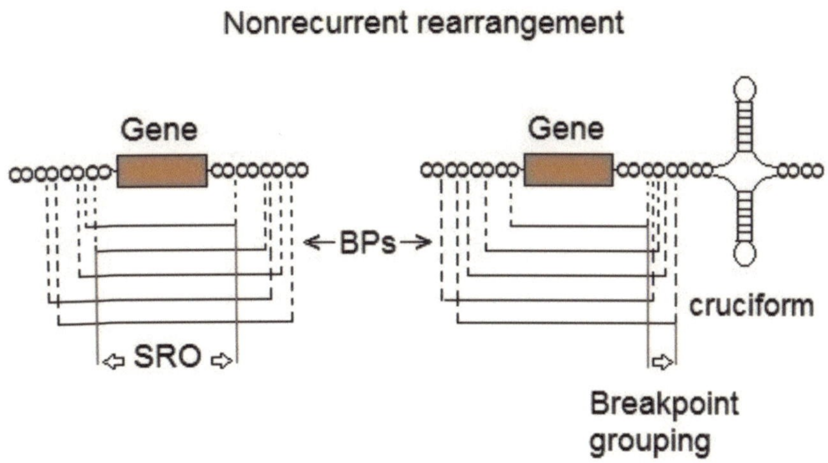

Figure 2. Nonrecurrent rearrangements share a smallest region of overlap (SRO). Dashed lines indicate the scattered breakpoints (BPs). In left side, a cruciform near the region containing the grouping of 3′ BPs is demonstrated.

Double strand breaks involving genomic rearrangements, translocations and deletions in neoplastic cells are usually joined by NHEJ [74]. NHEJ is active throughout the cell cycle, and its activity increases during transition from G1 to G2/M, whereas HR is most active in the S phase in human cells, concluding that normal human somatic cells also mostly utilised error-prone NHEJ at all cell cycle stages [75].

NHEJ mechanism tolerates nucleotide loss or addition at the rejoining site. This nonhomologous repair pathway requires three enzymatic activities (**Figure 3**), which involve the nucleases removing damaged DNA, the polymerases aiding in the repair and a ligase restoring the phosphodiester backbone [81].

Essential components of the canonical or classical NHEJ (c-NHEJ) include Ku70/80, DNA-PKcs and LIG4/XRCC4/XLF complex (**Figure 3a**), whereas the alternative forms of NHEJ, termed microhomology-mediated end joining (MMEJ), alt-NHEJ or A-EJ (**Figure 3b**, **c**), involves PARP1, MRN complex and its partner CtIP [77, 80, 82]. c-NHEJ actually plays a conservative role in genomic integrity but is versatile and adaptable in joining process of imperfect complementary DNA ends [83]. In other words, the accuracy of repair depends on the structure of DNA ends rather than c-NHEJ pathway [83].

A-EJ repairs the DSBs in the absence of key c-NHEJ proteins [84]. A-EJ is highly error-prone during end-joining process, leading to frequent DNA loss at the junctions and chromosomal rearrangements [79]. Other alternative end joining pathway, microhomology-mediated end joining (MMEJ), requires a microhomology of at least five nucleotides between DNA ends at the break sites and is independent of Ku70/80 and Ligase IV proteins of c-NHEJ but is dependent on MRN complex (Mre11, Rad50 and NBS1), Ligase III, XRCC1, FEN1 and PARP1 (**Figure 3b**), as compared to c-NHEJ that uses either no microhomology or sometimes terminal microhomology of 1–4 nucleotides between two ends [76, 78]. MMEJ can operate in where the microhomology is present, even in the presence of c-NHEJ in both cancer and normal cells [78].

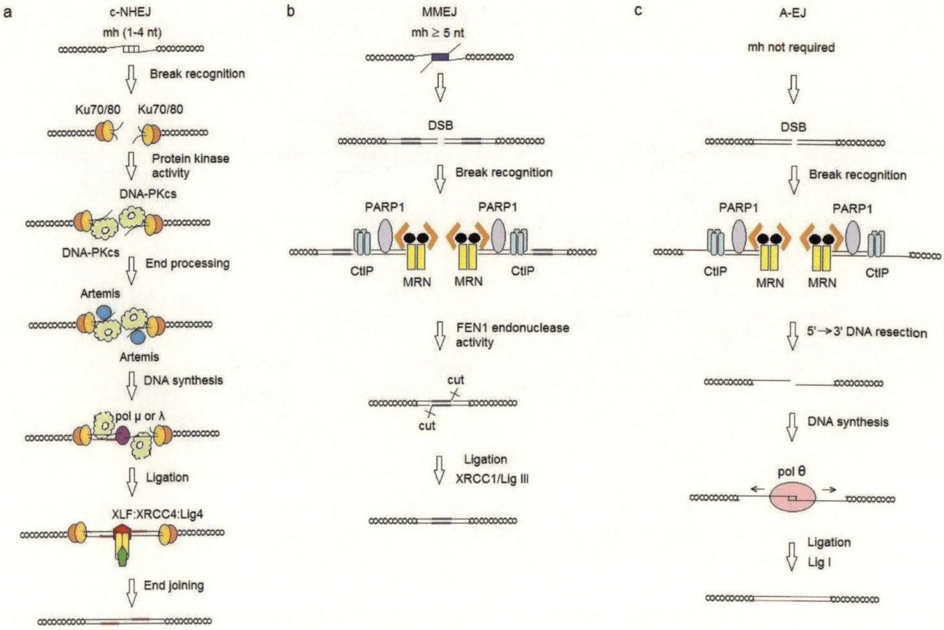

Figure 3. End joining mechanisms for repair of double-strand breaks. (**a**) Classical NHEJ (c-NHEJ) joins the DNA ends with microhomology (mh) of 1–4 nucleotides (nt) [76]. DNA break is recognised by Ku70/80, which recruits the DNA-dependent protein kinase catalytic subunit (DNA-PKcs). DNA-PKcs activates the Artemis that shows the endonuclease activity in both ends during end processing. DNA polymerase (pol µ or λ) performs the DNA synthesis, followed by ligation process (XLF:XRCC4:Lig4 complex) [77, 78]. (**b**) MMEJ joins the DNA ends with mh ≥5 nt. MRN complex and PARP1 recognise the DNA break, and CtIP starts the DNA resection. FEN1 endonuclease removes the flap, followed by ligation process with Ligase III (Lig III) [78, 79]. (**c**) A-EJ does not require the microhomology. A-EJ shares first step (break recognition) with MMEJ. But, A-EJ involves DNA synthesis with pol θ, followed by ligation with Lig I [79, 80].

In addition, replication-based mechanisms (**Figure 4**), FoSTeS and microhomology-mediated break-induced replication (MMBIR) for the formation of nonrecurrent rearrangements involving complex duplication and deletion, inversion, translocation, triplication and rolling circle were proposed [85, 86].

Taken together, the breakpoint analysis of structural chromosomal rearrangements in solid tumours shows that NHEJ, A-EJ and MMEJ are predominant mechanisms underlying these somatic aberrations; however, FoSTeS and MMBIR are responsible for a significant number of structural variations, in particular somatic complex deletions [87–89].

3.1.3. Translocations

Chromosomal translocations, which are one of the most common types of genetic rearrangements, generally arise from reciprocal exchange of heterologous chromosome fragments and can cause deregulation of gene expression through either juxtaposition of the oncogenes near promoter/enhancer elements or gene fusion [90]. Contrary to reciprocal translocations, Robertsonian translocations can be generated by joining between the long arms of two acrocentric chromosomes around a single centromeric region [91]. Reciprocal translocations can

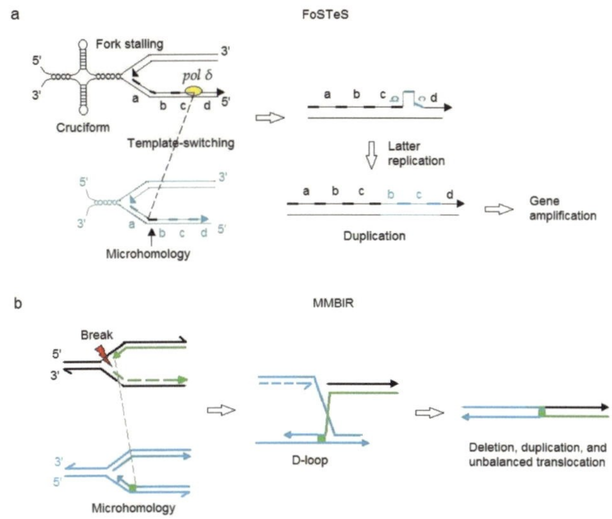

Figure 4. Replication-based mechanisms proposed for generating the nonrecurrent rearrangements. (**a**) A DNA lesion or a non-B DNA structure like cruciform can cause fork stalling during replication, stimulating the fork stalling and template switching (FoSTeS) mechanism [8, 85]. Lagging strand may then invade other fork via microhomology, leading to template-switching. By this way, duplication can arise after second round of replication. Successive template switching can result in gene amplification (see Section 3.1.7). (**b**) Microhomology-mediated break-induced replication (MMBIR) mechanism can be triggered by a single strand break, which gives rise to replication collapse [86]. The 3′ single strand overhang can invade a microhomology site at the other fork, and DNA polymerase restarts DNA synthesis through D-loop formation, resulting in deletion, duplication, and unbalanced translocation.

lead to balanced or unbalanced rearrangements. Balanced translocations do not cause the gain or loss of genetic material but can result in promoter swapping/substitution or loss of gene function, which was reported in some benign and malignant solid tumours [3], whereas unbalanced translocations result in a gain or loss, involving trisomy or monosomy in any chromosome segment, respectively [92].

Malignant solid tumours generally harbour non-recurrent balanced aberrations including many translocations rather than recurrent balanced ones; see **Table 1** in Ref. [3]. In addition, solid tumours show less often gene fusions compared to haematological disorders. Most of them, such as *EWSR1-POU5F1* (Bone sarcoma), *EWSR1-ERG* (Ewing sarcoma) and *PAX3-FOXO1A* (Rhabdomyosarcoma), were observed in sarcomas [3].

Many recurrent unbalanced translocations, such as der(1)t(1;1)(p36;q12) (Breast adenocarcinoma), der(3)t(3;6)(p11;p11) (Kidney adenocarcinoma), der(19)t(11;19)(q12;q13) (Lung squamous cell carcinoma) and der(12)t(11;12)(q12;q23) (Testis germ cell tumour), were detected in solid tumours [12].

Numerous inter-chromosomal and intra-chromosomal translocations in solid tumours were identified, and majority of these translocations were reported to form via NHEJ and A-EJ mechanisms (**Figure 5a**), while a small number of them was generated by FoSTeS/MMBIR [88]. A-EJ was more abundant in most cases. In addition, A-EJ is more significantly associated with breast tumours compared to other tumour types. Alt-NHEJ is also primary mediator of

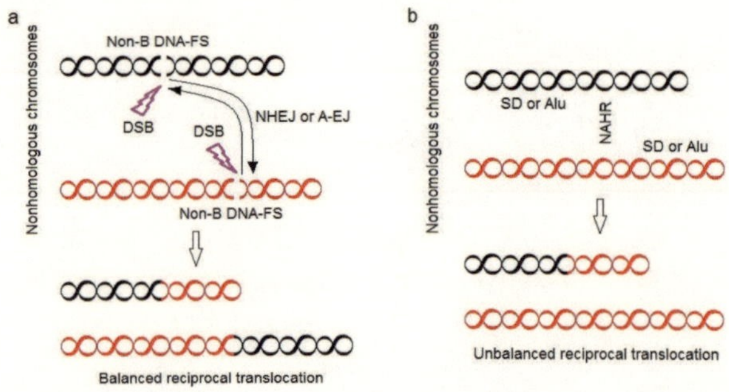

Figure 5. Reciprocal translocation mechanisms. (**a**) A balanced reciprocal translocation resulted from nonhomologous recombination. Random or a non-B DNA-forming sequence (Non-B DNA-FS) may induce the double-strand breaks on the nonhomologous chromosomes, stimulating NHEJ or A-EJ. (**b**) An unbalanced reciprocal translocation arose from nonallelic homologous recombination. Interchromosomal segmental duplications (SDs) or Alu interspersed elements may be mediator of NAHR [53–55, 93].

translocation formation in mammalian cells [94]. However, it was reported that c-NHEJ is the predominant mechanism for repair of the double-strand breaks, resulting in translocation formation in human cells [95].

On the other side, it was found that the breakpoint regions of recurrent translocations in solid tumours are flanked by segmental duplications and Alu element [93], suggesting that SD or Alu-mediated NAHR mechanism involves formation of recurrent translocations in solid tumours (**Figure 5b**).

In vertebrates, NHEJ is the main pathway for repair of DSBs, which is required for suppressing the chromosomal translocations [96]. However, the non-B DNA structures around breakpoint junctions can lead to chromosomal translocations (**Figure 5a**). Potential non-B DNA structure (e.g., hairpin/cruciform, triplex and quadruplex)-forming repeats such as inverted repeat, direct repeat, inversions of inverted repeat, (AT)n, (GAA)n, (GAAA)n, G4-DNA motifs and H-DNA are significantly associated with breakpoint regions of translocations in the cancers including solid tumours [97–99]. In addition, formation of *de novo* translocations between AT-rich repeats (PATRRs) was tested in cultured human cells. Contrary to *de novo* deletions, *de novo* translocations between PATRRs were not observed during both leading and lagging strand synthesis in the presence of slowed DNA replication. Kurahashi *et al.* thus proposed that translocation may be formed via a DNA replication-independent cruciform structure induced by PATRR [100].

3.1.4. Deletions

Chromosomal deletion is the most common structural aberration among recurrent unbalanced chromosomal abnormalities in solid tumours [12]. Chromosomal deletions are mainly classified into two groups as interstitial and terminal deletions. Interstitial deletion is formed by two breaks, whereas terminal deletion can occur due to one break near telomere [10].

Gross deletions can cause the loss of one or more genes in human-inherited diseases and cancers [71]. Heterozygous or homozygous deletions involving many tumour suppressor genes may play a major role in tumour initiation and progression. Interstitial heterozygous deletions within chromosome 3 common eliminated region I (C3CER I) including multiple genes such

http://dx.doi.org/10.5772/67733

as *LIMD1*, *LTF* and *TMEM7*, mapped to 3p21.3, are widespread in solid tumours, suggesting that C3CER I region may harbour some tumour suppressor genes, besides its LOH may be causative in tumour development rather than reflection of an unstable genome in tumour cells [101]. Another study suggests that homozygous deletion of *PTEN* locus may be associated with metastasis in prostate cancer [102].

Homozygous deletions observed in multiple different chromosomal loci, some of them encompass LRP1B, FHIT, PARK2, CDKN2A (p16), CDKN2B (p15), PTEN, and WWOX tumour suppressor genes were frequently found in many cancer cell lines, usually derived from a solid tumour [103].

Many model mechanisms can explain gross genomic deletions. But, formation mechanism of deletion remains to be clearly enlightened.

NAHR-mediated deletion (**Figure 1**) was reported in a limited number of solid tumours. A study indicated that large deletion of EXT1 and EXT2 genes in multiple osteochondromas families can be occurred by NAHR between *Alu* repeats as well as NHEJ [60].

The genomic rearrangements including deletions in solid tumours are predominantly caused by end-joining mechanisms, NHEJ, MMEJ or A-EJ; however, complex deletions are generally formed by FoSTeS/MMBIR [87–89].

In addition, gross deletions have been associated with non-B DNA structure-forming sequences in breakpoint regions, including direct repeats, inverted repeats, inversion of inverted repeats, long inverted repeats (LIRs), and *Alus* in the genomes of cancers including solid tumours [71, 72, 97–99].

Gordenin *et al.* [104] previously proposed that an inverted repeat can form a hairpin at the lagging strand during replication, causing a deletion via slippage of DNA polymerase between short direct repeats adjacent to both side of stem of a LIR or between smaller repeats within LIR (**Figure 6a**). Lobachev *et al.* [105] proposed that homologous recombination between sister chromatids will repair the DNA strand without deletion at the inverted repeat site. According to their model, if another inverted repeat is present on the other chromosome, recombination then could lead to a deletion.

Later, it was shown that a hairpin formed by inverted repeat stalled the replication fork in both prokaryotes and eukaryotes, indicating that DNA hairpins are formed likely during lagging strand synthesis [106]. Kurahashi *et al.* [100] demonstrated that deletions occurred within PATRRs due to slow replication and uncoupling of DNA polymerase and helicase complex respectively during the synthesis of both lagging and leading strands in human cells, suggesting that replication slippage caused deletion of the hairpins induced by PATRRs in leading and lagging strand (**Figure 6b**).

Akgün *et al.* [107] proposed that the break generated by a nicking endonuclease in the top of hairpin can stimulate the cellular repair mechanisms, resulting in one-sided (in only one of repeat units) or two-sided (in both of the repeat units) palindrome deletions (**Figure 6c**). Cunningham *et al.* [108] showed that a nicking near hairpin tips by endonuclease in a perfect palindrome can result in deletions at the center of palindrome after rejoining of the breaks by NHEJ (**Figure 6c**).

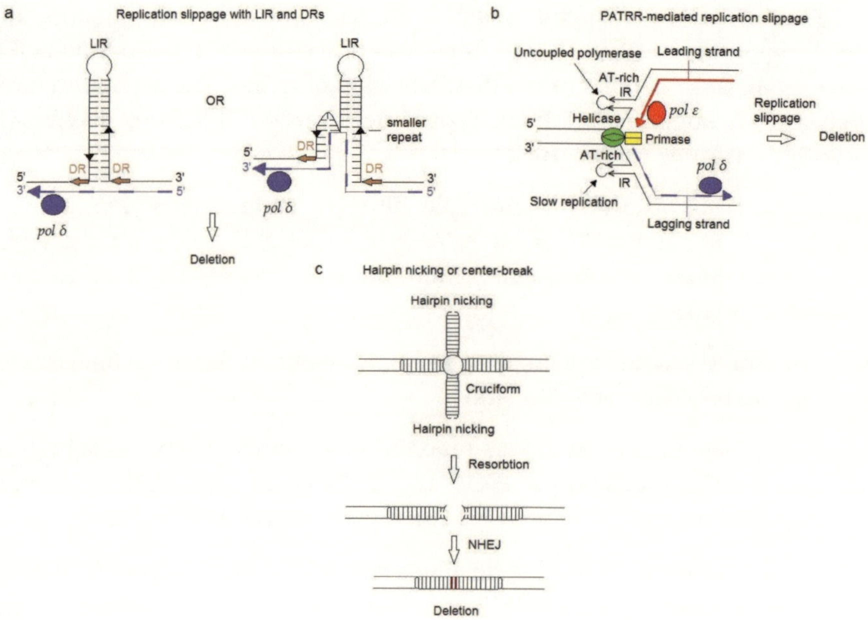

Figure 6. Chromosomal deletion mechanisms. (**a**) Replication slippage caused by a LIR in lagging strand during DNA replication. Direct repeats in both side of LIR and smaller repeats within LIR lead to deletions at entire LIR and a segment of LIR, respectively. (**b**) Replication slippage induced by palindromic AT-rich repeats (PATRRs). Deletion of both PATRRs in lagging and leading strand templates can form via slow replication and uncoupling of DNA polymerase and helicase complex, respectively. (**c**) Hairpin nicking or center-break mechanism. Hairpin nicking can result in deletion at the center or both sides of a cruciform. NHEJ rejoins double-strand break after resorbtion.

I previously found that LIRs are significantly associated with the breakpoint regions of gross deletions in human-inherited diseases and cancers [71]. Statistical analysis showed that a positive significant strong correlation was found between 5′ and 3′ LIR numbers. In addition, negative significant correlations were found between deletion size and the numbers of 5′ and 3′ LIRs. These results suggest that LIRs could be contributed to DNA sequence evolution in human genome. Statistical analyses also suggested that DNA strand is potentially broken in locations closer to bigger LIRs. Another analysis demonstrated that loop length and stem identity of 3′ LIRs were more important in larger deletions. In light of these findings, I proposed two model mechanisms involving LIR-mediated gene deletion (**Figure 7a, b**). In first mechanism, it was proposed that gross deletion can be generated by breaks formed near two LIRs at the 5′ and 3′ breakpoints, which are located two contiguous replication bubbles (**Figure 7a**). In second mechanism, it was proposed that back-folded stem loop structure can cause a second break at the 5′ breakpoint region after a break near 3′ LIR occurred during replication, resulting in gene deletion (**Figure 7b**). In this chapter, I also proposed a new modified model mechanism involving 5′ and 3′ LIRS within same replicon, adapted from other two ones (**Figure 7c**).

Hairpin structures were shown to form at an interrupted LIR with 111-bp stem and 24-bp spacer at the frequencies of 32–37% on both leading and lagging strand templates, respectively, suggesting that hairpins were extruded simultaneously by palindrome on both leading and lagging strand templates during replication [110]. However, another study showed that an

http://dx.doi.org/10.5772/67733

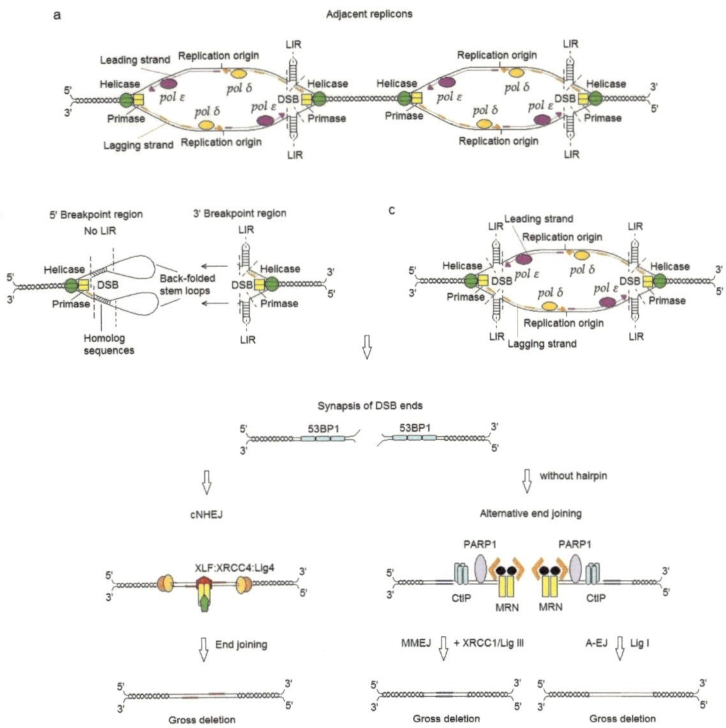

Figure 7. Model mechanisms of long inverted repeat (LIR)-mediated gene deletion during replication (adapted from Ref. [71]). (**a**) LIR-induced gene deletion between adjacent replicons. (**b**) Back-folded stem loop-mediated gene deletion within same replicon. (**c**) 5′ and 3′ LIRs-involved gene deletion within same replicon. Synapsis of DNA double-strand break (DSB) ends is performed by 53BP1 [109]. C-NHEJ can join DNA DSB ends with hairpin or no hairpin via Artemis—DNA-PKcs complex (see **Figure 3**) [74]. In alternative end joining mechanisms, hairpin-opening activity was not yet reported. According to these models proposed here, MMEJ and A-EJ can involve the joining of free DNA ends without hairpin.

interrupted palindrome with 230-bp stem and 20-bp spacer formed a hairpin only on the lagging-strand template in *Escherichia coli*, whereas perfect palindrome generated hairpin on both leading and lagging strand templates during replication [111].

53BP1 can combine free DNA ends between distant sites for repair of double-strand breaks by NHEJ [109]. Through a process dependent on 53BP1 and DNA ligase 4 that are the factors of c-NHEJ, double-strand breaks associated with DNA replication during S phase in BRCA1-deficient cells are aberrantly joined, leading to complex chromosome rearrangements [112]. The ablation of 53BP1 rescues genomic instability in mice expressing BRCA1 lacking N-terminal RING domain [113].

3.1.5. Duplication

Recurrent unbalanced duplications were considerably reported, even though deletions and unbalanced translocations were much more frequent among unbalanced abnormalities in solid tumours [12]. Identical copies of duplicated segments can be distributed as either tandem or interspersed in human genome [10, 114].

Most of germline duplication CNVs (83%) were found to be tandem duplications in direct orientation [115]. A tandem duplication of about 2 Mb at 7q34 produces a novel oncogenic *KIAA1549:BRAF* fusion gene capable of transformation in pilocytic astrocytomas [116]. Duplication or gain of chromosome 2p containing the *MYCN* locus by unbalanced translocations is often observed in neuroblastoma cell lines [117].

Segmental duplications (so called low copy repeats, LCRs) in direct or inverted orientation can lead to recurrent chromosomal abnormalities via NAHR mechanism in both germ line and somatic cells, as discussed in Section 3.1.1 (**Figure 1**). A total of approximately 4% of human genome contains segmental duplications, classified as intrachromosomal (2.64%) and interchromosomal (1.44%) duplications [118].

Gene duplication can be produced either by DNA-mediated mechanisms such as unequal crossing over, tandem segmental, chromosomal, and genome duplications or by RNA-based retroposition involving reverse transcription of RNAs from parental genes [119]. In addition, gene duplication can be formed by MMBIR mechanism (**Figure 8**), which is a replication-based mechanism [48].

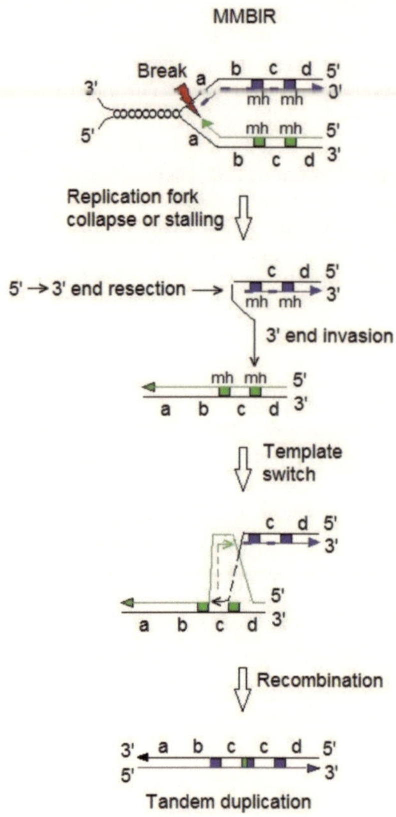

Figure 8. Tandem duplication via microhomology-mediated break-induced replication (MMBIR) mechanism. A single strand break during replication leads to fork collapse or stalling [48]. Then, free 3′ end invades a microhomology (mh) site on the other template, causing template switch. MMBIR results in tandem duplication.

http://dx.doi.org/10.5772/67733

Tandem duplications are often observed in solid tumours [87–89]. The breakpoints of tandem duplications in solid tumours have mostly no or short microhomology, indicating a template-switching mechanism that does not require microhomology or another non-homology–based mechanism underlying chromosomal duplications [88].

3.1.6. *Other chromosomal rearrangements*

Normal human genome contains recurrent DNA inversion rearrangements derived from NAHR in particular chromosomes 3, 15, and 19 [57]. The pericentric inv(1) has been more frequently observed in cancer patients (15%), as compared with normal population (4%) [43]. Inversions were much more common (54%) in solid tumours [89].

A small inversion within chromosome 2p generates the *EML4/ALK* fusion gene capable of transformation in non–small-cell lung cancer (NSCLC) cells [120]. Likewise, a pericentric inversion inv(10)(p11.22q11.21) gives rise to *KIF5B/RET* fusion gene that overexpresses chimeric RET receptor tyrosine kinase capable of cellular transformation in NSCLC cells [121].

Inversion is a balanced structural abnormality (**Figure 9a**) and recurs in chromosomes 2, 3, 6, 7, 10, 12, 16, 19 and X in solid tumours [12]. In addition, inversion of chromosome 1 was found in ovary carcinoma, breast carcinoma, seminoma and lymphosarcoma tumours [43].

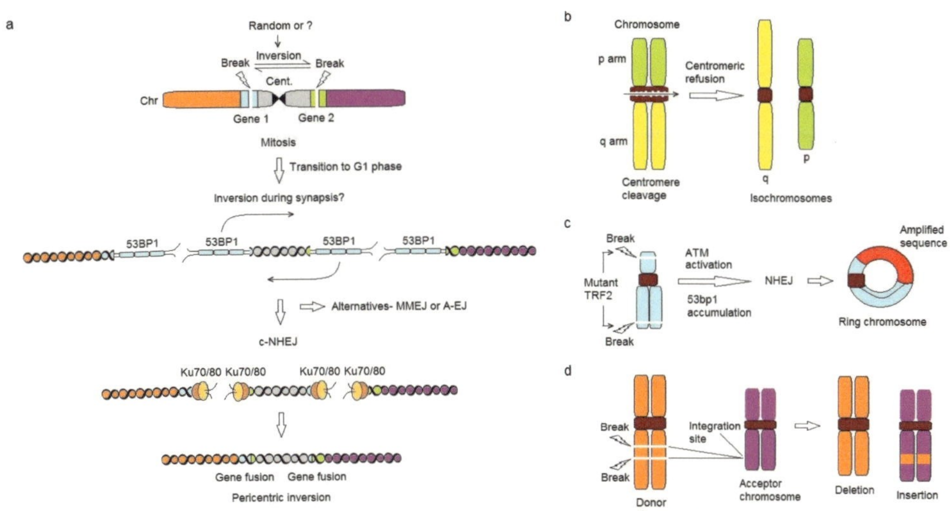

Figure 9. Model mechanisms for the formation of other chromosomal abnormalities observed in solid tumours. (**a**) Model mechanism of a pericentric inversion causing gene fusion is illustrated. NHEJ can result in inversion [49]. According to this model, two chromosomal breaks around centromere in mitosis lead to a pericentric inversion [121]. However, it is not clear how the inversion occurred in which phase of the cell cycle. DSBs occurring in mitosis are not repaired until cells will enter G1 phase [122]. Later, double-strand breaks can be rejoined by NHEJ in G1, see also **Figure 3a** [81], after synapsis of break ends with 53BP1 [109]. (**b**) A model mechanism involving centromere cleavage for isochromosome formation. (**c**) NHEJ-mediated ring chromosome formation. Mutant TRF2 leads to not protect telomeres from DSBs, and 53BP1 promotes NHEJ pathway, which joins the dysfunctional telomeres. (**d**) A chromosomal insertion occurred by three breaks. The fragment resulted from two breaks on the donor chromosome is inserted into integration site at the acceptor chromosome, resulting in an insertion.

An inversion can result from NAHR between inversely oriented LCRs in germ line and somatic cells; see Section 3.1.1 in this chapter (**Figure 1c**). The rearrangement junctions of inversions in breast cancer genomes contain mean 2.5-bp (range, 0–21) microhomology, suggesting that non-homologous end-joining DNA repair involves in formation of inversion [123].

Isochromosomes involving chromosomes 1–17, 21, 22, and X were reported in solid tumours [12]. The i(5p) is a specific chromosome change in bladder cancer, while the i(12p) is seen in almost all tumours of germ cell origin, including seminomas, embryonal cell tumours and teratocarcinomas [124]. Isochromosome 5q along with dmins and hsrs bears extra copies of DHFR gene in the amplified RAD54 deficient cells [125]. In 8% of non-*MYCN* amplified primary tumours, a small number of additional *MYCN* gene copies was shown to be gained through either formation of an isochromosome 2p, or an unbalanced translocation of chromosome 2p including *MYCN* gene, suggesting that isochromosome formation might be one of mediators of gene amplification [126].

For the formation of isochromosomes, multiple mechanisms such as centromeric cleavage, transverse division of the centromere, and NAHR between paralogous LCRs on the sister chromatids were proposed [52, 127, 128]. The centromeric cleavage among these mechanisms was presented (**Figure 9b**).

Constitutional ring chromosomes, 10, 11, 13, 17 and 22, including tumour suppressor gene, were reported in thyroid follicular adenocarcinoma, Wilms tumour, retinoblastoma, neurofibromatosis and meningioma, respectively [129].

Ring chromosomes can form by end-to-end reunion or fusion to other subtelomeric end of the breakage site(s) occurred on either both chromosome arms or one of them, respectively [130], as shown in **Figure 9c**. The ring chromosomes that are observed in atypical lipomatous tumours and other subtypes of mesenchymal neoplasms contain the amplified sequences, primarily from chromosome 12 [131]. In addition, deletion of the shelterin component TRF2 from mouse cells leads to not protect telomeres from DSBs, resulting in activation of ATM kinase and accumulation of 53BP1, promoting the joining of dysfunctional telomeres by NHEJ repair process [132]. NHEJ can generate either a circular chromosome or an unstable dicentric chromosome through a single end joining event between two telomeres [133]. These studies suggest that 53BP1-promoted NHEJ pathway can give rise to formation of a ring chromosome in the absence of TRF2 (**Figure 9c**).

Insertion can be produced by at least three chromosomal breaks, involving a non-reciprocal translocation either between two nonhomologous chromosomes (interchromosomal insertion) or between different regions of same chromosome (intrachromosomal insertion) [134]. During this abnormal process, a chromosomal segment, which is formed by two breaks in a donor chromosome, is inserted into an interstitial region of acceptor chromosome (**Figure 9d**). Large insertions can also be seen in solid tumours [88]. In addition, exonic insertion of L1 and Alu elements was identified in somatic or germline cells in epithelial ovarian cancers [135].

3.1.7. Gene amplification

A large number of oncogenes are amplified in many solid tumours [15, 136]. Amplification of various oncogenes located chromosomes 1–8, 11–14, 16–20 and X, which include AuroraA/AURKA

http://dx.doi.org/10.5772/67733

(bladder, breast and oesophageal), CCND1 (breast, lung, malignant melanoma and oral squamous cell carcinoma), EGFR (colorectal, glioma, lung and oesophageal), ERBB2 (bladder, breast, endometrial, gastric, oesophageal and ovarian), MDM2 (breast, glioma, lung, neuroblastoma and sarcoma), MYC (breast, colorectal, gastric, lung, medulloblastoma and prostate), MYCL1 (lung), *MYCN* (lung, neuroblastoma and rhabdomyosarcoma) and SKP2 (lung, oesophageal and soft tissue sarcoma) was reported in Ref. [15].

The copies of amplified genes are included on either hsrs or dmins [16]. The hsr and dmin are often observed in cell lines derived from solid tumours [137]. Amplicon size of hsr regions varies between 0.8 and 12.7 Mb [138]. The dmins are tiny spherical extrachromosomal structures lacking centromere and telomere, in size of a few Mb [139].

Gene amplification usually results in overexpression of amplified gene, but gene expression level and DNA amplification do not always show an exact match, suggesting that some driver genes can be overexpressed by different mechanisms in the absence of DNA amplification [15, 16]. Up to 44% of highly amplified genes were reported to be overexpressed in breast cancer cell lines, whereas only 10.5% of overexpressed genes demonstrated the increased copy number [140].

Many model mechanisms for the formation of gene amplification have been proposed. First model involves the breakage-fusion-bridge (BFB) cycle, which was first proposed by McClintock [141], between the sister chromatids in mitosis [142]. Lo *et al.* [142] demonstrated that spontaneous telomere loss on a marker chromosome 16 resulted in sister chromatid fusion in a human tumour cell line followed by the amplification of subtelomeric DNA, supporting BFB cycles-mediated gene amplification model (**Figure 10a**).

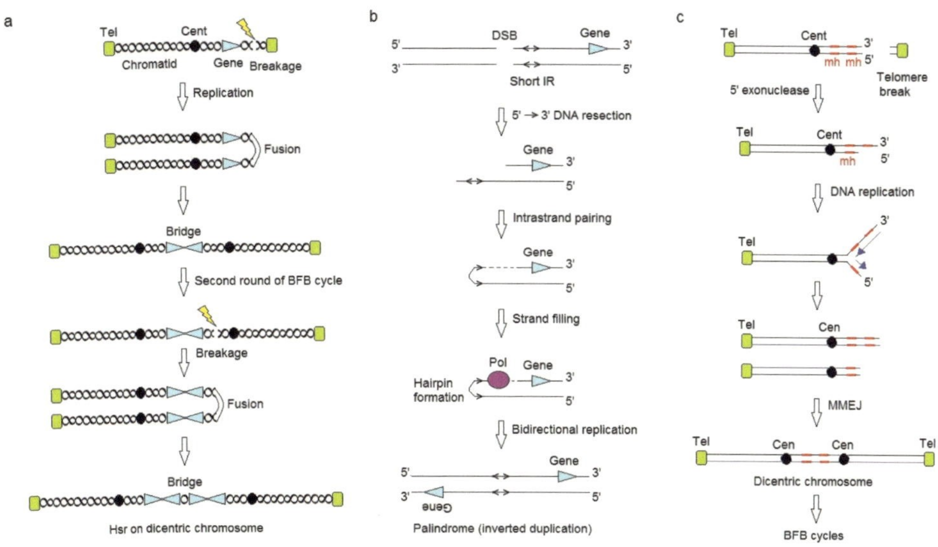

Figure 10. Model mechanisms of gene amplification producing the duplicated units in inverted orientation. (**a**) A gene amplification model involving BFB cycles resulted in hsr on the dicentric chromosome. (**b**) Short IR-mediated amplification model involving intrastrand pairing leading to hairpin formation followed by palindrome. (**c**) Microhomology-mediated gene amplification producing a dicentric chromosome followed by BFB cycles.

Tanaka *et al.* [143] showed that a short inverted repeat, which is introduced into the genome of Chinese hamster ovary cells, promoted the formation of a large DNA palindrome after an adjacent double-strand break. Therefore, the authors proposed an intramolecular recombination model initiating gene amplification through formation of head to head duplication (**Figure 10b**).

Okuno *et al.* [144] have sequenced the junction of head-to-head palindromes of an amplicon containing DHFR amplification in Chinese hamster ovary cells and showed that junction includes a 2-bp microhomology between sites separated by 4 kb. The authors thus proposed a microhomology-mediated recombination model for palindrome formation leading to dicentric chromosome, followed by BFB cycles that trigger the gene amplification (**Figure 10c**).

Difilippantonio *et al.*, [145] reported that a recombination activating gene (RAG)-induced DNA cleavage resulted in coamplification of *IgH* and c-*myc* genes after development of lymphoma in NHEJ DNA repair protein Ku and p53 tumour suppressor-deficient mice. The authors proposed a model mechanism involving RAG-induced translocation of *IgH* and c-*myc* in G1, followed by break-induced replication and c-*myc*/*IgH* amplification (head to head) after BFB cycles (**Figure 11**).

On the other side, the replication-based mechanisms for gene amplification were also proposed. Amler and Schwab [26] showed that neuroblastoma cell lines harboured multiple tandem arrays of DNA segments including *MYCN* gene, in head to tail orientation with sizes varying from 100 to 700 kb. The authors proposed that gene amplification may be involved in unscheduled DNA replication, recombination, and dmin formation followed by integration into a chromosome, resulting in subsequent *in situ* multiplication (**Figure 12a**). Schwab [146] also proposed an extra replication model involving excision of amplified segment, integration into a chromosome site, and *in situ* amplification, resulting in hsr (**Figure 12a**).

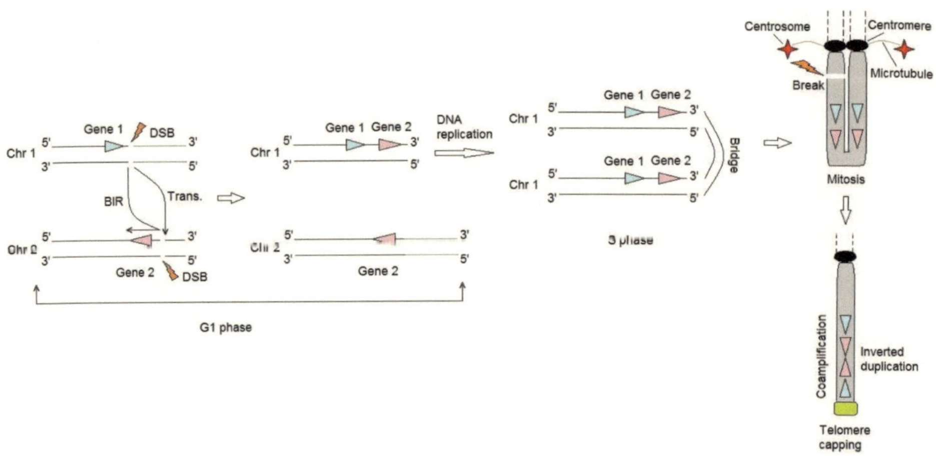

Figure 11. A gene amplification model triggered by double-strand breaks (DSBs). A DSB stimulates break-induced replication (BIR) and unbalanced translocation in G1, resulting in juxtaposition of two different genes. After DNA replication in S phase, BFB cycles cause gene duplication in inverted orientation, resulting in coamplification of two genes.

http://dx.doi.org/10.5772/67733

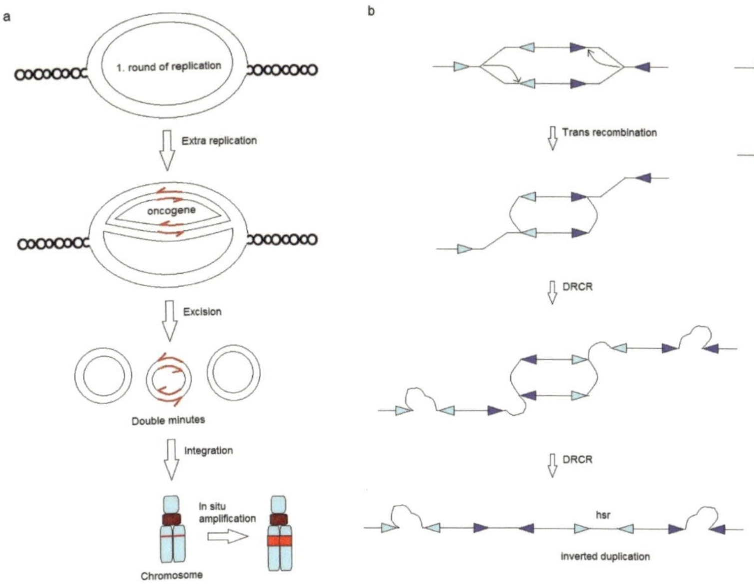

Figure 12. Replication-based mechanisms for gene amplification. (**a**) Extrareplication mechanism involving dmin formation followed by integration of dmin into a chromosome and *in situ* amplification. (**b**) Double rolling-circle replication (DRCR) model by *trans* and *cis* recombination producing hsr and dmin, respectively.

Tower [147] suggested that initial step in amplification of human oncogene and drug-resistant genes may be started by firing of DNA re-replication during S phase. Watanabe *et al.* [148] developed a gene amplification system based on double rolling-circle replication (DRCR) in yeast and mammalian cells, utilising a recombinational process induced by IRs coupled with replication, leading to hsrs and dmins (**Figure 12b**). In addition, Slack *et al.* [149] proposed the FoSTeS mechanism involving long-distance template switching for the gene amplification mechanism (**Figure 4a**).

3.2. Numerical chromosome abnormalities

Changes in chromosome number are frequently observed in particular solid tumours [4]; see **Table 1**. These changes can result from aneuploidy or polyploidy [150]. Aneuploidy refers to abnormal chromosome number deviated from euploidy that is defined as exact multiples of a haploid chromosome set [13, 150]. The chromosome sets in haploid and diploid number are cases of normal euploidy, whereas polyploidy reflects more than two sets of chromosomes, resulting in triploidy (3n), tetraploidy (4n), pentaploidy (5n), and so forth [150].

Aneuploidy involving gain or loss of whole chromosomes, at the same time, can result from some gross chromosomal structural abnormalities including deletion, duplication, unbalanced translocation, and overamplification, as described in other sections of this chapter. This type of aberrant ploidy regarding chromosomal parts is termed segmental or structural aneuploidy [151].

Near-diploid chromosome number (≤68) was predominant (71.8%) in solid tumours compared with near-tetraploid chromosome number (≥69) (19.3%) [13].

Aneuploidy is one of the main implications of chromosomal instability (CIN), leading to tumourigenesis in somatic cells [14]. Errors in cellular processes, such as chromosome condensation, chromatid cohesion, kinetochore assembly, and microtubule/centrosome formation as well as checkpoints, which involved in replication and segregation of chromosomes during mitosis, could lead to the CIN, resulting in chromosomal losses and gains in most cancers (**Figure 13a–d**) [25].

In addition, tetraploid cells can give rise to CIN and aneuploid cell populations *in vivo* (**Figure 13e**) [152]. Increased 4N (G2/tetraploid) fraction along with p53 inactivation during neoplastic progression of Barett's epithelial cells progressed to aneuploidy in Barrett's esophagus, which is a pre-malignant condition [153]. Studies in human cancer cell lines derived from glioblastoma, breast cancer, and melanoma showed direct relation between cell invasiveness and tumour-genome duplication (tetraploid) [154].

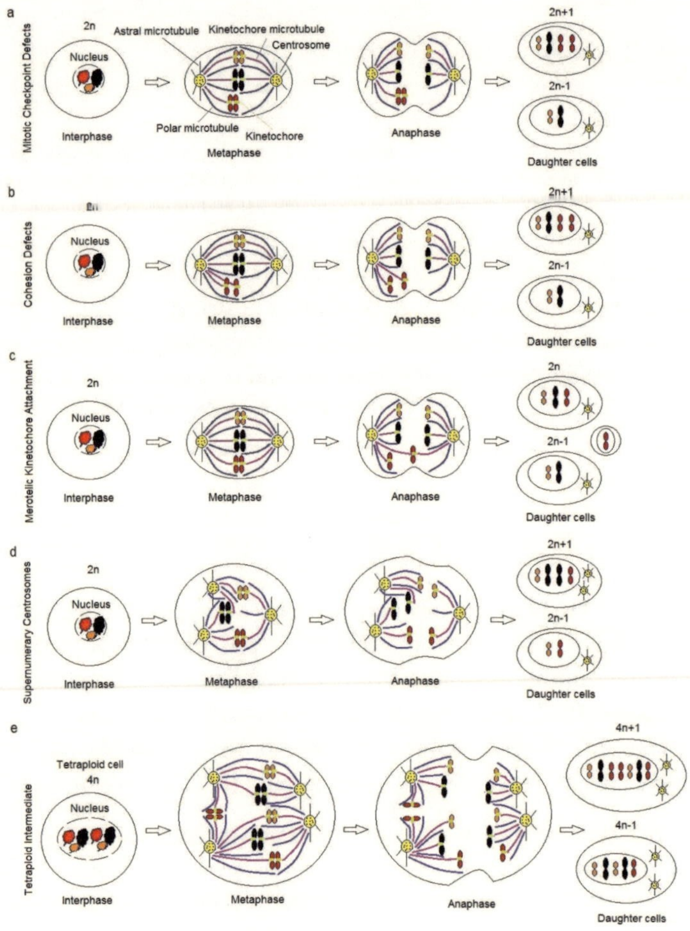

Figure 13. Formation mechanisms of aneuploidy. Errors in (**a**) mitotic checkpoint, (**b**) chromatid cohesion, (**c**) kinetochore attachment, and (**d**) centrosome formation can lead to aneuploidy. (**e**) In addition, tetraploid cells can cause aneuploid cell populations.

In addition, it was proposed that the acquisition of a single trisomy may initiate change from euploidy to aneuploidy as initial event in the development of all malignant solid tumours [155]. Aneuploidy was shown to arise from missegregation of tetraploid nuclei in yeast [156].

In addition, mice with reduced levels of CENP-E motor protein developed aneuploidy and chromosomal instability *in vitro* and *in vivo*, later formed spontaneous lymphomas and lung tumours by an increased rate of aneuploidy in aged animals, suggesting that aneuploidy drives tumourigenesis [157]. Transduction experiments between congenic euploid and trisomic fibroblasts with different oncogenes showed that nearly all aneuploid cell lines divided slowly *in vitro*, relative to matched euploid lines, suggesting that aneuploidy, particularly single-chromosome gains can reveal a tumour suppresive function, but at same time, may facilitate the development of high-complexity karyotypes, leading to advanced malignancies [158].

3.3. MYCN gene amplification in neuroblastoma

Neuroblastoma derived from primitive cells of the sympathetic nervous system is the most common malignancy among childhood cancers [159, 160]. Neuroblastoma is usually a sporadic disease that manifests many complex chromosomal abnormalities such as *MYCN* amplification, 1p deletion, 17q gain, unbalanced t(1;17) translocations, whole chromosome aneuploidies involving trisomies of chromosomes 6, 7, 19 and monosomies of 13, 22, X and Y, as well as LOH of chromosomes 2q, 3p, 4p, 9p, 11q, 14q, 16p and 18q observed in both primary tumours and cell lines [16, 42, 161–163].

MYCN amplification is observed in 18–38% of neuroblastoma cases and multiple neuroblastoma cell lines [45, 164–168]. *MYCN* amplification and 1p36 deletion are important poor prognostic factors in neuroblastoma [17, 164, 169]. We demonstrated that both 1p36 deletion and *MYCN* amplification are significant correlated with undifferentiated tumours [164]. Our group also showed that *MYCN* amplification and 1p36 deletion were associated with high tumour vascularity in neuroblastoma, suggesting close relation of *MYCN* amplification and 1p36 deletion with angiogenesis [170].

The causes and consequences of *MYCN* amplification have been widely studied, but the formation mechanism of *MYCN* amplification still remains to be completely explained. As presented in gene amplifications, some replication-based mechanisms involving the formation of *MYCN* amplification were described. In addition, multiple models of deletion including LIR-mediated gross deletion mechanism were argued in Section 3.1.4.

In this section of chapter, it was investigated the relation between LIRs and *MYCN* amplification. For this aim, LIR distribution in a genomic segment of 16,135,119 bp lying between chromosome 2p25.3 and 2p24.3 loci, including *MYCN* gene locus was first examined. In addition, LIRs were identified in the boundary sequences of amplicons containing *MYCN* gene reported in 14 neuroblastoma cell lines and 42 solid tumours. The results show that a significant association between LIRs and *MYCN* amplification loci. In addition, present data provide some insights into the *MYCN* amplification mechanism.

3.3.1. Material and methods

3.3.1.1. Bioinformatics data

In this study, the boundaries of amplicon units containing *MYCN* gene in 14 neuroblastoma cell lines (CHP134, KP-N-YS, IMR-5, SIMA, NB17, CHP-212, NB7, NB14, NB6, GOTO, NB1, NB5, NB10 and CHP-126) and 42 primary solid tumours (10 lungs, 6 endometriums, 4 bladders, 4 central nervous systems, 3 stomachs, 3 breasts, 2 heads and necks, 2 intestinals, 2 germ cells, 1 ovary, 1 liver, 1 skin, 1 oesaphagus, 1 cervix and 1 adrenal) were analyzed for LIR identification (**Table 2**). Boundary positions and their reference sequences were obtained from COSMIC database that is a catalogue of somatic mutations in cancer [171]. In addition,

Sample	Tumour	B Pos (Mb)	5′ LIR*	<2 kb	In/Out	3′ LIR**	<2 kb	In/Out	Mh
CHP134	NB	15.86–15.95	28	+	O	17	+	O	5
KPNYS	NB	15.47–15.97	6	+	I	18	+	O	5
IMR-5	NB	14.73–15.98	0	–	–	46	+	I	5
SIMA	NB	15.59–15.99	25	+	O	55	+	I	6
NB17	NB	15.61–16.80	8	+	O	1	>	Over	7
CHP212	NB	15.58–16.07	23	+	I	10	+	O	3
NB7	NB	15.66–15.96	3	>	O	12	>	O	5
NB14	NB	15.05–16.94	1	+	I	0	–	–	8
NB6	NB	15.89–15.96	10	+	I	14	+	O	5
GOTO	NB	15.82–15.95	15	+	I	17	+	I	6
NB1	NB	15.90–15.97	23	+	O	18	+	O	3
NB5	NB	15.16–16.26	0	–	–	0	–	–	2
NB10	NB	15.69–15.97	3	+	O	18	+	O	4
CHP126	NB	15.41–15.99	1	>	Over	46	+	O	2
1	EC	15.52–16.05	5	>	I	15	+	Over	2
2	BC	5.26–17.60	0	–	–	0	–	–	4

Sample	Tumour	B Pos (Mb)	5′ LIR*	<2 kb	In/Out	3′ LIR**	<2 kb	In/Out	Mh
3	LSCC	0.013–69.96	8	+	I	13	+	I	14
4	EC	7.06–17.55	1	>	Over	0	–	–	12
5	GLI	15.15–15.95	3	+	O	17	+	I	6
6	LAC	12.47–16.93	15	+	I	0	–	–	2
7	HNSCS	15.14–22.35	3	+	I	4	+	I	13
8	EC	15.72–16.05	2	>	I	10	+	I	5
9	CAC	15.93–16.09	44	+	O	37	+	I	3
10	OSC	6.04–20.35	0	–	–	26	+	O	6
11	BC	12.20–18.09	3	+	I	0	–	–	8
12	HCC	14.96–19.29	1	+	I	5	+	I	5
13	GLI	14.57–16.90	3	+	I	4	+	Over	8
14	LSCC	13.26–16.35	2	+	O	18	+	O	6
15	GLI	15.75–16.11	0	–	–	9	+	I	8
16	LAC	15.65–16.00	15	+	Over	21	+	I	4
17	MM	0.013–16.33	8	+	I	1	>	I	7
18	OC	15.92–16.98	35	+	I	10	+	I	2
19	SAC	13.84–17.27	2	+	I	0	–	–	7
20	CSCC	10.61–31.02	27	+	I	3	+	I	2
21	GLI	12.83–16.77	5	+	O	4	+	I	10
22	LAC	7.60–16.41	67	+	O	1	>	O	5
23	GCT	0.38–37.53	2	+	I	4	+	O	3
24	EC	0.013–19.41	8	+	I	7	+	Over	9
25	CAC	0.013–32.27	8	+	I	86	+	I	6

Sample	Tumour	B Pos (Mb)	5′ LIR*	<2 kb	In/Out	3′ LIR**	<2 kb	In/Out	Mh
26	BRC	13.15–15.95	0	–	–	17	+	I	5
27	BC	13.02–17.49	27	+	I	0	–	–	7
28	LAC	15.88–17.36	8	+	O	3	>	Over	5
29	HNSCC	4.03–64.05	1	>	O	35	+	I	4
30	LAC	0.013–25.64	8	+	I	19	+	O	2
31	LSCC	14.44–17.81	0	–	–	8	+	I	5
32	LSCC	15.84–16.98	10	+	I	10	+	I	4
33	BRC	5.56–16.48	3	>	Over	1	>	O	6
34	SAC	1.77–29.73	5	+	I	0	–	–	2
35	EC	15.69–15.98	7	+	Over	52	+	I	2
36	EC	15.61–17.52	9	+	O	1	+	I	4
37	BRC	0.013–31.19	8	+	I	1	>	I	5
38	SAC	14.93–16.74	2	+	I	1	+	I	3
39	BC	11.94–20.22	6	+	I	5	+	O	2
40	ACC	15.59–15.95	26	+	I	17	+	I	5
41	GCT	10.81–22.55	28	+	O	2	+	I	4
42	LAC	14.72–15.97	1	+	O	18	+	O	2
T: 56			T: 562	42 < 2 kb 75%	I: 28 O: 16	T: 757	40 < 2 kb 71.43%	I: 26 O: 16	M:5.18 (2–14)

[a]All amplicons including *MYCN* gene analyzed here are located at the short arm (p) of chromosome 2.

*$P < 0.05$, compared with control group.

**$P < 0.01$, compared with control group.

Abbreviations: ACC, adrenal cortical carcinoma; BC, bladder carcinoma; BRC, breast carcinoma; CAC, colon adenocarcinoma; CSCC, cervix squamous cell carcinoma; EC, endometrioid carcinoma; GCT, germ cell tumour; GLI, glioma; HNSCS, head and neck squamous cell carcinoma; LAC, lung adenocarcinoma; LSCC, lung squamous cell carcinoma; MM, malignant melanoma; NB, neuroblastoma; OC, oesophagus carcinoma; OSC, ovary serous carcinoma; SAC, stomach adenocarcinoma. B Pos, boundary position; In/Out, inside/outside the amplicon; LIR, long inverted repeat; M, mean; Mh, microhomology; Over, on the boundary of amplicon; T, total.

Table 2. Boundary positions, microhomology and LIR analyses at the amplicon units containing *MYCN* gene locus in neuroblastoma cell lines and other solid tumours[a].

contiq sequences (NCBI acc no: NT_005334.17) of *Homo sapiens* chromosome 2p containing *MYCN gene* for examining the LIR distribution were downloaded from NCBI website [172].

In addition, microhomology analysis between 150-bp DNA sequences spanning 5′ and 3′ boundaries was performed using Dialign software program [173].

3.3.1.2. LIR identification

LIRs with stem length ≥20 bp, stem identity ≥70%, and internal spacer (loop length) of 0–10 kb were identified at ±10 kb (a total of 20 kb) segments encompassing the rearrangement (boundary) sites of the amplicon units including *MYCN* gene, using the inverted repeat finder (IRF) software [174] in cell lines and primary tumours, as described in Ref. [71]. In addition, LIR distribution was determined in a genomic segment of 16,135,119 bp lying between chromosome 2p25.3 and 2p24.3 loci, including *MYCN* gene locus. LIRs with same features were also investigated at the DNA segments of 20 kb in control group (n = 61), including the randomly selected genes that were not shown to associate with any DNA amplification or deletion in literature and HGMD site, respectively [15, 136, 175]. Total LIR numbers of both amplification boundaries and control gene segments were determined (**Table 2**) and statistically compared with each other.

3.3.1.3. Statistical analysis

Mann-Whitney U test was used for statistical comparison of mean ranks of LIR numbers between test and control groups. Two-sided P values <0.05 were considered statistically significant. Analyses were performed using SPSS 11.0 software (Chicago, USA).

3.3.2. Results and discussion

We previously showed that Kelly neuroblastoma cell line harbours only one of chromosomes 2 in 23 metaphases using FISH method (Aygun N and Altungoz O, unpublished data). We also confirmed that *MYCN* locus is deleted on this unique chromosome 2, and hsrs containing *MYCN* amplification are located only two chromosomes 17 (**Figure 14**). In addition, I revealed a significant association between LIRs and breakpoint regions of gross deletions in human cancers and inherited diseases [71]. To investigate the relation between LIRs and mechanism of the *MYCN* gene amplification in this chapter, I examined the distribution of LIRs on a genomic segment of 16,135,119 bp lying between p25.3 and p24.3 loci of the short arm (p) of chromosome 2, which contains the *MYCN* gene (**Figure 15a**).

A total of 6839 LIRs with stem length ≥20 bp, stem identity ≥70% and internal spacer (loop length) of 0–10 kb were identified in this genomic segment (NCBI acc no: NT_005334.17), using IRF software (**Figure 15b**). Of these identified LIRs, 5155 (75.38%) are distributed along second half (9–17 Mb) of this segment (**Figure 15b**), containing *MYCN* locus at 2p24.3 (**Figure 15a**). Of second half LIRs, a total of 1751 (33.97%) have stem length ≥20 bp, stem identity ≥70% and loop length of 0–2 kb (**Figure 15c**). Of this second group LIRs, a total of 330 (18.85%) have stem length ≥20 bp, stem identity ≥85%, and loop length of 0–2 kb (**Figure 15d**), which may be potentially recombinogenic [177]. Second half of chromosome 2p25.3–2p24.3

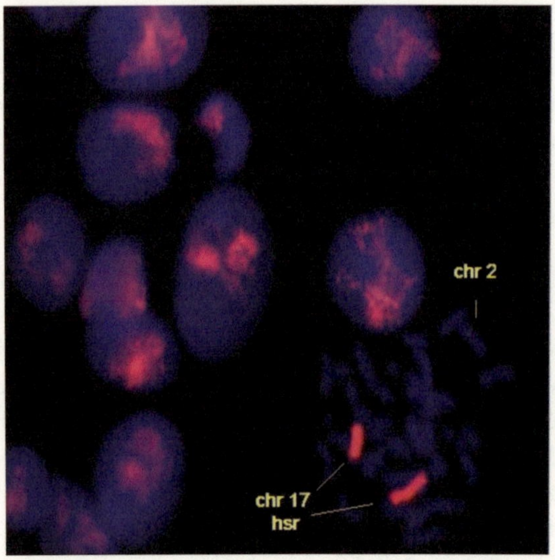

Figure 14. A metaphase demonstrating deleted 2p24 locus on single chromosome 2 and two hsrs including *MYCN* gene on chromosomes 17 in Kelly neuroblastoma cell line. Fluorescence *in situ* hybridization (FISH) probe: *MYCN* gene (2p24)/Chromosome 2 Alpha-Satellite (red/green, Qbiogene, cat. no., PONC0224).

also includes an SRO of ~68 kb (**Table 2**: 15,900,307–15,968,674, **Figure 15b**) between amplicon units analyzed here, all of them contain *MYCN* gene (NT_005334.17, 15,930,557–15,930,962).

It was found that two common fragile sites (cFS) spanning 747-kb *FRA2Ctel* and 746-kb *FRA2Ccen* at 2p24.3 and 2p24.2, respectively, are separated by a 2.8-Mb non-fragile region containing *MYCN* [178]. The authors also determined that 56.5% of *MYCN* amplicons from neuroblastoma cell lines and primary tumours are clustered in *FRA2C*, suggesting that *MYCN* amplicons could be formed due to extrareplication rounds of unbroken DNA secondary structures that accumulate at *FRA2C*.

To investigate significance of the association between LIRs and *MYCN* gene amplification, LIRs were identified at the ±10 kb segments encompassing both 5′ and 3′ rearrangement boundaries of amplicon units including *MYCN* gene, using IRF software in neuroblastoma cell lines and primary solid tumours. LIRs were also investigated at 20-kb segments of the genes in control group. In conclusion, statistical analysis showed that mean LIR number was significantly higher in both 5′ and 3′ rearrangement boundaries of the amplicon units including *MYCN* gene than in control group, respectively ($P < 0.025$; $P < 0.004$; **Table 2**). Of 5′ boundaries in 56 amplicon units, 49 (87.5%) have at least one LIR with stem length ≥20 bp, stem identity ≥70%, and loop length of 0–10 kb, while 47 (83.93%) of 3′ boundaries include at least one LIR with same features (**Table 2**). Of these 49 5′ LIRs and 47 3′ LIRs, 28 (57.14%) and 26 (55.32%) are inside the amplicon unit, respectively. In addition, 42 (85.71%) of 49 5′ LIRs have loop length <2 kb, while 40 (85.11%) of 47 3′ LIRs contain the loops <2 kb (**Table 2**). Of these 42 5′ and 40 3′ LIRs with loops <2 kb, 26 (61.9%) and 24 (60%) were found inside the amplicon

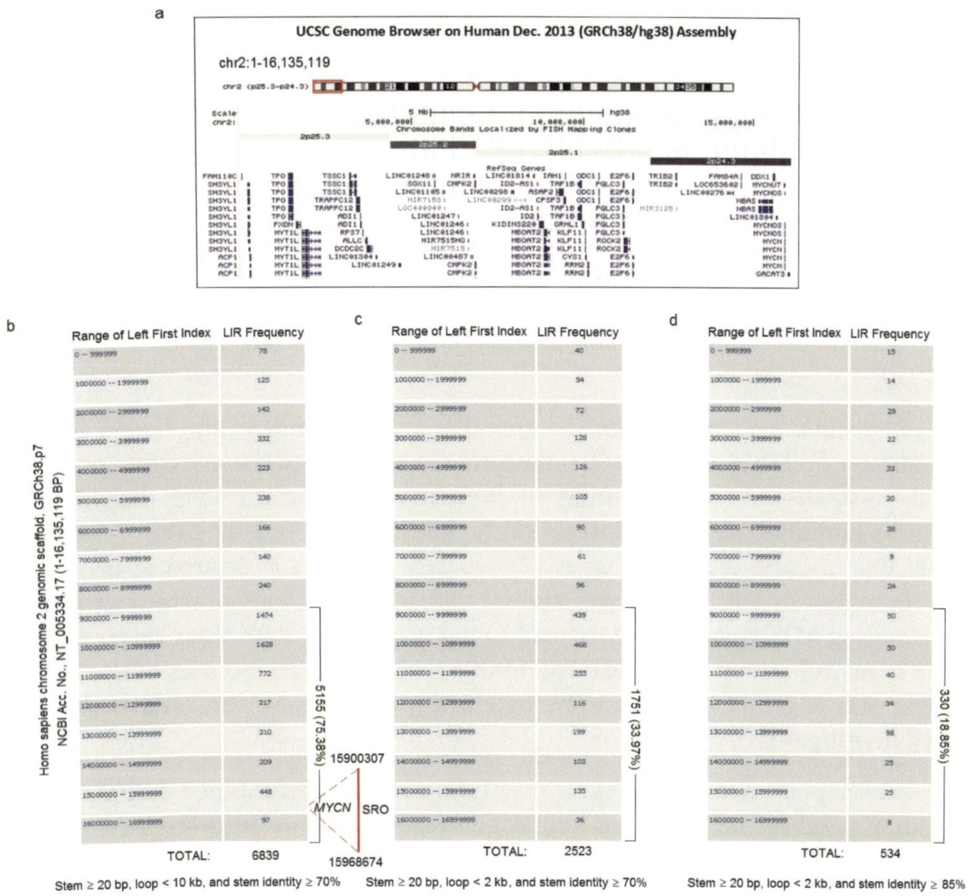

Figure 15. LIR identification in chromosome 2p containing *MYCN* gene. (**a**) LIR distribution was examined in a genomic segment (NT_005334.17) of 16,135,119 bp lying between chromosome 2p25.3-p24.3. Map of this chromosomal region was obtained from UCSC genome browser [176]. (**b**) LIR frequency with stem length ≥20 bp, stem identity ≥70%, and loop length <10 kb. (**c**) LIR frequency with stem length ≥20 bp, stem identity ≥70%, and loop length <2 kb. (**d**) LIR frequency with stem length ≥20 bp, stem identity ≥85%, and loop length <2 kb.

unit, respectively, suggesting that LIRs inside the amplicon unit could potentially generate a hairpin at single-stranded DNA and break the DNA strand during replication. Hairpin structure was shown to form at an interrupted LIR with 111-bp stem and 24-bp internal spacer on both leading and lagging strand templates during replication [110]. In addition, a single-strand DNA break may cause replication fork stalling or collapse [48]. However, LIRs outside a replicon, near the rearrangement boundaries, may also cause a replication fork stalling through formation of cruciform extrusion [110].

Of 49 5′ LIRs, 28 (57.14%) have stem length ≥20 bp, stem identity ≥75% (18 LIRs with stem identity ≥85% were found, 14 of them were inside the amplicon unit) and loop length of 0–2 kb, while 37 (78.72%) of 47 3′ LIRs have stem identity ≥75% (9 LIRs with stem identity ≥85% were found, six of them were inside the amplicon unit; data not shown in **Table 2**). LIRs with stem identity >85% were highly recombinogenic in human and other organisms [177]. In addition, the long Alu IRs with 75% stem identity can cause a mild replication blockage in *E. coli* [106]. Therefore, present data suggest that LIRs with 85 and 75% stem identities identified here in the boundaries of the amplicons including *MYCN* gene can be potentially recombinogenic or can lead to at least mild replication blockage, respectively.

Present results also showed that a microhomology of mean 5.18 bp ranging from 2 to 14 bp between sequences of 5′ and 3′ boundaries in the amplicons (**Table 2**). Microhomology between 0 and 15 bp can be a signature for NHEJ, MMEJ, MMBIR, or FoSTeS mechanisms [86, 149, 179].

On the other side, a recombination hotspot harbouring tandem amplicons in head to tail orientation at 17q21 that is not linked to common fragile sites, containing *ERBB2* gene locus, was discovered, indicating an alternative mechanism other than BFB model in oncogene amplification [180]. Interestingly, additional copies of *MYCN* oncogene in Kelly cell line are also integrated at 17q21 locus, whereas it is deleted at original 2p24 locus (**Figure 14**). In addition, it was shown that multiple tandem arrays of DNA segments including *MYCN* gene were in head to tail orientation with sizes varying from 100 to 700 kb in neuroblastoma cell lines [26]. In this chapter, the boundaries of the amplicons containing *MYCN* gene located 2p were analyzed for LIRs, however, LIRs at 17q21 locus remained investigated.

Taken together, present results suggest that LIRs could be contributed to induce *MYCN* amplification possibly through either replication fork stalling or break-induced replication dependent on microhomology during replication in chromosome 2p (**Figure 16**). In addition, LIRs may cause deletion of *MYCN* gene at 2p24 and trigger its insertion into chromosome 17q21 involving nonhomologous recombination in Kelly cell line. After insertion, 2p24 hsr including *MYCN* gene at 17q21 might be arisen from again replication fork stalling or break-induced replication dependent on microhomology.

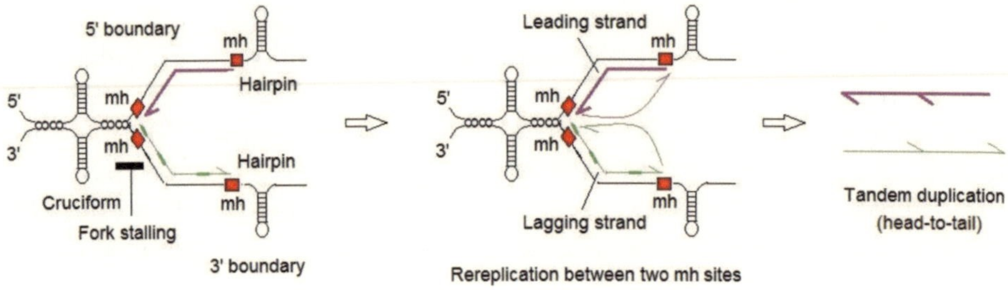

Figure 16. A model of long inverted repeat (LIR)-induced gene amplification. A cruciform near 5′ boundary of an amplicon unit can cause the fork stalling during replication. Hairpins formed at both leading and lagging strand templates may slow the DNA synthesis. Both cruciform and hairpin structures could trigger a rereplication between two microhomology (mh) sites located 5′ and 3′ boundaries of the amplicon, leading to the formation of head-to-tail tandem duplication.

Acknowledgements

I thank "Nature Publishing Group (NPG)" for reusing to be adapted without obtaining permission in this chapter (**Figure 7a–c**) of **Figures 6** and **7** in my article entitled "Correlations between long inverted repeat (LIR) features, deletion size and distance from breakpoint in human gross gene deletions" [71], published in Scientific Reports. NPG provides the right to reuse the figures without obtaining permission for the authors of previously published articles, which are licenced under a Creative Commons Attribution 4.0 International Licence (http://creativecommons.org/licenses/by/4.0).

Author details

Nevim Aygun

Address all correspondence to: nevim.aygun@gmail.com

Department of Medical Biology, Faculty of Medicine, Dokuz Eylul University, Inciralti, Izmir, Turkey

References

[1] Albertson DG, Collins C, McCormick F, Gray JW. Chromosome aberrations in solid tumors. Nat Genet. 2003;**34**:369-376. DOI: 10.1038/ng1215

[2] Barrett MT, Lenkiewicz E, Evers L, *et al*. Clonal evolution and therapeutic resistance in solid tumors. Front Pharmacol. 2013;**4**:2. DOI: 10.3389/fphar.2013.00002

[3] Mitelman F, Johansson B, Mertens F. The impact of translocations and gene fusions on cancer causation. Nat Rev Cancer. 2007;**7**:233-245. DOI: 10.1038/nrc2091

[4] Mitelman F, Johansson B, Mertens F (Eds.). Mitelman database of chromosome aberrations and gene fusions in cancer [Internet]. 2016. Available from: https://www.cgap.nci.nih.gov/Chromosomes/Mitelman [Accessed: 2016-10-15].

[5] Johansson B, Mertens F, Mitelman F. Primary vs. secondary neoplasia-associated chromosomal abnormalities–balanced rearrangements vs. genomic imbalances? Genes Chromosomes Cancer. 1996;**16**:155-163. DOI: 10.1002/(SICI)1098-2264(199607)16:3 <155::AID-GCC1>3.0.CO;2-Y

[6] Grade M, Difilippantonio MJ, Camps J. Patterns of chromosomal aberrations in solid tumors. Recent Results Cancer Res. 2015;**200**:115-142. DOI: 10.1007/978-3-319-20291-4_6

[7] Database: Atlas of genetics and cytogenetics in oncology and haematology [Internet]. 2016. Available from: https://www.atlasgeneticsoncology.org/Tumors/Tumorliste.html [Accessed: 2016-10-15]

[8] Gu W, Zhang F, Lupski JR. Mechanisms for human genomic rearrangements. Pathogenetics. 2008;**1**:4. DOI: 10.1186/1755-8417-1-4

[9] Shaw CJ, Lupski, JR. Implications of human genome architecture for rearrangement-based disorders: The genomic basis of disease. Hum Mol Genet. 2004;**13**:R57-R64. DOI: 10.1093/hmg/ddh073

[10] Mitelman F. ISCN (1995): An international system for human cytogenetic nomenclature. Mitelman F (ed). Basel: S. Karger Press; 1995. 114 p.

[11] Heng HH, Regan SM, Liu G, Ye CJ. Why it is crucial to analyze non clonal chromosome aberrations or NCCAs? Mol Cytogenet. 2016;**9**:15. DOI: 10.1186/s13039-016-0223-2

[12] Mitelman F, Mertens F, Johansson B. A breakpoint map of recurrent chromosomal rearrangements in human neoplasia. Volume is 15 (Spec No). Nature Genetics 15, 417 - 474 (1997) doi:10.1038/ng0497supp-417

[13] Weaver BA, Cleveland DW. Does aneuploidy cause cancer? Curr Opin Cell Biol. 2006;**18**: 658-667. DOI: 10.1016/j.ceb.2006.10.002

[14] Giam M, Rancati G. Aneuploidy and chromosomal instability in cancer: A jackpot to chaos. Cell Div. 2015;**10**:3. DOI: 10.1186/s13008-015-0009-7

[15] Santarius T, Shipley J, Brewer D, Stratton MR, Cooper CS. A census of amplified and overexpressed human cancer genes. Nat Rev Cancer. 2010;**10**:59-64. DOI: 10.1038/nrc2771

[16] Schwab M. Oncogene amplification in solid tumors. Semin Cancer Biol. 1999;**9**:319-325. DOI: 10.1006/scbi.1999.0126

[17] Seeger RC, Brodeur GM, Sather H, *et al*. Association of multiple copies of the N-myc oncogene with rapid progression of neuroblastomas. N Engl J Med. 1985;**313**:1111-1116. DOI: 10.1056/NEJM198510313131802

[18] Idbaih A, Crinière E, Marie Y, *et al*. Gene amplification is a poor prognostic factor in anaplastic oligodendrogliomas. Neuro Oncol. 2008;**10**:540-547. DOI: 10.1215/15228517-2008-022

[19] Bown NP. Chromosome studies of solid tumours. J Clin Pathol. 1992;**45**:556-560.

[20] Wan TS. Cancer cytogenetics: Methodology revisited. Ann Lab Med. 2014;**34**:413-425. DOI: 10.3343/alm.2014.34.6.413

[21] Bridge JA. Advantages and limitations of cytogenetic, molecular cytogenetic, and molecular diagnostic testing in mesenchymal neoplasms. J Orthop Sci. 2008;**13**:273-282. DOI: 10.1007/s00776-007-1215-1

[22] Lagos SMR, Jiménez NER. Cytogenetic analysis of primary cultures and cell lines: Generalities, applications and protocols. In: Tirunilai P (ed). Recent trends in cytogenetic studies-methodologies and applications. InTech; 2012. pp. 1-24. DOI: 10.5772/34200. Available from: http://www.intechopen.com/books/recent-trends-in-cytogenetic-studies-methodologies-and-applications/cytogenetic-from-primary-cultures-and-cell-lines-applications-protocols-and-nomenclature.

[23] Foijer F. Mouse models for chromosomal instability. In: Storchova Z, (ed). Aneuploidy in health and disease. InTech; 2012. pp. 59-78. DOI: 10.5772/48025. Available from: http://www.intechopen.com/books/aneuploidy-in-health-and-disease/mouse-models-for-chromosomal-instability

[24] Weinstock DM, Brunet E, Jasin M. Induction of chromosomal translocations in mouse and human cells using site-specific endonucleases. J Natl Cancer Inst Monogr. 2008;**39**:20-24. DOI: 10.1093/jncimonographs/lgn009

[25] Lengauer C, Kinzler KW, Vogelstein B. Genetic instabilities in human cancers. Nature. 1998;**396**:643-649. DOI: 10.1038/25292

[26] Amler LC, Schwab M. Amplified N-myc in human neuroblastoma cells is often arranged as clustered tandem repeats of differently recombined DNA. Mol Cell Biol. 1989;**9**:4903-4913.

[27] Strouhal E, Kritscher H. Neolithic case of a multiple myeloma from Mauer (Vienna, Austria). Anthropologie (Brno). 1990;**28**:79-87.

[28] Tsoucalas G, Sgantzos M. Hippocrates (ca 460-370 BC) on nasal cancer. J BUON. 2016;**21**:1031-1034.

[29] Faguet GB. A brief history of cancer: Age-old milestones underlying our current knowledge database. Int J Cancer. 2015;**136**:2022-2036. DOI: 10.1002/ijc.29134

[30] Saidi F. The historical basis for the esophageal cancer belt of South-Central Asia. Arch Iran Med. 1999;**2**:26-27.

[31] Karamanou M, Tsoucalas G, Saridaki Z, Iavazzo C, Androutsos G. Avenzoar's (1091-1162) clinical description of cancer. J BUON. 2015;**20**:1171-1174.

[32] Mendel G. Versuche über Plflanzen-hybriden. Verhandlungen des naturforschenden Ver-eines in Brünn, Bd. IV für das Jahr. Abhand-lungen. 1865;3-47. (English version: Mendel G. Experiments in plant hybridization (1865). Available from: http://www.mendelweb.org/Mendel.html)

[33] Moore JA. Darwin's theory of pangenesis. In: Moore JA, (ed). Heredity and development. 2nd ed. New York: Oxford University Press; 1972. pp. 7-18.

[34] Paweletz N. Walther Flemming: Pioneer of mitosis research. Nat Rev Mol Cell Biol. 2001;**2**:72-75. DOI: 10.1038/35048077

[35] Foijer F. CINister thoughts. Biochem Soc Trans. 2010;**38**:1715-1721. DOI: 10.1042/BST0381715

[36] Balmain A. Cancer genetics: From Boveri and Mendel to microarrays. Nat Rev Cancer. 2001;**1**:77-82. DOI: 10.1038/35094086

[37] Crow EW, Crow JF. 100 years ago: Walter Sutton and the chromosome theory of heredity. Genetics. 2002;**160**:1-4.

[38] Nowell PC, Hungerford DA. A minute chromosome in human chronic granulocytic leukemia. Science. 1960;**142**:1497.

[39] Spriggs AI, Boddington MM, Clarke CM. Chromosomes of human cancer cells. Br Med J. 1962;**2**:1431-1435.

[40] Rowley JD. A new consistent chromosomal abnormality in chronic myelogenous leukaemia identified by quinacrine fluorescence and Giemsa staining. Nature. 1973;**243**:290-293. DOI: 10.1038/243290a0

[41] Biedler JL, Spengler BA. A novel chromosome abnormality in human neuroblastoma and antifolate-resistant Chinese hamster cell lines in culture. J Natl Cancer Inst. 1976;**57**:683-695. DOI: 10.1093/jnci/57.3.683

[42] Brodeur GM, Sekhon GS, Goldstein MN. Chromosomal aberrations in human neuroblastomas. Cancer. 1977;**40**:2256-2263. DOI: 10.1002/1097-0142(197711)40:5<2256::AID-CNCR2820400536>3.0.CO;2-1

[43] Atkin NB, Baker MC. Pericentric inversion of chromosome 1: Frequency and possible association with cancer. Cytogenet Cell Genet. 1977;**19**:180-184. DOI:10.1159/000130807

[44] Bauman JG, Wiegant J, Borst P, van Duijn P. A new method for fluorescence microscopical localization of specific DNA sequences by in situ hybridization of fluorochromelabelled RNA. Exp Cell Res. 1980;**128**:485-490. DOI: 10.1016/0014-4827(80)90087-7

[45] Schwab M, Alitalo K, Klempnauer KH, *et al.* Amplified DNA with limited homology to myc cellular oncogene is shared by human neuroblastoma cell lines and a neuroblastoma tumour. Nature. 1983;**305**:245-248. DOI: 10.1038/305245a0

[46] Kallioniemi A, Kallioniemi OP, Sudar D, *et al.* Comparative genomic hybridization for molecular cytogenetic analysis of solid tumors. Science. 1992;**258**:818-821. DOI: 10.1126/science.1359641

[47] Schröck E, du Manoir S, Veldman T, *et al.* Multicolor spectral karyotyping of human chromosomes. Science. 1996;**273**:494-497. DOI: 10.1126/science.273.5274.494

[48] Carvalho CM, Lupski JR. Mechanisms underlying structural variant formation in genomic disorders. Nat Rev Genet. 2016;**17**:224-238. DOI: 10.1038/nrg.2015.25

[49] Chen JM, Cooper DN, Férec C, Kehrer-Sawatzki H, Patrinos GP. Genomic rearrangements in inherited disease and cancer. Semin Cancer Biol. 2010;**20**:222-233. DOI: 10.1016/j.semcancer.2010.05.007

[50] Stankiewicz P, Lupski JR. Genome architecture, rearrangements and genomic disorders. Trends Genet. 2002;**18**:74-82. DOI: 10.1016/S0168-9525(02)02592-1

[51] Sharp AJ, Locke DP, McGrath SD, *et al.* Segmental duplications and copy-number variation in the human genome. Am J Hum Genet. 2005;**77**:78-88. DOI: 10.1086/431652

[52] Liu P, Carvalho CM, Hastings PJ, Lupski JR. Mechanisms for recurrent and complex human genomic rearrangements. Curr Opin Genet Dev. 2012;**22**:211-220. DOI: 10.1016/j.gde.2012.02.012

[53] Ou Z, Stankiewicz P, Xia Z, *et al.* Observation and prediction of recurrent human translocations mediated by NAHR between nonhomologous chromosomes. Genome Res. 2011;**21**:33-46. DOI: 10.1101/gr.111609.110

[54] Robberecht C, Voet T, Zamani Esteki M, Nowakowska BA, Vermeesch JR. Nonallelic homologous recombination between retrotransposable elements is a driver of de novo unbalanced translocations. Genome Res. 2013;**23**:411-418. DOI: 10.1101/gr.145631.112

[55] Luo Y, Hermetz KE, Jackson JM, *et al.* Diverse mutational mechanisms cause pathogenic subtelomeric rearrangements. Hum Mol Genet. 2011;**20**:3769-3778. DOI: 10.1093/hmg/ddr293

[56] Turner DJ, Miretti M, Rajan D, *et al.* Germline rates of de novo meiotic deletions and duplications causing several genomic disorders. Nat Genet. 2008;**40**:90-95. DOI: 10.1038/ng.2007.40

[57] Flores M, Morales L, Gonzaga-Jauregui C, *et al.* Recurrent DNA inversion rearrangements in the human genome. Proc Natl Acad Sci U S A. 2007;**104**:6099-6106. DOI: 10.1073/pnas.0701631104

[58] Redon R, Ishikawa S, Fitch KR, *et al.* Global variation in copy number in the human genome. Nature. 2006;**444**:444-454. DOI: 10.1038/nature05329

[59] Darai-Ramqvist E, Sandlund A, Müller S, Klein G, Imreh S, Kost-Alimova M. Segmental duplications and evolutionary plasticity at tumor chromosome break-prone regions. Genome Res. 2008;**18**:370-379. DOI: 10.1101/gr.7010208

[60] Jennes I, de Jong D, Mees K, Hogendoorn PC, Szuhai K, Wuyts W. Breakpoint characterization of large deletions in EXT1 or EXT2 in 10 multiple osteochondromas families. BMC Med Genet. 2011;**12**:85. DOI: 10.1186/1471-2350-12-85

[61] Steinmann K, Cooper DN, Kluwe L, *et al.* Type 2 NF1 deletions are highly unusual by virtue of the absence of nonallelic homologous recombination hotspots and an apparent preference for female mitotic recombination. Am J Hum Genet. 2007;**81**:1201-1220. DOI: 10.1086/522089

[62] Zickler AM, Hampp S, Messiaen L, *et al.* Characterization of the nonallelic homologous recombination hotspot PRS3 associated with type-3 NF1 deletions. Hum Mutat. 2012;**33**:372-383. DOI: 10.1002/humu.21644

[63] Kehrer-Sawatzki H, Bengesser K, Callens T, *et al.* Identification of large NF1 duplications reciprocal to NAHR-mediated type-1 NF1 deletions. Hum Mutat. 2014;**35**:1469-1475. DOI: 10.1002/humu.22692.

[64] Bacolla A, Jaworski A, Larson JE, *et al.* Breakpoints of gross deletions coincide with non-B DNA conformations. Proc Natl Acad Sci U S A. 2004;**101**:14162-14167. DOI: 10.1073/pnas.0405974101

[65] Woodward KJ, Cundall M, Sperle K, *et al.* Heterogeneous duplications in patients with Pelizaeus-Merzbacher disease suggest a mechanism of coupled homologous and nonhomologous recombination. Am J Hum Genet. 2005;**77**:966-987. DOI: 10.1086/498048

[66] Bauters M, Van Esch H, Friez MJ, *et al.* Nonrecurrent *MECP2* duplications mediated by genomic architecture-driven DNA breaks and break-induced replication repair. Genome Res. 2008;**18**:847-858. DOI: 10.1101/gr.075903.107

[67] Vissers LE, Bhatt SS, Janssen IM, *et al.* Rare pathogenic microdeletions and tandem duplications are microhomology-mediated and stimulated by local genomic architecture. Hum Mol Genet. 2009;**18**:3579-3593. DOI: 10.1093/hmg/ddp306

[68] Kato T, Kurahashi H, Emanuel BS. Chromosomal translocations and palindromic AT-rich repeats. Curr Opin Genet Dev. 2012;**22**:221-228. DOI: 10.1016/j.gde.2012.02.004

[69] Verdin H, D'haene B, Beysen D, *et al.* Microhomology-mediated mechanisms underlie non-recurrent disease-causing microdeletions of the FOXL2 gene or its regulatory domain. PLoS Genet. 2013;**9**:e1003358. DOI: 10.1371/journal.pgen.1003358

[70] Bose P, Hermetz KE, Conneely KN, Rudd MK. Tandem repeats and G-rich sequences are enriched at human CNV breakpoints. PLoS One. 2014;**9**:e101607. DOI: 10.1371/journal.pone.0101607

[71] Aygun N. Correlations between long inverted repeat (LIR) features, deletion size and distance from breakpoint in human gross gene deletions. Sci Rep. 2015;**5**:8300 DOI: 10.1038/srep08300

[72] Lu S, Wang G, Bacolla A, Zhao J, Spitser S, Vasquez KM. Short inverted repeats are hotspots for genetic instability: Relevance to cancer genomes. Cell Rep. 2015;**10**:1674-1680. DOI: 10.1016/j.celrep.2015.02.039

[73] Inagaki H, Kato T, Tsutsumi M, Ouchi Y, Ohye T, Kurahashi H. Palindrome-mediated translocations in humans: A new mechanistic model for gross chromosomal rearrangements. Front Genet. 2016;**7**:125. DOI: 10.3389/fgene.2016.00125

[74] Lieber MR. The mechanism of double-strand DNA break repair by the nonhomologous DNA end-joining pathway. Annu Rev Biochem. 2010;**79**:181-211. DOI: 10.1146/annurev.biochem.052308.093131

[75] Mao Z, Bozzella M, Seluanov A, Gorbunova V. DNA repair by nonhomologous end joining and homologous recombination during cell cycle in human cells. Cell Cycle. 2008;**7**:2902-2906. DOI: 10.4161/cc.7.18.6679

[76] Lieber MR. The biochemistry and biological significance of nonhomologous DNA end joining: An essential repair process in multicellular eukaryotes. Genes Cells. 1999;**4**:77-85. DOI: 10.1046/j.1365-2443.1999.00245.x

[77] Li L, Robert C, Rassool FV. The role of error prone alternative non-homologous end-joining in genomic instability in cancer. In: Vengrova S, (ed). DNA repair and human health. InTech; 2011. pp. 93-120. DOI: 10.5772/24262. Available from: http://www.intechopen.com/books/dna-repair-and-human-health/the-role-of-error-prone-alternative-non-homologous-end-joining-in-genomic-instability-in-cancer

[78] Sharma S, Javadekar SM, Pandey M, Srivastava M, Kumari R, Raghavan SC. Homology and enzymatic requirements of microhomology-dependent alternative end joining. Cell Death Dis. 2015;**6**:e1697. DOI: 10.1038/cddis.2015.58

[79] Frit P, Barboule N, Yuan Y, Gomez D, Calsou P. Alternative end-joining pathway(s): Bricolage at DNA breaks. DNA Repair (Amst). 2014;**17**:81-97. DOI: 10.1016/j.dnarep.2014.02.007

[80] Dueva R, Iliakis G. Alternative pathways of non-homologous end joining (NHEJ) in genomic instability and cancer. Transl Cancer Res. 2013;**2**:163-177. DOI: 10.3978/j.issn.2218-676X.2013.05.02

[81] Lieber MR. The mechanism of human nonhomologous DNA end joining. J Biol Chem. 2008;**283**:1-5. DOI: 10.1074/jbc.R700039200

[82] Chiruvella KK, Liang Z, Wilson TE. Repair of double-strand breaks by end joining. Cold Spring Harb Perspect Biol. 2013;**5**:a012757. DOI: 10.1101/cshperspect.a012757

[83] Bétermier M, Bertrand P, Lopez BS. Is non-homologous end-joining really an inherently error-prone process? PLoS Genet. 2014;**10**:e1004086. DOI: 10.1371/journal.pgen.1004086

[84] Sharma S, Raghavan SC. Nonhomologous DNA end joining in cell-free extracts. J Nucleic Acids. 2010;**2010**:389129. DOI: 10.4061/2010/389129

[85] Lee JA, Carvalho CM, Lupski JR. A DNA replication mechanism for generating non-recurrent rearrangements associated with genomic disorders. Cell. 2007;**131**:1235-1247. DOI: 10.1016/j.cell.2007.11.037

[86] Hastings PJ, Ira G, Lupski JR. A microhomology-mediated break-induced replication model for the origin of human copy number variation. PLoS Genet. 2009;**5**:e1000327. DOI: 10.1371/journal.pgen.1000327

[87] Zhuang J, Weng Z. Local sequence assembly reveals a high-resolution profile of somatic structural variations in 97 cancer genomes. Nucleic Acids Res. 2015;**43**:8146-8156. DOI: 10.1093/nar/gkv831

[88] Yang L, Luquette LJ, Gehlenborg N, *et al.* Diverse mechanisms of somatic structural variations in human cancer genomes. Cell. 2013;**153**:919-929. DOI: 10.1016/j.cell.2013.04.010

[89] Malhotra A, Lindberg M, Faust GG, *et al.* Breakpoint profiling of 64 cancer genomes reveals numerous complex rearrangements spawned by homology-independent mechanisms. Genome Res. 2013;**23**:762-776. DOI: 10.1101/gr.143677.112

[90] Nambiar M, Raghavan SC. How does DNA break during chromosomal translocations? Nucleic Acids Res. 2011;**39**:5813-5825. DOI: 10.1093/nar/gkr223

[91] Bunting SF, Nussenzweig A. End-joining, translocations and cancer. Nat Rev Cancer. 2013;**13**:443-454. DOI: 10.1038/nrc3537

[92] Emanuel BS, Saitta SC. From microscopes to microarrays: Dissecting recurrent chromosomal rearrangements. Nat Rev Genet. 2007;**8**:869-883. DOI: 10.1038/nrg2136

[93] Daga A, Ansari A, Rawal R, Umrania V. Characterization of chromosomal translocation breakpoint sequences in solid tumours: "an in silico analysis". Open Med Inform J. 2015;**9**:1-8. DOI: 10.2174/1874431101509010001

[94] Simsek D, Jasin M. Alternative end-joining is suppressed by the canonical NHEJ component Xrcc4-ligase IV during chromosomal translocation formation. Nat Struct Mol Biol. 2010;**17**:410-416. DOI: 10.1038/nsmb.1773

[95] Ghezraoui H, Piganeau M, Renouf B, *et al*. Chromosomal translocations in human cells are generated by canonical nonhomologous end-joining. Mol Cell. 2014;**55**:829-842. DOI: 10.1016/j.molcel.2014.08.002

[96] Reid DA, Rothenberg E. Repair of chromosomal breaks by NHEJ. Oncotarget. 2015;**6**:15730-15731. DOI: 10.18632/oncotarget.4593

[97] Bacolla A, Tainer JA, Vasquez KM, Cooper DN. Translocation and deletion breakpoints in cancer genomes are associated with potential non-B DNA-forming sequences. Nucleic Acids Res. 2016;**44**:5673-5688. DOI: 10.1093/nar/gkw261

[98] Chuzhanova N, Abeysinghe SS, Krawczak M, Cooper DN. Translocation and gross deletion breakpoints in human inherited disease and cancer II: Potential involvement of repetitive sequence elements in secondary structure formation between DNA ends. Hum Mutat. 2003;**22**:245-251. DOI: 10.1002/humu.10253

[99] Abeysinghe SS, Chuzhanova N, Krawczak M, Ball EV, Cooper DN. Translocation and gross deletion breakpoints in human inherited disease and cancer I: Nucleotide composition and recombination-associated motifs. Hum Mutat. 2003;**22**:229-244. DOI: 10.1002/humu.10254

[100] Kurahashi H, Inagaki H, Kato T, *et al*. Impaired DNA replication prompts deletions within palindromic sequences, but does not induce translocations in human cells. Hum Mol Genet. 2009;**18**:3397-3406. DOI: 10.1093/hmg/ddp279

[101] Petursdottir TE, Thorsteinsdottir U, Jonasson JG, *et al*. Interstitial deletions including chromosome 3 common eliminated region 1 (C3CER1) prevail in human solid tumors from 10 different tissues. Genes Chromosomes Cancer. 2004;**41**:232-242. DOI: 10.1002/gcc.20072

[102] Yoshimoto M, Cunha IW, Coudry RA, *et al*. FISH analysis of 107 prostate cancers shows that PTEN genomic deletion is associated with poor clinical outcome. Br J Cancer. 2007;**97**:678-685. DOI: 10.1038/sj.bjc.6603924

[103] Abkevich V, Iliev D, Timms KM, *et al*. Computational method for estimating DNA copy numbers in normal samples, cancer cell lines, and solid tumors using array comparative genomic hybridization. J Biomed Biotechnol. 2010;**2010**:386870. DOI: 10.1155/2010/386870

[104] Gordenin DA, Lobachev KS, Degtyareva NP, Malkova AL, Perkins E, Resnick MA. Inverted DNA repeats: A source of eukaryotic genomic instability. Mol Cell Biol. 1993;**13**:5315-5322. DOI: 10.1128/MCB.13.9.5315

[105] Lobachev KS, Shor BM, Tran HT, *et al*. Factors affecting inverted repeat stimulation of recombination and deletion in *Saccharomyces cerevisiae*. Genetics. 1998;**148**:1507-1524.

[106] Voineagu I, Narayanan V, Lobachev KS, Mirkin SM. Replication stalling at unstable inverted repeats: Interplay between DNA hairpins and fork stabilizing proteins. Proc Natl Acad Sci U S A. 2008;**105**:9936-9941. DOI: 10.1073/pnas.0804510105

[107] Akgün E, Zahn J, Baumes S, *et al*. Palindrome resolution and recombination in the mammalian germ line. Mol Cell Biol. 1997;**17**:5559-5570. DOI: 10.1128/MCB.17.9.5559

[108] Cunningham LA, Coté AG, Cam-Ozdemir C, Lewis SM. Rapid, stabilizing palindrome rearrangements in somatic cells by the center-break mechanism. Mol Cell Biol. 2003;**23**:8740-8750. DOI: 10.1128/MCB.23.23.8740-8750.2003

[109] van Gent DC. Reaching out for the other end with p53-binding protein 1. Trends Biochem Sci. 2009;**34**:226-229. DOI: 10.1016/j.tibs.2009.01.009

[110] Lai PJ, Lim CT, Le HP, *et al*. Long inverted repeat transiently stalls DNA replication by forming hairpin structures on both leading and lagging strands. Genes Cells. 2016;**21**:136-145. DOI: 10.1111/gtc.12326

[111] Azeroglu B, Lincker F, White MA, Jain D, Leach DR. A perfect palindrome in the *Escherichia coli* chromosome forms DNA hairpins on both leading- and lagging- strands. Nucleic Acids Res. 2014;**42**:13206-13213. DOI: 10.1093/nar/gku1136

[112] Bunting SF, Callén E, Wong N, *et al*. 53BP1 inhibits homologous recombination in Brca1-deficient cells by blocking resection of DNA breaks. Cell. 2010;**141**:243-254. DOI: 10.1016/j.cell.2010.03.012.

[113] Li M, Cole F, Patel DS, *et al*. 53BP1 ablation rescues genomic instability in mice expressing 'RING-less' BRCA1. EMBO Rep. 2016;**17**:1532-1541. DOI: 10.15252/embr.201642497

[114] Alkan C, Coe BP, Eichler EE. Genome structural variation discovery and genotyping. Nat Rev Genet. 2011;**12**:363-376. DOI: 10.1038/nrg2958

[115] Newman S, Hermetz KE, Weckselblatt B, Rudd MK. Next-generation sequencing of duplication CNVs reveals that most are tandem and some create fusion genes at breakpoints. Am J Hum Genet. 2015;**96**:208-220. DOI: 10.1016/j.ajhg.2014.12.017

[116] Jones DT, Kocialkowski S, Liu L, *et al*. Tandem duplication producing a novel oncogenic BRAF fusion gene defines the majority of pilocytic astrocytomas. Cancer Res. 2008;**68**:8673-8677. DOI: 10.1158/0008-5472.CAN-08-2097

[117] Van Roy N, Van Limbergen H, Vandesompele J, *et al*. Chromosome 2 short arm translocations revealed by M-FISH analysis of neuroblastoma cell lines. Med Pediatr Oncol. 2000;**35**:538-540. DOI: 10.1002/1096-911X(20001201)35:6<538::AID-MPO8>3.0.CO;2-C

[118] Cheung J, Estivill X, Khaja R, *et al*. Genome-wide detection of segmental duplications and potential assembly errors in the human genome sequence. Genome Biol. 2003;**4**:R25. DOI: 10.1186/gb-2003-4-4-r25

[119] Kozlov AP. Expression of evolutionarily novel genes in tumors. Infect Agent Cancer. 2016;**11**:34. DOI: 10.1186/s13027-016-0077-6

[120] Soda M, Choi YL, Enomoto M, *et al*. Identification of the transforming EML4-ALK fusion gene in non-small-cell lung cancer. Nature. 2007;**448**:561-566. DOI: 10.1038/nature05945

[121] Ju YS, Lee WC, Shin JY, *et al*. A transforming KIF5B and RET gene fusion in lung adenocarcinoma revealed from whole-genome and transcriptome sequencing. Genome Res. 2012;**22**:436-445. DOI: 10.1101/gr.133645.111

[122] Lees-Miller SP. DNA double strand break repair in mitosis is suppressed by phosphorylation of XRCC4. PLoS Genet. 2014;**10**:e1004598. DOI: 10.1371/journal.pgen.1004598

[123] Stephens PJ, McBride DJ, Lin ML, *et al*. Complex landscapes of somatic rearrangement in human breast cancer genomes. Nature. 2009;**462**:1005-1010. DOI: 10.1038/nature08645.

[124] Sandberg AA, Turc-Carel C. The cytogenetics of solid tumors. Relation to diagnosis, classification and pathology. Cancer. 1987;**59**:387-395. DOI: 10.1002/1097-0142(19870201)59:3<387::AID-CNCR2820590306>3.0.CO;2-X

[125] Ruiz-Herrera A, Smirnova A, Khouriauli L, Nergadze SG, Mondello C, Giulotto E. Gene amplification in human cells knocked down for RAD54. Genome Integr. 2011;**2**:5. DOI: 10.1186/2041-9414-2-5

[126] Valent A, Le Roux G, Barrois M, *et al*. MYCN gene overrepresentation detected in primary neuroblastoma tumour cells without amplification. J Pathol. 2002;**198**:495-501. DOI: 10.1002/path.1244

[127] Jin Y, Jin C, Salemark L, Martins C, Wennerberg J, Mertens F. Centromere cleavage is a mechanism underlying isochromosome formation in skin and head and neck carcinomas. Chromosoma. 2000;**109**:476-481. DOI: 10.1007/s004120000107

[128] Horsthemke B, Greger V, Becher R, Passarge E. Mechanism of i(6p) formation in retinoblastoma tumor cells. Cancer Genet Cytogenet. 1989;**37**:95-102. DOI: 10.1016/0165-4608(89)90079-4

[129] Tommerup N, Lothe R. Constitutional ring chromosomes and tumour suppressor genes. J Med Genet. 1992;**29**:879-882. DOI: 10.1136/jmg.29.12.879

[130] Guilherme RS, Meloni VF, Kim CA, *et al*. Mechanisms of ring chromosome formation, ring instability and clinical consequences. BMC Med Genet. 2011;**12**:171. DOI: 10.1186/1471-2350-12-171

[131] Gisselsson D, Höglund M, Mertens F, *et al*. The structure and dynamics of ring chromosomes in human neoplastic and non-neoplastic cells. Hum Genet. 1999;**104**:315-325. DOI: 10.1007/s004390050960

[132] Dimitrova N, Chen YC, Spector DL, de Lange T. 53BP1 promotes non-homologous end joining of telomeres by increasing chromatin mobility. Nature. 2008;**456**:524-528. DOI: 10.1038/nature07433

[133] Marcand S. How do telomeres and NHEJ coexist? Mol Cell Oncol. 2014;**1**:e963438. DOI: 10.4161/23723548.2014.963438

[134] Gu S, Szafranski P, Akdemir ZC, *et al*. Mechanisms for complex chromosomal insertions. PLoS Genet. 2016;**12**:e1006446. DOI: 10.1371/journal.pgen.1006446

[135] Hayano T, Yamada S, Hosomichi K, *et al*. Identification of novel exonic mobile element insertions in epithelial ovarian cancers. Hum Genome Var. 2015;**2**:15030. DOI: 10.1038/hgv.2015.30

[136] Amplified and overexpressed genes in cancer (AOGIC) [Internet]. 2016. Available from: http://www.amplicon.icr.ac.uk/index.php [Accessed: 2016-11-05]

[137] Storlazzi CT, Lonoce A, Guastadisegni MC, *et al*. Gene amplification as double minutes or homogeneously staining regions in solid tumors: Origin and structure. Genome Res. 2010;**20**:1198-1206. DOI: 10.1101/gr.106252.110

[138] Bignell GR, Santarius T, Pole JC, *et al*. Architectures of somatic genomic rearrangement in human cancer amplicons at sequence-level resolution. Genome Res. 2007;**17**:1296-1303. DOI: 10.1101/gr.6522707

[139] Gebhart E. Double minutes, cytogenetic equivalents of gene amplification, in human neoplasia - a review. Clin Transl Oncol. 2005;**7**:477-485. DOI: 10.1007/BF02717000

[140] Hyman E, Kauraniemi P, Hautaniemi S, *et al*. Impact of DNA amplification on gene expression patterns in breast cancer. Cancer Res. 2002;**62**:6240-6245.

[141] McClintock B. The stability of broken ends of chromosomes in Zea mays. Genetics. 1941;**26**:234-282.

[142] Lo AW, Sabatier L, Fouladi B, Pottier G, Ricoul M, Murnane JP. DNA amplification by breakage/fusion/bridge cycles initiated by spontaneous telomere loss in a human cancer cell line. Neoplasia. 2002;**4**:531-538. DOI: 10.1038/sj.neo.7900267

[143] Tanaka H, Tapscott SJ, Trask BJ, Yao MC. Short inverted repeats initiate gene amplification through the formation of a large DNA palindrome in mammalian cells. Proc Natl Acad Sci U S A. 2002;**99**:8772-8777. DOI: 10.1073/pnas.132275999

[144] Okuno Y, Hahn PJ, Gilbert DM. Structure of a palindromic amplicon junction implicates microhomology-mediated end joining as a mechanism of sister chromatid fusion during gene amplification. Nucleic Acids Res. 2004;**32**:749-756. DOI: 10.1093/nar/gkh244

[145] Difilippantonio MJ, Petersen S, Chen HT, *et al*. Evidence for replicative repair of DNA double-strand breaks leading to oncogenic translocation and gene amplification. J Exp Med. 2002;**196**:469-480. DOI: 10.1084/jem.20020851

[146] Schwab M. Human neuroblastoma: From basic science to clinical debut of cellular oncogenes. Naturwissenschaften. 1999;**86**:71-78. DOI: 10.1007/s001140050574

[147] Tower J. Developmental gene amplification and origin regulation. Annu Rev Genet. 2004;**38**:273-304. DOI: 10.1146/annurev.genet.37.110801.143851

[148] Watanabe T, Tanabe H, Horiuchi T. Gene amplification system based on double rolling-circle replication as a model for oncogene-type amplification. Nucleic Acids Res. 2011;**39**:e106. DOI: 10.1093/nar/gkr442

[149] Slack A, Thornton PC, Magner DB, Rosenberg SM, Hastings PJ. On the mechanism of gene amplification induced under stress in *Escherichia coli*. PLoS Genet. 2006;**2**:e48. DOI: 10.1371/journal.pgen.0020048

[150] Orr B, Godek KM, Compton D. Aneuploidy. Curr Biol. 2015;**25**:R538-R542. DOI: 10.1016/j.cub.2015.05.010

[151] Storchova Z. The causes and consequences of aneuploidy in eukaryotic cells. In: Storchova Z, (ed). Aneuploidy in health and disease. InTech; 2012. pp. 1-22. DOI: 10.5772/45781. Available from: http://www.intechopen.com/books/aneuploidy-in-health-and-disease/the-effect-of-aneuploidy-on-physiology-of-eukaryotic-cell

[152] Storchova Z, Kuffer C. The consequences of tetraploidy and aneuploidy. J Cell Sci. 2008;**121**:3859-3866. DOI: 10.1242/jcs.039537

[153] Galipeau PC, Cowan DS, Sanchez CA, *et al.* 17p (p53) allelic losses, 4 N (G2/tetraploid) populations, and progression to aneuploidy in Barrett's esophagus. Proc Natl Acad Sci U S A. 1996;**93**:7081-7084. DOI: 10.1073/pnas.93.14.7081

[154] Mercapide J, Anzanello F, Rappa G, Lorico A. Relationship between tumor cell invasiveness and polyploidization. PLoS One. 2012;**7**:e53364. DOI: 10.1371/journal.pone.0053364

[155] Atkin NB. Aneuploidy in carcinomas may be initiated by the acquisition of a single trisomy. Cytogenet Genome Res. 2003;**101**:99-102. DOI: 10.1159/000074162

[156] Harrison BD, Hashemi J, Bibi M, *et al.* A tetraploid intermediate precedes aneuploid formation in yeasts exposed to fluconazole. PLoS Biol. 2014;**12**:e1001815. DOI: 10.1371/journal.pbio.1001815

[157] Weaver BA, Silk AD, Montagna C, Verdier-Pinard P, Cleveland DW. Aneuploidy acts both oncogenically and as a tumor suppressor. Cancer Cell. 2007;**11**:25-36. DOI: 10.1016/j.ccr.2006.12.003

[158] Sheltzer JM, Ko JH, Burgos NCH, *et al.* Single-chromosome aneuploidy commonly functions as a tumor suppressor. bioRxiv. 2016;1-42. DOI: 10.1101/040162

[159] Gurney JG, Ross JA, Wall DA, Bleyer WA, Severson RK, Robison LL. Infant cancer in the U.S.: Histology-specific incidence and trends, 1973 to 1992. J Pediatr Hematol Oncol. 1997;**19**:428-432. DOI: 10.1097/00043426-199709000-00004

[160] Brodeur GM. Neuroblastoma: Biological insights into a clinical enigma. Nat Rev Cancer. 2003;**3**:203-216. DOI: 10.1038/nrc1014

[161] Van Roy N, Laureys G, Cheng NC. 1;17 translocations and other chromosome 17 rearrangements in human primary neuroblastoma tumors and cell lines. Genes Chromosomes Cancer. 1994;**10**:103-114. DOI: 10.1002/gcc.2870100205

[162] Meddeb M, Danglot G, Chudoba I, *et al.* Additional copies of a 25 Mb chromosomal region originating from 17q23.1-17qter are present in 90% of high-grade neuroblastomas. Genes Chromosomes Cancer. 1996;**17**:156-165. DOI: 10.1002/(SICI)1098-2264(199611)17:3<156::AID-GCC3>3.0.CO;2-3

[163] Savelyeva L, Corvi R, Schwab M. Translocation involving 1p and 17q is a recurrent genetic alteration of human neuroblastoma cells. Am J Hum Genet. 1994;**55**:334-340.

[164] Altungoz O, Aygun N, Tumer S, Ozer E, Olgun N, Sakizli M. Correlation of modified Shimada classification with MYCN and 1p36 status detected by fluorescence in situ hybridization in neuroblastoma. Cancer Genet Cytogenet. 2007;**172**:113-119. DOI: 10.1016/j.cancergencyto.2006.10.005

[165] Brodeur GM, Seeger RC, Schwab M, Varmus HE, Bishop JM. Amplification of N-myc in untreated human neuroblastomas correlates with advanced disease stage. Science. 1984;**224**:1121-1124. DOI: 10.1126/science.6719137

[166] Bartram CR, Berthold F. Amplification and expression of the N-myc gene in neuroblastoma. Eur J Pediatr. 1987;**146**:162-165. DOI: 10.1007/BF02343225

[167] Valent A, Guillaud-Bataille M, Farra C, *et al*. Alternative pathways of MYCN gene copy number increase in primary neuroblastoma tumors. Cancer Genet Cytogenet. 2004;**153**:10-15. DOI: 10.1016/j.cancergencyto.2003.12.007

[168] Edsjö A, Nilsson H, Vandesompele J, *et al*. Neuroblastoma cells with overexpressed MYCN retain their capacity to undergo neuronal differentiation. Lab Invest. 2004;**84**:406-417. DOI: 10.1038/labinvest.3700061

[169] Maris JM, Matthay KK. Molecular biology of neuroblastoma. J Clin Oncol. 1999;**17**:2264-2279. DOI: 10.1200/JCO.1999.17.7.2264

[170] Ozer E, Altungoz O, Unlu M, Aygun N, Tumer S, Olgun N. Association of MYCN amplification and 1p deletion in neuroblastomas with high tumor vascularity. Appl Immunohistochem Mol Morphol. 2007;**15**:181-186. DOI: 10.1097/01.pai. 0000210 418.38246.58

[171] COSMIC database. The catalogue of somatic mutations in cancer [Internet]. 2016. Available from: http://cancer.sanger.ac.uk/cosmic [Accessed: 2016-11-13]

[172] NCBI website. The National Center for Biotechnology Information advances science and health by providing access to biomedical and genomic information [Internet]. 2016. Available from: http://www.ncbi.nlm.nih.gov [Accessed: 2016-12-01]

[173] Dialign software program for multiple sequence alignment [Internet]. 2016. Available from: https://bibiserv.cebitec.uni-bielefeld.de/dialign [Accessed: 2016-12-12]

[174] IRF software program for finding the inverted repeats [Internet]. 2016. Available from: https://tandem.bu.edu/cgi-bin/irdb/irdb.exe [Accessed: 2016-11-12]

[175] HGMD database. The human gene mutation database [Internet]. 2016 Available from: http://www.hgmd.cf.ac.uk/ac/index.php [Accessed: 2016-12-17]

[176] UCSC genome browser [Internet]. 2016. Available from: https://genome.ucsc.edu/cgi-bin [Accessed: 2016-12-15].

[177] Wang Y, Leung FC. Long inverted repeats in eukaryotic genomes: Recombinogenic motifs determine genomic plasticity. FEBS Lett. 2006;**580**:1277-1284. DOI: 10.1016/j.febslet.2006.01.045

[178] Blumrich A, Zapatka M, Brueckner LM, Zheglo D, Schwab M, Savelyeva L. The FRA2C common fragile site maps to the borders of MYCN amplicons in neuroblastoma and is associated with gross chromosomal rearrangements in different cancers. Hum Mol Genet. 2011;**20**:1488-1501. DOI: 10.1093/hmg/ddr027

[179] Conrad DF, Bird C, Blackburne B, *et al*. Mutation spectrum revealed by breakpoint sequencing of human germline CNVs. Nat Genet. 2010;**42**:385-391. DOI: 10.1038/ng.564

[180] Kuwahara Y, Tanabe C, Ikeuchi T, *et al*. Alternative mechanisms of gene amplification in human cancers. Genes Chromosomes Cancer. 2004;**41**:125-132. DOI: 10.1002/gcc.20075

Chapter 4

Chromosome Abnormalities and Hematopoietic Stem Cell Transplantation in Acute Leukemias

Tatiana L. Gindina, Nikolay N. Mamaev and Boris V. Afanasyev

Additional information is available at the end of the chapter

http://dx.doi.org/10.5772/67802

Abstract

The chapter considers specific treatment options, including allogeneic hematopoietic stem cell transplantation (allo-HSCT) in acute myeloid leukemia (AML) and acute lymphoblastic leukemia (ALL), in patients with some prognostically proven cytogenetic variants as monosomal ones, complex and hyperdiploid karyotypes, like chromosomal translocations t(v;11)(v;q23), t(3;3)/inv(3); t(8;21), t(9;22), etc. Important prognostic role of additional chromosome abnormalities was shown for the patients with t(8;21) and t(9;22). Hence, it is evident that allo-HSCT in patients with poor risk cytogenetic variant must be performed as early as possible, i.e., during first complete remission.

Keywords: leukemia, cytogenetic abnormalities, prognosis, allo-HSCT

1. Introduction

Acute leukemias represent a mixed group of malignant diseases with heterogeneous morphology, cytogenetics, and prognosis. From a genetic point of view, acute myeloid leukemias (AML) and acute lymphoblastic leukemias (ALL) consist of patients with favorable-, intermediate-, and poor-risk cytogenetic variants. A group of AML patients with favorable cytogenetics traits include those with translocations t(15;17), inv(16)/t(16;16), and t(8;21), whereas t(12;21) and high hyperdiploid karyotypes are associated with better prognosis in ALL patients. Currently, the group of AML patients with poor-risk cytogenetics includes cases with -7/7q-, -5/5q-, -17/17p-, t(3;3), t(6;9), t(v;11)(v;q23), monosomal, and complex karyotypes, whereas those with ALL exhibit mainly t(4;11) and t(9;22). Since a great part of AML and ALL patients are not cured by single chemotherapy, they need allogeneic hematopoietic stem cell transplantation (allo-HSCT). So far, the results of allo-HSCT in patients with poor-risk and favorable-risk leukemias were analyzed in common cohorts [1, 2]. The aim of our work is to compare clinical outcomes of allo-HSCT for the patients with distinct cytogenetic variants.

2. Acute myeloid leukemia

2.1. AML with monosomal karyotype

One of the poor-risk chromosome abnormalities in AML patients is monosomal karyotype (MK), which is defined by the presence of one single autosomal monosomy in association with, at least, one additional autosomal monosomy or one structural chromosomal abnormality except for marker and ring chromosomes (**Figure 1**). MK is associated with a dismal prognosis and seems to be prognostically important even in complex karyotype AML. Breems et al. [3] were the first who have noted clinical significance of this finding. More recently, a strong association with *TP53* mutations was shown to be an important feature of this malignancy. Although *TP53* is only rarely affected in AML, it is the most frequently altered gene in complex and monosomal AML karyotypes. Hence, a conclusion was drawn that the loss-of-function of *TP53* might cause cytogenetic instability with subsequent development of complex karyotype alterations, but not *vice versa* [4]. Meanwhile, 5-year survival of the patients with this pathology did not exceed 5% [5], though 3-year survival in this group of AML patients may be increased from 5 to 19% following allo-HSCT [6]. A more favorable 4-year survival was achieved in a quarter of treated AML patients, if HSCT was performed at the first remission [7–9]. Additional analysis showed that the 5-year overall survival (OS) in transplanted patients was longer, as compared to those treated with single chemotherapy or by autologous transplantation (19% vs. 9%, respectively; $P = 0.02$). A similar trend seems to exist with respect

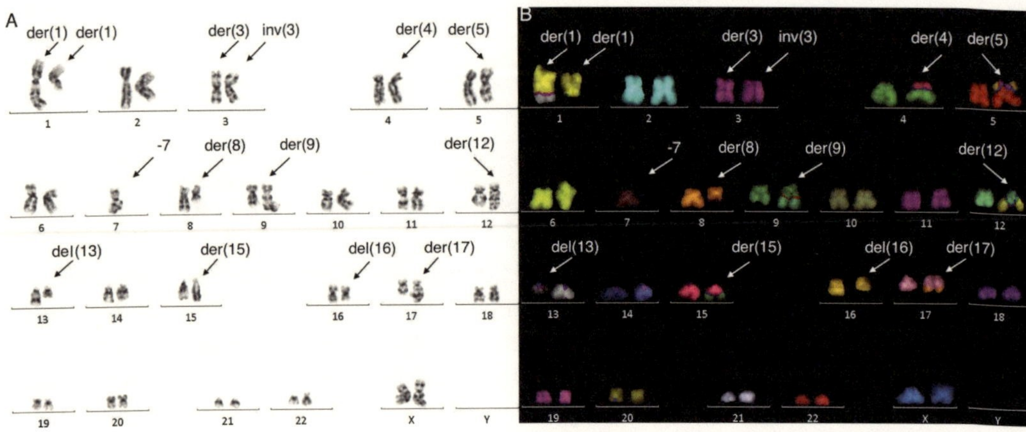

Figure 1. GTG-banded (A) and multicolor FISH (B) karyograms of bone marrow cells with complex and monosomal karyotype in acute myeloid leukemia patient. Karyotype: 45,XX,t(1;13)(q23;q14), der(1)t(1;9)(q21;?), der(3)t(3;5)(q?;?), inv(3)(q21q26),t(4;15)(p12;q22), der(5)t(5;16)(p?;q?)ins(5;3)(?;??),–7,t(8;17)(q22;q25), der(9)t(9;12)(q22;q13),der(12)t(1;12)(q21;q22) ins(12;9)(?;??),del(13)(q14),del(16)(q22).

to 5-year disease-free survival (DFS) or EFS (17% vs. 7%, $P = 0.003$). Multivariate analysis of these data revealed a strong correlation between lower relapse rates and prolonged EFS ($P < 0.001$). On the other hand, there was an only minimal difference in results of multivariate and intergroup analyses of posttransplant relapses and EFS between the groups with monosomal karyotypes and with other poor-risk cytogenetic aberrations. We have observed only eight patients with MK+, including 5q- and -7/7q-, in whom a 3-year disease-free survival was significantly lower than in MK− patients (13% vs. 27%, $P = 0.009$) [10]. Impact of MK upon the outcomes allo-HSCT performed at first remission was evaluated in 263 patients with AML [5]. First, there was a highly significant difference in 5-year OS ranging between 67%, for the most favorable, and 32%, for the poorest risk group ($P = 0.001$). Second, patients with non-MK abnormalities (MK−) and cytogenetically normal cases showed identical incidence of 5-year relapse (24%). Third, multivariate analysis revealed MK to be an independent prognostic factor, which was able to successfully predict OS (hazard ratios (HR) 3.74, $P = 0.01$) and relapse incidence (HR 3.74, $P = 0.005$), as compared to some other criteria, including those of SWOG/ECOG. Finally, subgroup analysis revealed prognostic ability of MK-based classification to be highly efficient in the patients treated with standard myeloablative conditioning prior to allo-HSCT ($P = 0.0011$ for OS, $P = 0.0007$ for relapse). However, the MK-based grouping failed to predict OS or incidence of relapse in HSCT patients treated with reduced intensity conditioning (RIC).

2.2. AML with complex karyotype

The interest to AML with CK as a distinct biological entity has appeared recently [7–11]. This anomaly is defined as three and more structural and numerical chromosome aberrations per metaphase (**Figure 1**), when excluding such recurring abnormalities, as t(8;21), inv(16)/t(16;16), t(15;17), or 11q23/MLL rearrangements [11–14]. Nowadays, it accounts for 10–20% of AML cases and increases sharply with age [15]. Despite intensive treatment, including allo-HSCT, median OS for these patients was <6 months and less than 10% patients achieved long-term survival [16]. It has been also established that incidence of CK+ cases in AML may increase after chemotherapy [17] and HSCT [18–20]. However, some recent data [21] suggested that a 90% CR rate was achieved for these poor-risk patients, if allo-HSCT was performed within 80–100 days after diagnosis even in active phase of the disease. A hypothetic explanation is that poor prognosis of AML patients with CK may be associated with a chromosomal instability which, in turn, is directly related to clonal evolution, selection, and adaptation of leukemic cells [3].

2.3. AML with hyperdiploid karyotype

Patients with hyperdiploid karyotypes (HDK) are not so rare in AML too, revealing many in common with aforementioned CK (**Figure 2**). For instance, in cases of sole chromosomes 8, 21, and 13 trisomies, these cases are classified as intermediate risk group. On the other hand, a new heterogeneous group with high hyperdiploidy and modal chromosome numbers from 49 to 65 has been recently described in about 2% of poor-risk AML patients [22], which was prognostically poor. Finally, cases with near triploid/tetraploid karyotype, especially associated

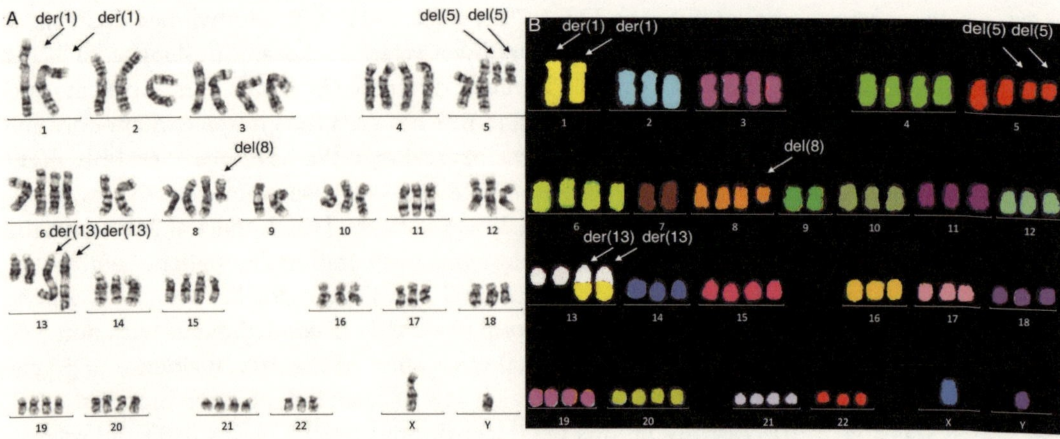

Figure 2. GTG-banded (A) and multicolor FISH (B) karyograms of bone marrow cells with hyperdiploid karyotype and adverse chromosome abnormality 5q− in acute myeloid leukemia patient relapsing after allo-HSCT. Karyotype: 75,<3n>,XY,−X,−1,der(1)del(1)(p32)ins(1;1)(q21;p32p36)x2,+3,+4,+5,del(5)(q13q33)x2,+6,−7,+8,del(8)(q11q23),−9,+13, der(13)t(1;13)(q21;q34)x2,+15,−17,+19,+20,+21,+22.

with structural chromosome anomalies are encountered not so often [23, 24]. Since there are no available publications concerning of allo-HSCT results in AML patients with HDK, we presented here our data on the topic in details [25]. Study group enrolled 47 AML patients (21 females, 26 males, aged 1–58 years; median age 23.9 years), in whom allo-HSCT was performed at our university during 2008–2015 years. Cytogenetic evaluation included standard GTG differential staining of chromosomes as well as Multicolor FISH (M-FISH), which were carried out according to standard manufacturer recommendations. Criteria for defining aberrations and nomenclature for description of the cytogenetic findings were in accordance to the international system for human cytogenetic nomenclature (ISCN) [26]. Allo-HSCT was performed in 13/47 (28%) patients in the first complete remission (CR), in 7/47 (15%) patients in the second CR, whereas 27/47 (57%) patients were transplanted in active disease. Sources of stem cells for the patients were as follows: bone marrow (n = 23; 49%) or peripheral blood stem cells (*n* = 21; 45%), while both were used in three (6%) patients. Reduced-intensity conditioning (RIC) regimen, including fludarabine, busulfan, and/or cyclophosphamide, as well as myeloablative regimen was used in 31 (66%) and 16 (34%) patients, respectively. HLA-related and nonrelated donors were used for nine (19%) and 32 (68%) patients, respectively. At the same time, related haploidentical allo-HSCT was performed for six (13%) patients. Thirty-one of 47 (66%) patients with HDK contained karyotypes with modal chromosome numbers of 47–48. A phenomenon of hyperdiploidy (49–65 chromosomes per metaphase) was revealed in 13/47 (28%) patients. At the same time in 3/47 (6%) patients, the modal numbers were near triploid and near tetraploid. Structural chromosome aberrations were revealed in 23/47 (49%) patients. Complex karyotypes with three or more chromosome anomalies were found in 19/47 (40%) patients, whereas the adverse chromosome abnormalities were registered in nine cases (19%). Numerical chromosomal anomalies were nonrandom. Trisomy 8 was the most common, being revealed in 22 patients (50%) patients excluding those with triploid and tetraploid karyotypes. It was as a single finding in seven (32%) patients while being combined with other structural and numerical chromosome anomalies in 15 (68%) patients. In some patients, trisomy 8 was associated with t(6;9), monosomy 7, and abn(3q26), thus allowing to include them into the poor-risk cytogenetic group. The second position in the rate of trisomy incidence takes chromosome 21, which was revealed in 14 (32%) patients. It was observed as a single abnormality in seven (50%) patients, whereas in seven other cases (50%), the combination with additional chromosome abnormalities was noted. Of note, one patient exhibited a tetraploid set of chromosome 21. This is followed by chromosome 13 and 22 trisomies, which were revealed in seven patients each (16%). Trisomy 22 was found as single finding in two (29%) patients, in combination with the other chromosome abnormalities in five (71%) patients. Moreover, combination of trisomy 21 and del(11p) was noticed in one patient. Trisomy 13 was not presented alone, having been combined with other chromosome aberrations, with trisomy 19 and additional X chromosome in six (14%) and five (11%) patients, respectively. Numerical aberrations of chromosome 4 were less common, being revealed in four patients (9%), with a tetrasomic set in one case. Moreover, trisomy 7 and trisomy 6 were revealed in three (7%) and two (5%) patients, respectively. Finally, single findings of trisomy 3, 5, 9, 11, 12, 15, and 18 chromosomes as well as double Y were also documented. Chromosomal monosomy in AML patients with HDK was rare. Meanwhile, monosomy 18 was revealed in three (7%) patients from this subgroup. Three other patients had monosomies 2, 7, and 21. According to common classification the karyotypes of 19/47 (40%) may be designated as CK. They exhibited three or more chromosomal abnormalities coupled with, at least, one structural aberration. Poor-risk cytogenetic aberrations, e.g., -7/7q-, 5q-, anomalies 3q26, and 17p were revealed in 9/47 (19%) patients. This may be exemplified by a patient with tetraploid chromosome set associated with structural rearrangements including 5q- and other anomalies. Univariate analysis showed that OS and DFS after allo-HSCT significantly depend on clinical status of the patients' status at allo-HSCT ($P = 0.003$ and $P = 0.002$, respectively) as well as on the presence of adverse chromosome aberrations ($P = 0.002$ and $P = 0.01$, respectively). A significant difference in OS and DFS were revealed also in patients who were transplanted in the first or second remissions ($P = 0.04$ and $P = 0.04$, respectively). At the same time, the results of allo-HSCT did not depend on AML variant, patients' gender, donor's type, conditioning regime, source of HSC, as well as on modal number of chromosomes and presence or absence of structural rearrangements and complex aberrations in HDK. Using multivariate analysis, we have shown independent predictors for improved OS and DFS in AML patients with HDK, as following: (a) remission at allo-HSCT ($P = 0.003$ and $P = 0.021$, respectively); and (b) the absence of adverse chromosome aberrations ($P = 0.002$ and $P = 0.005$, respectively).

2.4. AML with *KMT2A (MLL)* rearrangement

AML with 11q23/*KMT2A* rearrangement is rare, and about 85 genes may be involved as partners for fusion with *KTM2A*. Most of these cytogenetic subtypes, except translocation of t(9;11)(p22;q23) [27], are classified into poor-risk cytogenetic group [28]. Predictive ability of this marker in HSCT setting was recently discussed [29, 30]. One of such recent studies [28] enrolled 138 patients with 11q23/*KMT2A*-rearranged AML, who were allografted in first or second CR. The cohort consisted of patients with t(9;11), t(11;19), t(6;9), and t(10;11) translocations. Two-year OS, leukemia-free survival, relapse incidence, and nonrelapse mortality were 56 ± 4%, 51 ± 4%, 31 ± 3%, and 17 ± 4%, respectively. The 11q23.3 rearrangements causing *KMT2A (MLL)* exchanges of gene are revealed in about 3–7% of adult AML patients. Higher efficiency of allo-HSCT over chemotherapy alone in the treatment of AML patients with *KMT2A (MLL)* rearrangements seems to be evident [31].

2.5. AML with t(3;3)(q21;q26.2)/inv(3)(q21q26.2)

AML with inv(3)(q21q26.2)/t(3;3)(q21;q26.2) is a distinct subtype of AML with recurrent genetic abnormalities. It is commonly refractory to conventional chemotherapy due to *EVI1* gene overexpression, thus being associated with poor prognosis [32–36]. Isolated inv(3)/t(3;3) were revealed in 43.7% of such patients [33]. The most frequently observed additional cytogenetic abnormalities were: −7/del(7q) (37.3%), complex chromosome abnormality, and sometimes Ph+ chromosome [33]. Monosomy 7 is reported in approximately 40–60% of inv(3)/t(3;3) AML patients and associated with dismal prognosis [33–35]. Of interest is that AML and MDS patients with inv(3)/t(3;3) regardless of blast number have both similar clinical and pathological characteristics and short OS. Complex and monosomal karyotypes were also considered independent negative prognostic factors in AML patients with inv(3)/t(3;3) [36]. Due to low incidence of this poor-risk AML subtype, efficacy of HSCT is still subject to small clinical studies [34–36], mainly, with poor results. As an example of treatment failure in such cases, we presented a clinical case of a young female with inv(3)(q21q26.2), −7. The patient underwent a quantitative monitoring with serial expressions of *WT1* and *EVI* gene levels, as reported earlier [35]. The last large investigation in the field has been published recently [36]. It enrolled 32 transplanted patients in the first remission with overexpression of *EVI1* gene, induced by aberrations of 3q26 and 11q23 loci, and 119 control patients with low *EVI1* expression. The study showed much higher *EVI1*+ frequency in adverse-risk group, as compared with intermediate-risk group (53% vs. 19%, $P = 0.005$). The results of DFS and OS in 24 months of the *EVI1*+ cohort were shorter (52.6% vs. 71.0%, $P = 0.02$ and 52.8% vs. 72.4%, $P = 0.01$, respectively), whereas cumulative incidence of relapse was higher (39.5% vs. 22.5%, $P = 0.01$). Multivariate analysis revealed that low *EVI1* expression as an independent prognostic factor favoring DFS (HR = 0.47, 95% CI 0.26–0.86, $P = 0.01$) but not OS. These results indicated that high *EVI1* expression might predict high risk of relapse in AML patients undergoing myeloablative allo-HSCT in CR1.

2.6. AML with t(8;21)(q22;q22) *RUNX1/RUNX1T1*, inv(16)(p13q22)/t(16;16) *CBFβ/MYH11*

In view of the data concerning poor-risk AML groups, it would be interesting to discuss clinical outcomes after allo-HSCT in cohorts with favorable-risk cytogenetics. Several such studies should be mentioned [37–39]. The data revealed by Yoon et al. [40] consist of 264 adult patients with CBF-positive AML, where 206 of whom were in CR. Allo-HSCT was performed in 115 patients, whereas other patients were treated either by auto-HSCT ($n = 72$) or chemotherapy alone ($n = 19$). There was no difference in OS in groups of patients with *CBFβ/MYH11* ($n = 62$) and *RUNX1/RUNX1T1* ($n = 144$). Meanwhile, it was noted that OS was better in the patients treated by auto-HSCT, compared to those treated by either allo-HSCT or chemotherapy alone ($P = 0.001$). According to cytogenetic data, OS seems to be longer in patients with inv(16), which is not accompanied by trisomy. On the other hand, OS terms were shorter in patients with t(8;21) accompanied by additional chromosome aberrations.

It should be mentioned that these findings were not supported by multivariate analysis. Molecular monitoring showed that OS was lower but incidence of posttransplant relapses proved to be higher in those patients with detectable minimal residual disease (MRD). Some other groups have recently reported on high number of additional chromosome and genetic abnormalities in patients with t(8;21), thus suggesting an impact on clinical outcome [41, 42]. We have recently yielded similar results in allo-HSCT patients with t(8;21) [43]. The study enrolled 25 *RUNX1-RUNX1T1*-positive AML patients (10 females and 15 males, age 2–58 years, a median of 20.2 years). The additional cytogenetic abnormalities were detected in 13 (52%) patients before the transplantation (**Figure 3**). CK with three or more chromosomal abnormalities were noticed in nine (69%) patients. The median follow-up was 566 (8–2127) days. Overall survival (OS) was 33% (95% CI 14–53) and relapse-free survival (RFS) was 26%

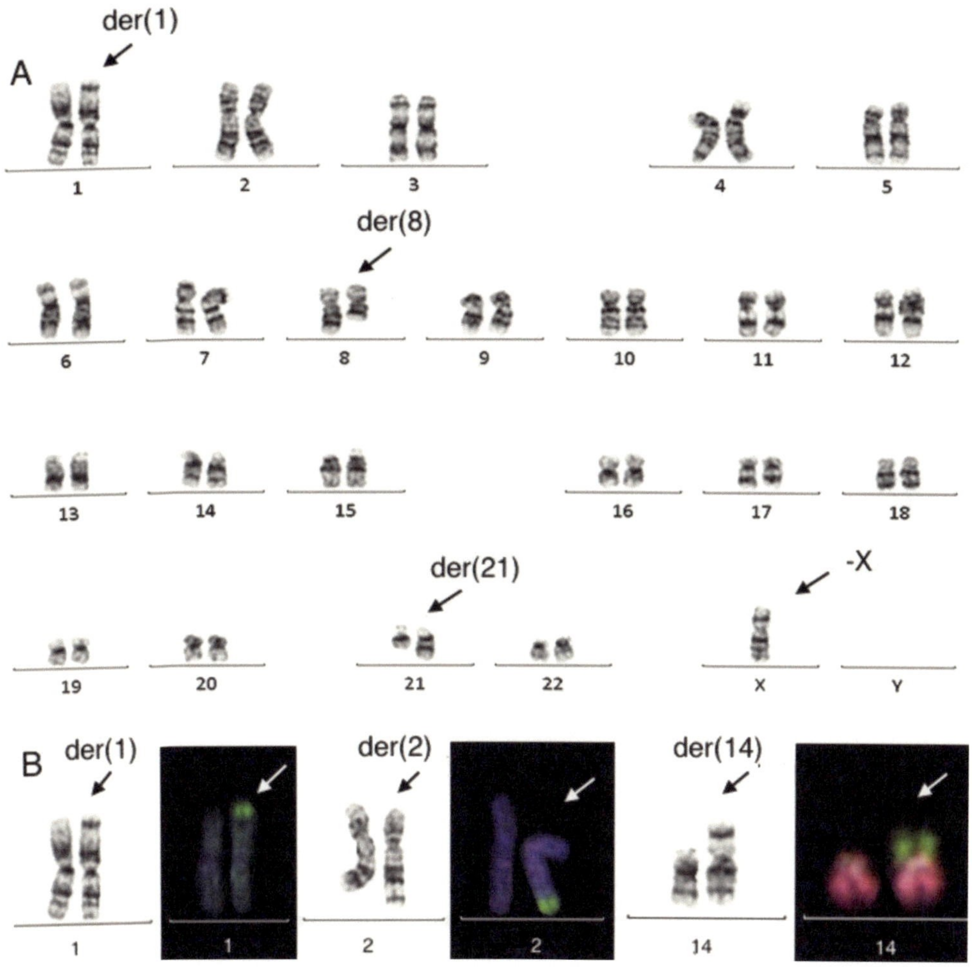

Figure 3. GTG-banded (A) and partial multicolor FISH (B) karyograms of bone marrow cells from AML patient demonstrate reciprocal translocation t(8;21)(q22;q22) and additional chromosome abnormalities, including "jumping" translocation 17q21-17qter followed by the production of derivative chromosomes #1, #2, #14. Karyotype: 45,X,-X,der(2)t(2;17)(q37;q21),t(8;21)(q22;q22)/45,X,-X, t(8;21),der(14)t(14;17)(p13;q21)/45,X,-X,der(1)t(1;17)(p36;q21),t(8;21).

(95% CI 9–45) at 4 years estimated with Kaplan-Meier method. The following factors predictive in univariate analysis for increased OS and RFS were: patients' age (>18 vs. <18 years; $P = 0.03$ and $P = 0.0006$, respectively), donor type (matched related/matched unrelated vs. haploidentical; $P = 0.0003$, $P = 0.02$, respectively), the disease status at transplant (complete remission vs. active disease; $P = 0.0002$ and $P = 0.005$, respectively), time interval from diagnosis to transplant (<360 vs. >360 days; $P = 0.008$, only for OS), ACA (ACA− vs. ACA+; $P = 0.02$ and $P = 0.009$, respectively), complex karyotype (CK− vs. CK+ ; $P = 0.004$ and $P = 0.0003$, respectively). In multivariate analysis, the ACA (HR 13.5; $P = 0.04$), the donor type (HR 6.86; $P = 0.01$), and time interval from diagnosis to HSCT (HR 6.80; $P = 0.02$) remained statistically significant for OS. Moreover, age (HR 0.11; $P = 0.004$) and the donor type (HR 4.16; $P = 0.04$) were independent predictors for RFS. On the basis of these findings, a conclusion may be drawn that AML with t(8;21)(q22;q22)/*RUNX1/RUNX1T1* translocation is a heterogeneous disease. The prognosis in patients with the additional cytogenetic abnormalities, especially in those with the CK, is worse both after the standard chemotherapy (i.e., before allo-HSCT) and after allo-HSCT as well.

3. Acute lymphoblastic leukemia

3.1. ALL with translocation t(9;22)(q34;q11.2) *BCR/ABL1*

Philadelphia-positive acute lymphoblastic leukemia (Ph+ ALL) has been regarded for decades as the ALL subgroup with inferior outcome. However, introduction of tyrosine kinase inhibitors (TKI) in the induction treatment provided complete hematologic remissions (CHRs) in nearly all patients [44–51], thus allowing to recommend them as gold for Ph+ ALL patient's treatment. Together, these findings show that complete response to the therapy, including molecular remission, were achieved earlier in TKI-treated cohorts of ALL patients, whereas OS and DFS in these patients lasted longer than in a cohort that avoided TKI, regardless of their combinations with auto- or allo-HSCT. It has been also noticed that additional chromosome aberrations may be a poor predictor for the treatment results [51]. Three-year leukemia-free survival (79.8% vs. 39.5%, $P = 0.01$) and 3-year OS (83% vs. 45.6%, $P = 0.02$) were superior in the Ph+ only cohort compared with the ACA cohort ($n = 12$). Our recent data are in a good accordance with the above results, and supported the aforementioned opinion. The study was performed in 65 patients with Ph-positive ALL (26 female and 39 males aged 5–48 years, a mean of 26.2 years). Thirty-one (48%) and 20 (31%) patients were transplanted in the first or the second remissions, respectively, whereas 14 (21%) patients received transplant in active disease. The stem cell sources were bone marrow ($n = 31$; 49%) and peripheral blood cells ($n = 32$; 49%) or both ($n = 2$; 3%). Reduced-intensity conditioning regimen (RIC) was used in 36 (55%) patients, whereas myeloablative conditioning was applied in 29 (45%) patients. Cytogenetic evaluation at diagnosis was carried out in 53 (80%) patients. Ph-chromosome as a sole karyotype anomaly was detected in 33 (62%) patients. Due to high number of additional chromosomal changes (≥3) in a quarter of this group, they are described as "complex karyotypes" (**Figure 4**). HLA-related siblings were donors for 18 recipients (38%), whereas stem cells

http://dx.doi.org/10.5772/67802

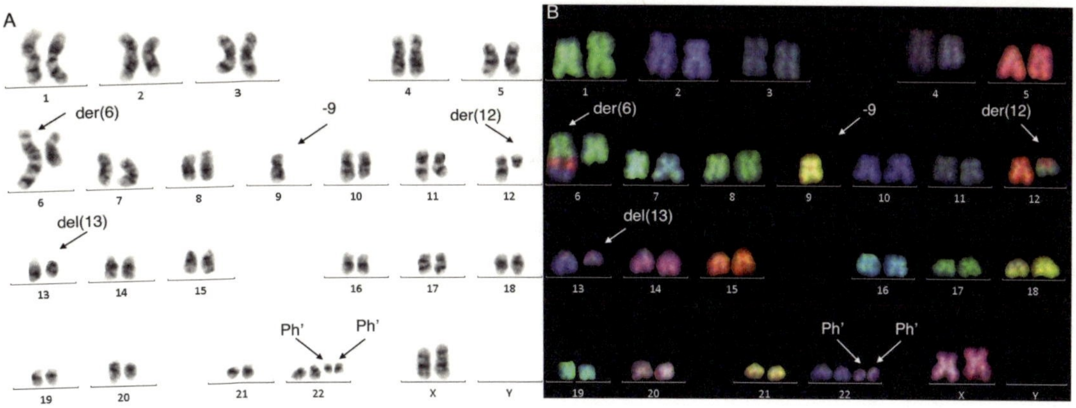

Figure 4. GTG-banded (A) and multicolor FISH (B) karyograms of bone marrow cells with translocation t(9;22)(q34;q11) and additional cytogenetic abnormalities in acute lymphoblastic leukemia patient relapsing after autological HSCT. Karyotype: 47,XX,der(6)t(6;13)(q23;q1?)ins(6;12)(q23;q13q24),-9,der(12) t(6;12)(q23;q13), del(13)(q1?),+22,+der(22)t(9;22)(q34;q11).

from HLA-matched nonrelated donors were used in 42 patients (65%). Moreover, five patients (7%) were transplanted with CD34+ cells from haploidentical family members. The number of CD34+ transfused cells ranged from 1.3 to 12.2 (mean 5.03) per kg of weight body. The study showed that additional chromosomal changes in Ph+ ALL were represented by numeric and/or structural abnormalities. Numeric changes were observed in 12 (60%) patients, affecting chromosomes 1, 2, 7, 8, 9, 10, 17, 19, and 22. Trisomy 1, 10, 22, and monosomy 7 were revealed in two patients each, whereas trisomy 2, 17, and 19 were revealed in single cases. The patterns and incidence of structural chromosome changes were as follows: deletions and translocations, involving 9p (n = 4; 20%); reciprocal translocations of 7p (n = 3; 15%), interstitial deletions/translocations of 5q (n = 4; 20%), deletions and translocations of chromosome 1 (n = 3; 15%) and 2 (n = 4; 20%), and structural aberrations of chromosome 17 (n = 2), including i(17q). Moreover, a double derivative of chromosome 22 was an additional chromosome abnormality in two patients. Univariate analysis revealed that 5-year OS was longer, when allo-HSCT was performed from HLA-matched related and unrelated donors (P = 0.02), when the patients had neither additional chromosome abnormalities in karyotypes (P = 0.04) nor primarily "complex" karyotypes (P = 0.01). On the other hand, DFS was longer in patients transplanted in the first remission (P = 0.01) with CD34-positive cells from completely matched donors (P = 0.02).

3.2. ALL patients with *KMT2A (MLL)* gene rearrangements

Structural rearrangements of 11q23.3 caused by inducing exchanges of *KMT2A (MLL)* gene are revealed in about 3–7% ALL patients, with up to 70–80% in newborn patients [28]. The main of these translocations—t(4;11)(q21;q23) *KMT2A/AFF1* [52]—occurs in 8–10% of ALL cases with a peak of incidence in infants. Despite generally poor prognosis for ALL with t(4;11) in all pediatric patients, it is the worst for infants [53–55]. Because of absent for this category of patient a targeted drug, allo-HSCT remains a single curative treatment [53]. According to recent findings, 5-year OS reached 67.4% in newborns with *KMT2A*+ ALL, subjected to earlier performed allo-HSCT in first remission [56–58]. Such curative effect did not depend on patient's age, initial leukocytosis, cytogenetic findings, donor type, and options of conditioning regimen, although myeloablative conditioning with Busulfan seems to be preferable in these cases. Multivariate analysis showed the number of transfused mononuclear donor cells to be a basic predictor for longer OS ($P = 0.04$). To our knowledge, only one survey concerned results of allo-HSCT in adult patients with t(4;11) [31]. In general, allo-HSCT was performed in 56 patients, including 46 patients over 15 years old, and 10 children. Twenty-nine patients (7–64 years old) were enrolled for autologous HSCT or chemotherapy alone, as a comparison group. Despite it, all tested patients showed myeloid engraftment. Overall, posttransplant relapses were diagnosed in 12 transplanted patients after a median of 208 days, reaching a cumulative incidence of hematological relapse of 25.3% at 3 years. Additional analysis showed that 6/41 (14.6%) transplanted in CR1 and 6/15 (40%) patients with non-CR1 status at transplantation relapsed after HSCT ($P = 0.04$). Univariate analysis showed that the 3-year CIR was 48.1 and 17.9% for the patients transplanted in CR1 and non-CR1 status, respectively ($P = 0.03$). In multivariate analysis, CR1 status at transplantation proved to be the only predictor of lower relapse rate ($P = 0.018$). Noteworthy, 37 patients were alive at the last follow-up, with a median survival time of 742 (range 172–1866) days after HSCT without recurrence of the disease. The probabilities for OS and DFS were 61.8 and 56.3% at 3 years, respectively, after HSCT. Adults and children had comparable OS and DFS rates. The patients who received nucleated cells above the median level had higher OS than the recipients transplanted at smaller cell doses (72.2% vs. 39.2%, $P = 0.02$). The predictive value of MNC numbers was mainly attributed to peripheral blood graft. Specifically, since patients receiving more nucleated cells in peripheral blood graft had higher OS than the patients, who received lower MNC quantities (65.8% vs. 42.9%, $P = 0.03$). In multivariate analysis higher MNC doses were found to be the only predictor for higher OS with hazard ratio (HR) of 0.34 (95% CI, 0.12–0.98, $P = 0.04$). In our recent study, HSCT was performed at the first or the second remissions in 11 (44%) and three (12%) patients, respectively, whereas 11 (44%) patients were transplanted in relapse state. This group included 21 patients with t(4;11)(q21;q23) *KMT2A/AFF1* and four recipients with variant translocations at 11q23 locus. Translocation t(4;11)(q21;q23) was the "sole" finding only in 10 (48%) patients. In 11 patients (52%), it was associated with other structural changes, i.e., del(1), del(3p), i(7q), i(17q), and der(19p). It should be also mentioned that seven patients had each ≥3 chromosome aberrations, thus allowing to place them to the group with "complex" karyotype. Rearrangements of chromosomes 1, 7, and 3 should be mentioned as additional chromosomal aberrations (in 5, 4, and 3 patients, respectively). Stem cells sources were bone marrow (n = 7), peripheral blood (n = 17), or both ($n = 1$). Reduced-intensity ($n = 13$; 52%) or myeloablative ($n = 12$; 48%) conditioning regimens were used for HSCTs. Donors were HLA-matched related or matched unrelated (6 and 11 patients, respectively). On the other hand, in eight (32%) patients haploidentical transplantation was performed. Univariate analysis confirmed the existing view that OS and DFS of patients with KMT2A involvement was significantly longer, when HSCT was performed in complete remission regardless of the first or the second remission ($P = 0.0001$), and if other sources than peripheral blood were used for HSCT ($P = 0.01$ and $P = 0.07$ for OS and DFS, respectively). Finally, DFS was shorter in patients with additional chromosome abnormalities in karyotypes ($P = 0.05$), especially with CK ($P = 0.01$). Data from multivariate analysis supported conclusions drawn by previous investigators demonstrating a favorable influence of CR status on HSCT outcomes only on outcome of HSCT in adult ALL patients with 11q23 abnormality.

4. Conclusion

Analysis of the HSCT results in patients with prognostically different cytogenetic variants of acute leukemias showed that this approach may be efficient in all the tested patients and that it can be effective enough in all tested cohorts, including patients with the most poor-risk leukemias with monosomal and complex karyotypes, as well as those with translocations t(4;11)(q21;q23), t(9;22)(q34;q11.1), t(3;3)(q21;q26.2), etc. The situation can be dramatically changed with the introduction of highly effective targeted drugs, e.g., TKIs, into therapeutic protocols for Ph-positive leukemias.

Acknowledgements

The authors would like to acknowledge the assistance of Professor Alexei Chukhlovin in the preparation of this manuscript.

Author details

Tatiana L. Gindina*, Nikolay N. Mamaev and Boris V. Afanasyev

*Address all correspondence to: gindinatl@spb-gmu.ru

Department of Hematology, Transfusiology and Transplantaion, R.M. Gorbacheva Memorial Institute of Oncology, Hematology and Transplantation, Pavlov First Saint-Petersburg State Medical University, Saint-Petersburg, Russian Federation

References

[1] Armand P, Kim HT, De Angelo DJ, et al. Impact of cytogenetics on outcome of de novo and therapy-related AML and MDS after allogeneic transplantation. Biol Blood Marrow Transplant. 2007:13:655-664. DOI: 10.1016/jbbmt.2007.01.079

[2] Nahi H, Remberger M, Machaczka M, et al. Different impact of intermediate and unfavorable cytogenetics at the time of diagnosis of de novo AML after allo-SCT: a long-term retrospective analysis from a single institution. Med Oncol. 2012;29:2348-2358. DOI: 10.1007/s12032-011-0155-y

[3] Breems DA, Van Putten WLL, De Greef GE, et al. Monosomal karyotype in acute myeloid leukemia: a better indicator of poor prognosis than a complex karyotype. J Clin Oncol. 2008;26:4791-4797. DOI: 10.1200/jco.2008.16.0259

[4] Bochtler T, Fröhling S, Krämer A, et al. Role of chromosomal aberrations in clonal diversity and progression of acute myeloid leukemia. Leukemia. 2015;29:1243-1252. DOI: 10.1038/leu.2015.32

[5] Hemmati PG, Schulze-Luchkov A, Terwey ThN, et al. Cytogenetic risk grouping by the monosomal karyotype classification is superior in predicting the outcome of acute myeloid leukemia undergoing allogeneic stem cell transplantation in complete remission. Eur J Haematol. 2013;92:102-110. DOI: 10.1111/ejh.12216

[6] Oran B, Dolan M, Cao Q, et al. Monosomal karyotype provides better prognostic prediction after allogeneic stem cell transplantation in patients with acute myelogenous leukemia. Biol Blood Marrow Transplant. 2011;17:356-364. DOI: 10.1016/j.bbmt.2010.05.012

[7] Fang M, Storer B, Estey E, et al. Outcome of patients with acute myeloid leukemia with monosomal karyotype who undergo hematopoietic stem cell transplantation. Blood 2011;118:1490-1494. DOI: 10.1182/blood-2011-02-339721

[8] Cornelissen JJ, Breems D, van Putten WL, et al. Comparative analysis of the value of allogeneic hematopoietic stem-cell transplantation in acute myeloid leukemia with monosomal karyotype versus other cytogenetic risk categories. J Clin Oncol. 2012;30:2140-2146. DOI: 10.1200/jco.2011.39.6499

[9] Pasquini M, Zhang M-J, Medeiros BC, et al. Hematopoietic cell transplantation outcomes in monosomal karyotype myeloid malignancies. Biol Blood Marrow Transplant. 2016;22:248-257. DOI: 10.1016/j.bbmt.2015.08.024

[10] Gindina TL, Mamaev NN, Bondarenko SN, et al. Allogeneic hematopoietic stem cell transplantation in acute myeloid leukemias: prognostic significance of complex karyotype including del(5q), -7, del(7q) abnormalities. Clin Oncohematol. 2016;9:271-278. DOI: 10.21320/2500-2139-2016-9-3-271-278 [In Russ].

[11] Schoch C, Kern W, Kohlmann A, et al. Acute myeloid leukemia with a complex aberrant karyotype is a distinct biological entity characterized by genomic imbalance and a special gene expression profile. Genes Chromosomes Cancer. 2005;43:227-238. DOI: 10.1002/gcc.20193

[12] Mrozek K. Cytogenetic, molecular genetics, and clinical characteristics of acute myeloid leukemia with a complex karyotype. Semin Oncol. 2008;358:365-377. DOI: 10.1053/j.seminoncol.2008.04.007

[13] Dobbelstein C, Dammann E, Weissinger E, et al. Prognostic impact a newly defined structurally complex karyotype in patients with AML and MDS after allogeneic stem cell transplantation [abstract]. Blood. (Ash Ann. Meet. Abstr.) 2013;122:3362-3363.

[14] Gindina TL, Mamaev NN, Bondarenko SN, et al. Complex chromosomal aberrations in patients with post-transplantation relapses of acute leukemias: clinical and theoretical aspects. Clin Oncohematol. 2015;5:69-77 [In Russ].

[15] Fleischman EW, Sokova OI, Popa AV, et al. Complex karyotype in paediatric acute myeloid leukemia. Clin Oncohematol. 2015;8:151-160 [In Russ].

[16] Zaccaria A, Rosti G, Testoni N, et al. Chromosome studies in patients with nonlymphocytic or acute lymphocytic leukemia submitted to bone marrow transplantation – results of European cooperative study. Cancer Genet Cytogenet. 1987;26:51-58. DOI: 10.1016/0165-4608(87)90132-4

[17] Schmidt-Hieber M, Blau IW, Richter G, et al. Cytogenetic studies in acute leukemia patients relapsing after allogeneic stem cell transplantation. Cancer Genet Cytogenet. 2010;198:135-143. DOI: 10.1016/j.cancergencyto. 2010.01.005

[18] Gindina TL, Mamaev NN, Barkhatov IM, et al. Complex chromosome damages in patients with recurrent acute leukemias after allogeneic hematopoietic stem cell transplantation. Ther Arkhiv. 2012;8:61-66 [In Russ].

[19] Chi H.S, Cho YU, Park SH, et al. Comparative analysis of cytogenetic evolution patterns during relapse in the hematopoietic stem cell transplantation and chemotherapy settings of patients with acute leukemia [abstract]. Blood. (Ash Ann. Meet. Abstr.) 2013;122:1320-1320.

[20] Yuasa M, Uchida M, Kaji D, et al. Prognostic significance of the cytogenetic evolution after the hematopoietic stem cell transplantation in adult acute myeloid leukemia [abstract]. Blood. (Ash Ann. Meet. Abstr.) 2013;122:1391-1391.

[21] Schmid C, Schleuning M, Tischer J, et al. Early allo-SCT for AML with a complex aberrant karyotype – results from a prospective pilot study. Bone Marrow Transplant. 2012;47:46-53. DOI: 10.1038/bmt.2011.15

[22] Chilton L, Hills RK, Harrison CJ, et al. Hyperdiploidy with 49-65 chromosomes represents a heterogeneous cytogenetic subgroup of acute myeloid leukemia with differential outcome. Leukemia. 2013;28:321-328. DOI: 10.1038/leu.2013.198

[23] Lazarus HM, Litzow MR. AML cytogenetics: the complex just got simpler. Blood. 2012;120:2357-2358. DOI: 10.1182/blood-2012-08-448555

[24] Pang CS, Pettenati MJ, Pardee TS, et al. Clinicopathological analysis of near-tetraploidy/tetraploidy acute myeloid leukemia. J Clin Pathol. 2015;68:236-240. DOI: 10.1136/clinpathol-2014-202697

[25] Gindina TL, Mamaev NN, Nikolaeva ES, et al. Outcome of allogeneic hematopoietic stem cell transplantation in acute myeloid leukemias with hyperdiploid karyotype. Clin Oncohematol. 2016;9:383-390. DOI: 10.21320/2500-2139-2016-9-4-383-390 [In Russ].

[26] Schaffer LG, McGovan-Jordan J, Schmid M. ISCN. An International System for Human Cytogenetic Nomenclature. Basel: Karger, 2013: 140 p.

[27] Mrozek K, Heinonen K, Lawrence D, et al. Adult patients with de novo acute myeloid leukemia and t(9;11)(p22q23) have a superior outcome to patients with other translocations involving band 11q23: a cancer and a leukemia group B study. Blood. 1997;90: 4532-4538.

[28] Wang Y, Liu QF, Qin YZ, et al. Improved outcome with hematopoietic stem cell transplantation in a poor prognostic subgroup of patients with mixed-lineage-leukemia-rearranged acute leukemia: results from a prospective, multicenter study. Am J Hematol. 2014;89:130-136. DOI: 10.1002/ajh.23593

[29] Chen Y, Kantarjian H, Pierce S, et al. Prognostic significance of 11q23 aberrations in adult acute myeloid leukemia and the role of allogeneic stem cell transplantation. Leukemia. 2013;27:836-842. DOI: 10.1038/leu.2012.319

[30] Pigneux A, Labopin M, Maertens J, et al. Outcome of allogeneic hematopoietic stem-cell transplantation in adult patients with AML and 11q23/MLL rearrangement (MLL-r-AML). Leukemia. 2015;29:2375-2381. DOI: 10.1038/leu.2015.143

[31] Yang H, Huang S, Zhu C-Y, et al. The superiority of allogeneic hematopoietic stem cell transplantation over chemotherapy alone in the treatment of acute myeloid leukemia patients with mixed lineage leukemia (MLL) rearrangements. Med Sci Monit. 2016;22:2315-2323. DOI: 10.12659/MSM.899186

[32] Lugthart S, Groeschel S, Beverloo HB, et al. Clinical, molecular, and prognostic significance of WHO type inv(3)(q21q26.2)/t(3;3)(q21;q26.2) and various other 3q abnormalities in acute myeloid leukemia. J Clin Oncol. 2010;28:3890-3898. DOI: 10.1200/JCO.2010.29.2771

[33] Rogers HJ, Vardiman JW, Anastasi J, et al. Complex or monosomal karyotype and not blast percentage is associated with poor survival in acute myeloid leukemia and myelodysplastic syndrome patients with inv(3)(q21q26.2)/t(3;3)(q21;q26.2): a Bone Marrow Pathology Group study. Haematologica. 2014;99:821-829. DOI: 10.3324/Haematol.2013.096420

[34] Mamaev NN, Gorbunova AV, Gindina TL, et al. Leukemias and myelodysplastic syndromes with high *EVI1* gene expression: theoretical and clinical aspects. Clin Oncohematol. 2012;5:361-364 [In Russ].

[35] Mamaev NN, Gorbunova AV, Gindina TL, et al. Stable donor hematopoiesis reconstitution after post-transplanation relapse of acute myeloid leukemia in patient with inv(3)(q21q26),–7 and EVI1 overexpression treated by donor lymphocyte infusions and hypomethylating agents. Clin Oncohematol. 2014;7:71-76 [In Russ].

[36] He X, Wang Q, Cen J, et al. Predictive value of high *EVI1* expression in AML patients undergoing myeloablative allogeneic hematopoietic stem cell transplantation in first CR. Bone Marrow Transplant. 2016;51;921-927. DOI: 10.1038/bmt.2016.71

[37] Schlenk RF, Pasquini MC, Perez WS, et al. HLA-identical sibling allogeneic transplant versus chemotherapy in acute myelogenous leukemia with t(8;21) in first complete remission : collaborative study between the German AML intergroup and CIBMTR. Biol Blood Marrow Transplant. 2008;14:187-196. DOI: 10.1016/j.bbmt.2007.10.006

[38] Kuwatsuka Y, Miyamura K, Suzuki R, et al. Hematopoietic cell transplantation for core binding factor acute myeloid leukemia; t(8;21) and inv(16) represent different clinical outcomes. Blood. 2009;113:2096-2103. DOI: 10.1182/blood-2008-03-145862

[39] Numata A, Fujimaki K, Aoshima T, et al. Retrospective analysis of treatment outcomes in 70 patients with t(8;21) acute myeloid leukemia. Rinsho Ketsueki. 2012;53:698-704.

[40] Yoon JH, Kim HJ, Kim JW, et al. Identification and cytogenetic risk factors for unfavorable core-binding factor–positive adult AML with post-remission treatment outcome analysis including transplantation. Bone Marrow Transplant. 2014;49:1466-1474. DOI: 10.1038/bmt.2014.180

[41] Krauth MT, Eder C, Alpermann T, et al. High number of additional genetic lesions in acute myeloid leukemia with t(8;21)/RUNX1-RUNX1T1: frequency and impact on clinical outcome. Leukemia. 2014;28:1449-1458. DOI: 10.1038/leu.2014.4

[42] Klein K, Kaspers G, Harrison CJ, et al. Clinical impact of additional cytogenetic aberrations, cKIT and RAS mutations and treatment elements in paediatric t(8;21)-AML: results from an international retrospective study by the international Berlin-Frankfurt-Munster study group. J Clin Oncol. 2015;33:4247-4258. DOI: 10.1200/jco.2015.61.1947

[43] Gindina TL, Mamaev NN, Bondarenko SN, et al. Results of allogeneic hematopoietic stem cell transplantation in patients with acute myeloid leukemia with t(8;21)(q22;q22)/*RUNX-RUNX1t1* and additional cytogenetic abnormalities. Clin Oncohematol. 2016;9:148-154. DOI: 10.21320/2500-2139-9-2-148-154 [In Russ].

[44] Parma M, Vigano C, Fumagalli M, et al. Good outcome for very risk adult B-cell acute lymphoblastic leukemia carrying genetic abnormalities t(4;11)(q21;q23) or t(9;22)(q34;q11), if promptly submitted to allogeneic transplantation after obtaining a good molecular remission. Mediterr J Hematol Infect Dis. 2015;7:e2015041. DOI: 10.4084/MJHID.2015.041

[45] Ribera JM, Oriol A, Gonzalez M, et al. Concurrent intensive chemotherapy and imatinib before and after stem cell transplantation in newly diagnosed Philadelphia chromosome-positive acute lymphoblastic leukemia: final results of the CSTIBES02 trial. Haematologica 2010;95:87-95. DOI: 10.3324/haematol.2009.011221

[46] Ribera JM, García O, Montesinos P, et al. Treatment of young patients with Philadelphia chromosome-positive acute lymphoblastic leukaemia using increased dose of imatinib and deintensified chemotherapy before allogeneic stem cell transplantation. Br J Haematol. 2012;159:78-81. DOI: 10.1111/j.1365-2141.2012.09240.x

[47] Kebriaei P, Saliba R, Rondon G, et al. Long-term follow-up of allogeneic hematopoietic stem cell transplantation for patients with Philadelphia chromosome positive acute lymphoblastic leukemia: impact of tyrosine kinase inhibitors on treatment outcomes. Biol Blood Marrow Transplant. 2012;18:584-592. DOI: 10.1016/j.bbmt.2011.08.011

[48] Armand P, Kim HT, Zhang MJ, et al. Classifying cytogenetics in patients with acute myelogenous leukemia in complete remission undergoing allogeneic transplantation: a Center for International Blood and Marrow Transplant Research study. Biol Blood Marrow Transplant. 2012;18:280-288. DOI: 10.1016/j.bbmt.2011.07.024

[49] Fielding AK, Rowe JM, Buck G, et al. UKALLXII/ECOG2993: addition of imatinib to a standard treatment regimen enhances long-term outcomes in Philadelphia positive acute lymphoblastic leukemia. Blood. 2014;123:843-850. DOI: 10.1182/blood-2013-09-529008

[50] Chiaretti S, Foa R. Management of adult Ph-positive acute lymphoblastic leukemia. Hematology. Am Soc Hematol Educ Prog. 2015;2015:406-415. DOI: 10.1182/asheducation-2015.1.406

[51] Aldoss I, Stiller T, Cao TM, et al. Impact of additional cytogenetic abnormalities in adults with Philadelphia chromosome-positive acute lymphoblastic leukemia undergoing allogeneic hematopoietic cell transplantation. Biol Blood Marrow Transplant. 2015;21:1326-1329. DOI: 10.1016/j.bbmt.2015.03.021

[52] Sanjuan-Pla A, Bueno C, Prieto C, et al. Revisiting the biology of infant t(4;11)/MLL-AF41 B-cell acute lymphoblastic leukemia. Blood. 2015;126:2676-2685. DOI: 10.1182/blood-2015-09-967378

[53] Kosaka Y, Koh K, Kinukawa N, et al. Infant acute lymphoblastic leukemia with MLL gene arrangements: outcome following intensive chemotherapy and hematopoietic stem cell transplantation. Blood. 2004;104:3527-3534. DOI: 10.1182/blood-2004-04-1390

[54] Mann G, Attarbaschi A, Schrappe M, et al. Improved outcome with hematopoietic stem cell transplantation in a poor prognostic subgroup of infants with mixed-lineage-leukemia (MLL)-rearranged acute lymphoblastic leukemia: results from the Interfant-99 Study. Blood. 2010;116:2644-2650. DOI: 10.1182/blood-2010-03-0273532

[55] Dreyer ZE, Dinndorf PA, Camitta B, et al. Analysis of the role of hematopoietic stem-cell transplantation in infants with acute lymphoblastic leukemia in first remission and MLL gene rearrangements: a report from the Children's Oncology Group. J Clin Oncol. 2011;29:214-222. DOI: 10.1200/jco.2009.26.8938

[56] Tomizava D, Kato M, Takahashi H, et al. Favourable outcome in non-infant children with MLL-AF4-positive acute lymphoblastic leukemia: a report from the Tokyo Children's Cancer Study Group. Int J Hematol. 2015; 102:602-610. DOI: 10.1007/s12185-015-1869-y

[57] Kato M, Hasegawa D, Koh K, et al. Allogeneic haematopoietic stem cell transplantation for infant acute lymphoblastic leukemia with KMT2A (MLL) rearrangements: a retrospective study from the pediatric acute lymphoblastic leukemia working group of the Japan Society for Haematopoietic Cell Transplantation. Br J Haematol. 2014;4:564-570. DOI: 10.1111/bjh.13174

[58] Koh K, Tomozawa D, Saito AM, et al. Early use of allogeneic hematopoietic stem cell transplantation for infants with MLL gene rearrangement-positive acute lymphoblastic leukemia. Leukemia. 2015;29:290-296. DOI: 10.1038/leu.2014.172

Chapter 5

Does Aneuploidy in the Brain Play a Role in Neurodegenerative Disease?

Hilda van den Bos, Diana C.J. Spierings,
Floris Foijer and Peter M. Lansdorp

Additional information is available at the end of the chapter

http://dx.doi.org/10.5772/67886

Abstract

Aneuploidy, a state in which cells exhibit copy number changes of (parts of) chromosomes, is a hallmark of cancer cells and, when present in all cells, leads to miscarriages and congenital disorders, such as Down syndrome. In addition to these well-known roles of aneuploidy, chromosome copy number changes have also been reported in some studies to occur in neurons in healthy human brain and possibly even more in Alzheimer's disease (AD). However, the studies of aneuploidy in the human brain are currently under debate as earlier findings, mostly based on in situ hybridization approaches, could not be reproduced by more recent single cell sequencing studies with a much higher resolution. Here, we review the various studies on the occurrence of aneuploidy in brain cells from normal individuals and Alzheimer's patients. We discuss possible mechanisms for the origin of aneuploidy and the pros and cons of different techniques used to study aneuploidy in the brain, and we provide a future perspective.

Keywords: Alzheimer's disease, aneuploidy, brain, neurodegeneration, single cell sequencing

1. Introduction

Aneuploidy is a state in which cells have an abnormal and unbalanced number of chromosomes. An aneuploid cell can have one or more extra chromosomes, called hyperploid, or it could have lost one or more chromosomes, which is called hypoploid. Following this definition of aneuploidy, a cell that has doubled its complete genome without dividing is called tetraploid and not aneuploid, because a balanced genome is still present.

Aneuploidy is well known from cancer and systemic trisomies such as Down syndrome. Indeed, at least two out of three cancers exhibit aneuploidy [1–3]. Although it has been shown that aneuploidy causes stress and reduces cellular fitness [4–7], cancer cells have somehow found a way to cope with aneuploidy and manage to proliferate despite the detrimental consequences of aneuploidy. This is known as the aneuploidy paradox [6]. Perhaps by selecting numerical chromosomal abnormalities that promote tumor progression in addition to other structural genomic rearrangements, cancer cells can survive and keep growing [8, 9]. The profound effect that aneuploidy has on healthy cells is emphasized by the fact that, besides sex-chromosome abnormalities, in humans, only three systemic autosomal trisomies are compatible with life: trisomy 21 causing Down syndrome, trisomy 13 causing Patau's syndrome and trisomy 18 causing Edward's syndrome [10–12]. The viability of these systemic aneuploidies can probably be explained by the fact that these three chromosomes contain the lowest number of genes of all human autosomes. Even though these trisomies can be compatible with life, the majority of such trisomic pregnancies end with a miscarriage, and the children that do survive until birth suffer from severe cognitive and developmental defects [13].

But what is the origin of aneuploid cells? Aneuploidy is the result of chromosomal instability (CIN) and can arise when errors occur during DNA replication or mitosis. To prevent such errors, cells have evolved many checkpoints and mechanisms that ensure faithful replication of DNA and proper chromosome segregation. One of these checkpoints, the spindle assembly checkpoint (SAC), ensures that chromosome segregation is prevented until all chromosomes are properly attached to the mitotic spindle. Therefore, when the SAC fails, daughter cells can end up with gained or lost chromosomes. Furthermore, merotelic attachments—chromosome attachments where one of the sister chromatids is attached to both spindle poles—can result in aneuploidy even with a functional SAC. Finally, several other mechanisms, such as cohesion defects, multipolar spindles and lagging chromosomes, can all lead to incorrect chromosome segregation and thus aneuploidy [14].

Many tumor cells have inactivated the tumor suppressor p53, a key transcription factor in the DNA damage response and other cell cycle checkpoints. When functional, stresses such as DNA damage lead to activation of p53. P53 then induces a cell cycle arrest and activates DNA repair or induces apoptosis when the damage cannot be repaired. Loss of p53 makes cells more tolerant of aneuploidy [15] and allows them to propagate despite DNA damage or short telomeres [16].

When telomeres become too short, following proliferation or due to defects in telomere function, cells exit the cell cycle [17]. Loss of p53 overcomes this tumor suppression mechanism and allows cells to proliferate with critically short telomeres. This results in end-to-end fusion of sister chromatid telomeres, resulting in dicentric chromosomes. Dicentric chromosomes are likely to missegregate during mitosis, thus resulting in aneuploidy and DNA breaks. Such broken chromosomes can trigger a so-called breakage-fusion-bridge (BFB) cycle, which can continue over many cell divisions, leading to large duplications and deletions and very heterogeneous aneuploidy in cells [18]. Altogether, many processes, alone or in combination, can yield cells with whole chromosome or segmental chromosomal changes.

http://dx.doi.org/10.5772/67886

2. Aneuploidy during development and aging

Studying aneuploidy in the brain is complicated by the largely postmitotic state of adult neurons, limiting the methods that can be used. Therefore, many studies have used methods like interphase FISH, or DNA dyes such as DAPI or PI in combination with, for example, flow cytometry to determine the DNA/genome content of individual cells. Given the detrimental effect that aneuploidy has on cells, one would expect somatic cells of the brain to be perfectly euploid. A publication by Rehen et al. in 2001 challenged this view [19]. In this study, the authors quantified aneuploidy in embryonic mouse neuroblasts, adult cortex and lymphocytes using spectral karyotyping (SKY) and fluorescence in situ hybridization (FISH). They found ~33% of the 220 mouse neuroblast metaphase cells studied to be aneuploid as assessed by SKY, the great majority of which was hypoploid (98%). In contrast, of the adult mouse lymphocytes only 3% of the metaphase cells were identified as being aneuploid. In the same study, X and Y chromosome aneuploidy was assessed using FISH in adult mouse brain. They found X or Y chromosome aneuploidy occurring in 1.2% of the brain cells examined. The same rate of aneuploidy was found when comparing total adult nuclei with nuclei ≥10 μm, which are likely to be neurons. In comparison, the rate of X and Y chromosome aneuploidy in the mouse neuroblasts was ~10% (of which ~8% loss and 2% gain) [19]. In summary, these results suggest a high rate of aneuploidy in the developing mouse brain, and a much lower but still significant number of aneuploid cells in the adult mouse brain [20, 21]. A number of other studies reported similar aneuploidy rates in the developing human brain using interphase FISH. Aneuploidy rates up to 30–35% in the (developing) human brain were found, some studies reporting mainly chromosome losses [22, 23], another mainly chromosome gains [21]. The cause of aneuploidy in the developing brain was speculated to be mitotic segregation defects, since in dividing mouse neuronal progenitor cells lagging chromosomes and multipolar spindles have been found [24]. In contrast, there is little consistency in the aneuploidy rates reported in adult human brain. For example, the percentages of aneuploidy range from 0 up to 40: no aneuploidy was found in 2 normal brains (n = 200/chromosome/sample) [25], ~4% aneuploidy of chromosome 21 (n = 500–1000 per sample) [26], 1.3–7.0% aneuploidy per chromosome (n ≥ 500 for adult and ≥1000 for embryonic samples for each chromosome) [22] and 40% aneuploidy in the normal human brain (n = NA) [27]. All of these studies used FISH to count the chromosomes. A study performed by the group of Rehen, which combined several techniques, reported that aneuploid neurons seem to be integrated into the brain circuity like euploid cells and that aneuploid neurons can be activated and seem to be functional [28]. Taken together, although the rate of aneuploidy reported varies widely, most reports state that, especially in the developing brain, aneuploid cells are present at detectable frequencies in the normal brain.

But if aneuploid cells are present in large numbers in the developing brain, and in lower quantities in the adult human brain, what happens during aging? An increase in aneuploidy for chromosome 17 and 21 was found in the hippocampus of aged individuals compared to young controls [29]. In sharp contrast, another study determined the number of cells with a DNA content above the diploid level in brain samples ranging from 30 to 90 years of age. They found a decrease in the number of cells exceeding the diploid level with age [30], but suggested that this might be due to a biased selection of "healthy aging" brains. Taken together, there appears to be little consensus on whether aneuploid cells are present in adult brains, their frequency, and changes during aging. An overview of previous studies on aneuploidy in the brain is shown in **Table 1**. To explain the high rates of aneuploidy in the brain, several of the above-discussed studies hypothesized that aneuploidy in fact might contribute to neuronal diversity.

Species/cell type	Technique(s) used	Chromosomes studied	Main conclusions	Reference
Mouse neuroblasts and adult cortical cells	SKY, FISH, FACS	All chromosomes	~33% aneuploidy in neuroblasts, of which 98% hypoploidy, 1.2% X/Y aneuploidy in adult cortical cells	Rehen et al. [19]
Undiseased human prefrontal cortical (area 10) neurons	FISH	1, 7, 8, 13, 16, 18, 21, 22, X and Y	No aneuploidy found	Yurov et al. [25]
Human hippocampal pyramidal cells of AD patients and age matched controls	FISH	11, 18 and 21	3 or 4 hybridization spots in 3.7% of cells in AD, no cells with more than 2 hybridization spots in controls	Yang et al. [51]
Mouse neuronal progenitor cells	SKY	All chromosomes	33.2% aneuploidy	Yang et al. [37]
Mouse subventricular zone (SVZ) cells	DAPI staining, SKY	All chromosomes	33% aneuploidy in SVZ cells, of which ~76% hypoploidy with the majority having lost multiple chromosomes	Kaushal et al. [24]
Human neurons and nonneuronal brain cells	FISH	21	4% aneuploidy of chromosome 21, mean chromosome number of 2.05, no difference between neurons and nonneuronal cells	Rehen et al. [26]
Mouse cortical neurons	FISH	X and Y	~0.2% combined hyperploidy	Kingsbury et al. [28]
Human (undiseased and AD) and mouse neurons	FISH	Not stated	43% (32–53%) aneuploidy in AD neurons, 40% (38–47%) in undiseased neurons, similar degree in murine neurons (data not shown)	Pack et al. [27]
Human brain cells from fetal tissue (medulla oblongata) and adult cortex (area 10)	FISH	1, 13/21, 18, X and Y	0.6–3.0% aneuploidy per chromosome in fetal brain cells, 0.1–0.8% aneuploidy per chromosome in adult brain cells	Yurov et al. [22]

Species/cell type	Technique(s) used	Chromosomes studied	Main conclusions	Reference
Human entorhinal cortical neurons from patients with AD and controls	SBC, CISH	Overall DNA content and 17	Increased hyperploidy in AD, increased hybridization spots for chromosome 17 in AD	Mosch et al. [41]
Human fetal brain	FISH	1, 9, 15, 16, 17, 18, X and Y	1.25–1.45% aneuploidy per chromosome	Yurov et al. [23]
Human buccal and hippocampal cells from AD patients and controls	FISH	17 and 21	Increased aneuploidy in buccal cells of AD patients but not in hippocampus	Thomas et al. [29]
Mouse NPCs and human and mouse cerebellum	DAPI staining, FISH	Mouse: 16 and X Human: 6 and 21	15.3% aneuploidy in mouse NPCs at P0, 20.8% at P7, 0.5–1.0% aneuploidy per chromosome in adult mouse and human NeuN+ and NeuN− cerebellar nuclei	Westra et al. [88]
Cerebral cortex of normal human brain and AD patients	FISH	1, 7, 11, 13, 14, 17, 18, 21, X and Y	0.5% aneuploidy per chromosome in normal and AD brain, except increased chromosome 21 aneuploidy in AD: 6–15%	Iourov et al. [64]
Cortical and hippocampal nuclei of normal human brain and AD patients	FISH	4, 6 and 21	0.4–3.5% tetrasomy in nonneuronal cells No difference in normal and AD brain in nonneuronal cells, no tetrasomy in neurons	Westra et al. [52]
Entorhinal cortex of normal, preclinical AD, mild AD and severe AD patients	SBC, FISH, CISH	Overall DNA content and 17	10% hyperploidy in normal brain, ~27% in preclinical AD, ~35% in mild AD and ~23% in severe AD	Arendt et al. [63]
Cerebral and cerebellar cortex of young and old mice	FISH	1, 7, 14, 15, 16, 18, 19 and Y	1% aneuploidy per chromosome in cerebral cortex of young mice, 2.3% in old mice, no increase in aneuploidy with age in cerebella	Faggioli et al. [20]
Neurons and NPCs derived from human induced pluripotent stem cells and normal human frontal cortex	Single cell sequencing, FISH	All chromosomes 20 and X with FISH	27.5% aneuploidy in hiPSC-derived neurons, 5% in hiPCS-derived NPCs, 2.7% aneuploidy in normal frontal cortex	McConnell et al. [82]

Species/cell type	Technique(s) used	Chromosomes studied	Main conclusions	Reference
Prefrontal cortex of normal brain and AD patients	FISH	1, 7, 11, 16, 17, 18 and X	Increased X chromosome aneuploidy in AD (1.16–1.74% in controls, 2.78–4.92% in AD)	Yurov et al. [65]
Human cortical neurons	Single cell sequencing	All chromosomes	5% aneuploidy in normal human cortical neurons	Cai et al. [81]
Mouse embryonic NPCs and adult brain, human frontal cortex	Single cell sequencing	All chromosomes	No aneuploidy in mouse NPCs and neurons, 2.3% aneuploidy in adult mouse brain, 2.2% aneuploidy in human brain	Knouse et al. [87]
Mouse embryonic and adult cerebral and cerebellar cortex	FISH	1, 7, 18	~1% (cerebral) and 0.1% (cerebellar) aneuploidy per chromosome in 14 weeks and 6-month-old mice, ~30% aneuploidy per chromosome (chr. 1 and 18) in embryonic mouse brain	Andriani et al. [21]
Prefrontal cortical neurons of normal brain and AD patients	Single cell sequencing	All chromosomes	No increased aneuploidy in AD: 0.7% aneuploidy in controls, 0.6% in AD	van den Bos et al. [66]

Table 1. Overview of studies on aneuploidy in the brain.

The human brain consists of approximately 100 billion neurons forming an estimated 0.15 quadrillion (10^{15}) synapses, and there is a very high diversity of neurons [31]. Human brains have a high level of cellular heterogeneity, and it has been estimated that our brains might have as many as 10,000 different types of neurons [32]. All these different neurons work together to allow us to perform complex tasks. It is suggested that the presence of aneuploid neurons could be one of the mechanisms providing more variability and complexity to the human brain [14, 32–34].

3. Origin of aneuploid cells in the brain

If our brain indeed contains aneuploid cells, where do they originate? As discussed above, aneuploid cells are usually formed when something goes wrong with DNA replication or in mitosis. Aneuploid cells could therefore be generated during early development when there is a high rate of cell division, or later in life during normal or abnormal cell division. We can think of a number of explanations. First, since especially in the developing brain high rates of aneuploid cells have been found, defective clearance of these cells could explain their presence in the adult brain [35]. During brain development, many more cells are formed than end up in the adult brain suggesting the existence of strong selection for certain cell types [36]. This process possibly includes negative selection for aneuploid cells, which could explain the much lower rate of aneuploidy reported in the adult brain than in the developing brain. Failure to select for diploid cells during this selection could result in aneuploid cells being present in the adult brain [37, 38]. Indeed, in vitro experiments have shown that the differentiation of pluripotent stem cells into neural progenitor cells by retinoic acid (RA) is accompanied by increased levels of aneuploidy and micronuclei [39]. Second, it has been hypothesized that cell cycle reentry and failure to complete the cell cycle of neurons might be involved in neurodegeneration [40–43]. Neurons might attempt to reenter the cell cycle, replicate their DNA but fail to complete cell division. The main evidence for this hypothesis is the observation that postmitotic neurons in AD brains sometimes stain positive for cell cycle markers such as PCNA, cyclins and cyclin depended kinases (CDKs) [44–50]. As a consequence of reentering the cell cycle, the presence of tetraploid cells in the brain is expected. These cells have completed DNA replication but are unable to complete mitosis. But whether tetraploid cells are indeed present in the brain is still under debate [51, 52]. By counting fluorescent signals from probes directed at either chromosome 11, 18 or 21, Yang et al., found that 3.7% of the hippocampal cells in six AD brains have displayed three or four fluorescent signals. Although the fluorescent probes were not combined on individual cells, no distinction was made between three and four fluorescent signals, and no neuronal marker or DNA counter stain was used; the researchers conclude from these results that 3.7% of the hippocampal cells in these AD brains have a fully or partially replicated genome. But these results can also reflect single chromosome aneuploidies [51]. In contrast, a study performed by Westra et al. failed to find any tetraploid neurons in the cells studied [52], the only cells with four fluorescent signals were nonneuronal, and no difference was found between AD and control samples. Also, this hypothesis of aberrant cell cycle reentry is not supported by the single chromosome aneuploidies found of which, in most cases, only one copy of one chromosome is lost or gained in a cell. Third, the limited amount of neurogenesis taking place in the adult brain could potentially be a source of aneuploid neurons [39, 53]. In summary, aneuploid neurons in the adult brain can have originated in the developing brain and escaped clearing mechanisms, or formed due to cell cycle reentry and failed mitosis of adult neurons although the evidence for this hypothesis is contrasting.

4. Aneuploidy in neurodegeneration

Because human brain tissue is inaccessible in vivo, many researchers used peripheral cells, such as lymphocytes and fibroblasts, to study the correlation between genomic damage and neurodegenerative diseases such as AD. Several studies with conflicting results have been published: some show a correlation between AD and increased peripheral aneuploidy [54–58], while others report no difference [59, 60]. Counting the presence of micronuclei is a way to assess genome stability. Micronuclei are formed when chromosome segregation is flawed, causing a part of or a whole chromosome to end up outside of the nucleus in a so-called micronucleus. Therefore, the number of micronuclei present is a marker for chromosome missegregation. Interestingly, AD patients were found to have increased numbers of micronuclei in their lymphocytes, mostly containing whole chromosomes [61]. More specifically, AD patients were reported to have increased rates of trisomy 21 in lymphocytes, while missegregation rates for chromosome 13 were unaltered, when compared to healthy controls [62]. Similarly, patients suffering from AD were found to exhibit frequent copy number changes for chromosomes 17 and 21 in buccal cells [29].

Since neurons are postmitotic, methods requiring dividing cells to determine chromosome copy numbers cannot be used when studying aneuploidy in neurons. Most studies therefore make use of fluorescence in situ hybridization (FISH)-based methods to count chromosomes in brain cells. When comparing control brain with early and late AD samples using slide-based cytometry (SBC), PCR amplification of *alu* repeats, and chromogenic in situ hybridization (CISH), a twofold increase in neurons with a DNA content between 2 and 4 n was found [41]. Also in preclinical stages of AD, an increased number of neurons with a more than diploid DNA content have been reported [63]. Iourov et al. found no overall significant difference in aneuploidy rates when looking at copy number changes of seven autosomes (chromosomes 1, 7, 11, 13, 14, 17 and 18) and the X and Y chromosome. But a specific increase in chromosome 21 aneuploidy in neurons of AD brain samples was identified, of which 60% where gains and 40% loss of chromosome 21 [64]. On the other hand, in a recent study, a twofold increase in X chromosome aneuploidy was found in AD neurons when compared to age matched controls [65]. To summarize, although again the rates of aneuploidy and which chromosomes are affected differ between studies, the overall trends suggest that aneuploidy might be increased in AD [66].

5. The possible link between Down syndrome and Alzheimer's disease

Down syndrome is the most common autosomal systemic aneuploidy. Besides the observation of increased levels of trisomy 21 in the brains of AD patients, Down syndrome and AD have more in common. First, Down syndrome patients are much more likely to develop AD and at an earlier age than genetic euploid individuals [67]. This could be related to the fact that the amyloid precursor protein (APP) gene, mutations in which are known to cause early onset AD, is located on chromosome 21 [68]. Also, in the brains of individuals with Down syndrome over 40 years of age protein aggregates, plaques and tangles, are present in amounts that are also observed in AD patients brains [69]. On the other hand, not all patients with trisomy 21 over 40 develop AD, although all of them develop plaques and tangles [70]. Second, it has been found that young mothers (<35 years) of a child with Down syndrome have increased chromosomal instability, as shown by having more micronuclei [71], and more chromosomal missegregation events in their lymphocytes [72]. In the great majority of cases (95%) the extra chromosome 21 originates from a maternal nondisjunction event [73, 74]. Moreover, Schupf et al. found that young mothers of a child with Down syndrome have a fivefold increased risk to develop AD, while the risk was not increased in mothers who had a child with Down syndrome at a later age (>35 years). It is therefore hypothesized that some women might have a genetic susceptibility to chromosome nondisjunction, increasing the risk of both getting a child with Down syndrome as well as developing AD [75, 76]. Lastly, also mouse models for Down syndrome display characteristics of AD [67]. For example, the widely used mouse model Ts65Dn, which has an extra copy of a large part of Mmu16, the mouse homolog of a large part human chromosome 21 including *APP*, displays increased levels of APP and Aβ, as well as progressive memory decline and neurodegeneration in adult mice [77–79].

6. How can aneuploid cells play a role in neurodegeneration?

Aneuploidy was shown to reduce cellular fitness [80]. It was therefore suggested that aneuploid cells might be selectively affected by cell death in the brains of AD patients. According to this hypothesis, a decrease in aneuploidy rates might be expected as the disease progresses. This is in line with the observation by Arendt et al. of decreased hyperploidy in severe AD compared to mild AD [63]. It must be noted that in this study, the total amount of DNA was studied with a DNA dye, rather than the rate of aneuploidy. On the other hand, if aneuploid cells remain present in the aging brain, aneuploidy could contribute to neurodegenerative diseases through proteotoxic stress. Misfolding of proteins leads to proteotoxic stress, the formation of protein aggregates and possibly neurodegeneration. Being aneuploid is a heavy burden for a cell. Having an extra copy of a chromosome generally means that the genes on this chromosome are transcribed and translated at the same rate compared to the two "normal" copies. Therefore, the cell has to deal with this 50% extra mRNA and protein [4, 7]. All these extra proteins have to be folded into the right conformation or processed by the protein degradation machinery. This leads to increased pressure on chaperones and the protein degradation machinery [5, 6]. Since protein aggregates are thought to play an important role in the development and progression of many neurodegenerative diseases, their formation might be stimulated by excess proteins that overload the protein folding and degradation machinery. Trisomy 21 has been reported to be more prevalent in the brains of AD patients. The extra copy of the APP gene on chromosome 21, which encodes the β-amyloid protein, could trigger the formation of amyloid plaques resulting in proteotoxic stress and ultimately cell death [68].

7. Low levels of aneuploidy found in the brain using single cell sequencing

Recently, it became possible to use single cell next generation sequencing (NGS) to look at aneuploidy in individual cells (**Figure 1**) [81, 82]. Compared to the classic method for measuring aneuploidy using FISH, single cell sequencing has some important advantages [83].

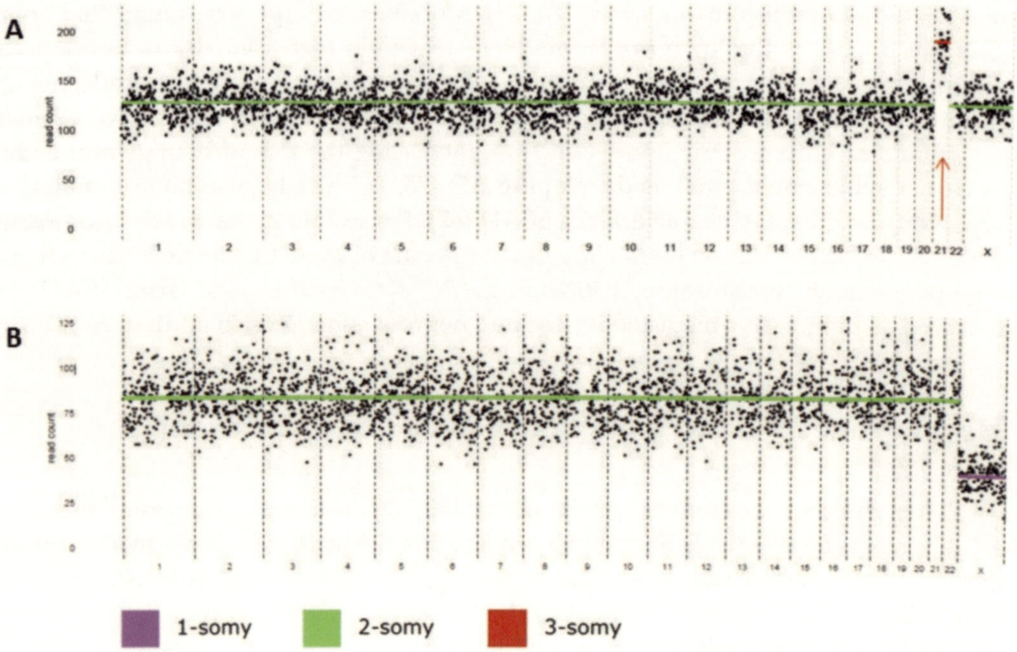

Figure 1. Single cell sequencing of a female cell with trisomy of chromosome 21 (A) and a male diploid cell (B). Plots are made using Aneufinder [89].

First, FISH studies are in most cases limited to examining only a few chromosomes per cell. Therefore, the total rate of aneuploidy is usually determined by extrapolating the aneuploidy rates of the few chromosomes that are studied, possibly resulting in an over- or underestimation of the frequency of aneuploidy. With single cell sequencing, the copy number of all chromosomes in each single cell can be determined more accurately. Each chromosome is sampled thousands of times, whereas with FISH the chromosomes are usually measured only once or twice. Although spectral karyotyping (SKY) can also be used to count all chromosomes within a cell, this method requires metaphase chromosomes and thus dividing cells, while single cell sequencing can be performed on nondividing cells [84]. Moreover, SKY is more likely to overestimate chromosome loss, due to chromosomes being washed away from the slide onto which they were dropped. This could explain the high rates of hypoploid cells found using SKY [19]. Second, since with FISH the karyotype is determined by simply counting the number of fluorescent spots, in several ways this can lead to errors in chromosome counts. Failure of the probe to hybridize can lead to underestimation, while nonspecific binding results in overestimation of aneuploidy rates.

Fortunately, the development of single cell sequencing protocols has allowed studies of all chromosomes in single, nondividing cells. For this approach, libraries are made of individual cells or nuclei. In most cases, library preparation starts with a whole genome amplification step. This can be problematic because uneven amplification of genomic DNA may result in a sequencing bias. Next, the DNA is fragmented either mechanically, such as by sonication, or enzymatically, for example with restriction enzymes. To enable binding of the fragments to the sequencing flow cell, adapters are ligated to either end of the fragmented DNA. Also, individual barcodes can be introduced to allow pooling (multiplexing) of more than one library on a flow cell, thus significantly reducing sequencing costs. After sequencing, the individual reads are split into libraries for each individual cell based on the cellular barcode (demultiplexing), and the copy numbers of individual chromosomes can be determined by comparing the read density on each chromosome. An extra copy of a chromosome is expected to result in 50% increase in read density, while loss of a chromosome leads to a 50% reduction of the read density on that chromosome [66, 85, 86]. Depending on the sequencing depth, single cell sequencing can, in addition to whole chromosome aneuploidies, also reveal smaller copy number changes. Since single cell sequencing is often combined with FACS sorting of single nuclei, micronuclei will be lost when sorting nuclei. Also, this method is relatively expensive and thereby limits large-scale sequencing projects. Even though only few studies so far used next generation sequencing based on karyotype cells, the results are contrasting some of the earlier FISH-based findings in that the rate of aneuploidy found was in general much lower than was reported previously. For instance, Knouse et al. identified one aneuploid brain cell of the 43 sequenced cells, and all of the nine neurons sequenced were euploid [87]. Another study found five neurons to be aneuploid out of the 100 neurons that passed the quality criteria [81]. Also, only one chromosomal gain and 2 losses were identified in 110 sequenced frontal cortex neurons of 3 individuals [82]. Finally, the largest study determined aneuploidy rates in postmortem frontal cortex neurons of normal human brain and samples from patients affected with AD. Interestingly, a very limited number of aneuploid neurons was found; <1% aneuploidy both in controls and AD [66]. All of these single cell sequencing studies use cells of which the chromosome copy numbers are known as validation of the method: human male trisomy 21 fibroblasts [82], human male trisomy 18 neurons [81], mouse trisomy 16 brain cells [87] and human female trisomy 21 neurons [66]. In each case, the known aneuploidy as well as the correct number of X chromosomes, male or female, was detected with 100% accuracy, confirming the sensitivity of single cell sequencing. Studying aneuploidy in the developing human brain with single cell sequencing remains to be done. But also here, the lack of aneuploidy reported in the 36 mouse neuronal progenitor cells sequenced might be an indication that also the embryonic aneuploidy levels have been overestimated [87]. Taken together, the results of single cell sequencing studies are in sharp contrast to the previously reported aneuploidy rates. How can these conflicting results obtained with different techniques be explained? As mentioned before, studies of aneuploidy in the human brain are complicated. Selecting a tissue or cell type as valid control is difficult, as no tissue is similar to brain tissue. Usually, lymphocytes are used as control. This potentially introduces problems, as the isolation of cells or nuclei from such very different sources requires very different experimental approaches: lymphocytes are isolated as single, unattached cells, while brain tissue needs some sort of mechanical or enzymatic dissociation to obtain individual cells or nuclei. On the other hand, brain tissue sections can also be used, but in this case, the inevitable cuts through nuclei can give rise to incorrect chromosome counts. While differences in handling of the tissue or cells may explain some of the reported differences, this explanation does not apply when comparing aneuploidy in normal and diseased brain samples.

8. Conclusion

The frequency of neuronal aneuploidy in the normal healthy brain remains a matter of debate. Although many studies report a certain level of aneuploidy, this is not confirmed by more recent reports using single cell sequencing. Whether the number of aneuploid cells is increased or decreased with aging and in neurodegenerative diseases remains to be conclusively shown. Aneuploid neurons could be involved in neurodegeneration because an incorrect karyotype could cause proteotoxicity via protein misfolding and aggregation. Single cell sequencing is a promising tool to address questions about aneuploidy in the brain and should provide more definite answers in the years to come.

Author details

Hilda van den Bos[1], Diana C.J. Spierings[1], Floris Foijer[1] and Peter M. Lansdorp[1,2,3]*

*Address all correspondence to: p.m.lansdorp@umcg.nl

1 European Research Institute for the Biology of Ageing, University Medical Centre Groningen, University of Groningen, Groningen, The Netherlands

2 Terry Fox Laboratory, British Columbia Cancer Agency, Vancouver, BC, Canada

3 Department of Medical Genetics, University of British Columbia, Vancouver, BC, Canada

References

[1] Duijf PHG, Benezra R. The cancer biology of whole-chromosome instability. Oncogene. 2013 Oct;32(40):4727-36.

[2] Weaver BAA, Cleveland DW. Does aneuploidy cause cancer? Curr Opin Cell Biol. 2006 Dec;18(6):658-67.

[3] Duijf PHG, Schultz N, Benezra R. Cancer cells preferentially lose small chromosomes. Int J Cancer. 2013 May;132(10):2316-26.

[4] Oromendia AB, Dodgson SE, Amon A. Aneuploidy causes proteotoxic stress in yeast. Genes Dev. 2012;26(24):2696-708.

[5] Oromendia AB, Amon A. Aneuploidy: implications for protein homeostasis and disease. Dis Model Mech. 2014;7(1):15-20.

[6] Sheltzer JM, Amon A. The aneuploidy paradox: costs and benefits of an incorrect karyotype. Trends Genet. 2011;446-53.

[7] Siegel JJ, Amon A. New insights into the troubles of aneuploidy. Annual Review of Cell and Developmental Biology. 2012;28:189-214.

[8] Negrini S, Gorgoulis VG, Halazonetis TD. Genomic instability—an evolving hallmark of cancer. Nat Rev Mol Cell Biol. 2010;11(3):220-8.

[9] Hanahan D, Weinberg RA. Hallmarks of cancer: the next generation. Cell. 2011;144(5): 646-74.

[10] Neri G, Opitz JM. Down syndrome: comments and reflections on the 50th anniversary of Lejeune's discovery. Am J Med Genet Part A. 2009 Dec;149(12):2647-54.

[11] Patau K, Smith D, Therman E, Inhorn S, Wagner H. Multiple congenital anomaly caused by an extra autosome. Lancet. 1960;275(7128):790-3.

[12] Edwards J, Harnden D, Cameron A, Mary Crosse V, Wolf O. A new trisomic syndrome. Lancet. 1960;275(7128):787-90.

[13] Houlihan, Orla a O'noghue K. The natural history of pregnancies with a diagnosis of trisomy 18 or trisomy 13; a retrospective case series. BMC Pregnancy Childbirth. 2013;13:209.

[14] Faggioli F, Vijg J, Montagna C. Chromosomal aneuploidy in the aging brain. Mech Ageing Dev. 2011 Aug;132(8-9):429-36.

[15] Fujiwara T, Bandi M, Nitta M, Ivanova E V, Bronson RT, Pellman D. Cytokinesis failure generating tetraploids promotes tumorigenesis in p53-null cells. Nature. 2005;437(7061):1043-7.

[16] Aylon Y, Oren M. P53: Guardian of ploidy. Mol Oncol. 2011;5(4):315-23.

[17] Hayflick L. The limited in vitro lifetime of human diploid cell strains. Exp Cell Res. 1965;37:614-36.

[18] Bailey SM, Murnane JP. Telomeres, chromosome instability and cancer. Nucleic Acids Res. 2006;34(8):2408-17.

[19] Rehen SK, McConnell MJ, Kaushal D, Kingsbury M a, Yang a H, Chun J. Chromosomal variation in neurons of the developing and adult mammalian nervous system. Proc Natl Acad Sci U S A. 2001 Nov;98(23):13361-6.

[20] Faggioli F, Wang T, Vijg J, Montagna C. Chromosome-specific accumulation of aneuploidy in the aging mouse brain. Hum Mol Genet. 2012;21(24):5246-53.

[21] Andriani GA, Faggioli F, Baker D, Dollé MET, Sellers RS, Hébert JM, et al. Whole chromosome aneuploidy in the brain of Bub1bH/H and Ercc1-/Δ7 mice. Hum Mol Genet. 2016;25(4):755-65.

[22] Yurov YB. The variation of aneuploidy frequency in the developing and adult human brain revealed by an interphase FISH study. J Histochem Cytochem. 2005;53 (3):385-90.

[23] Yurov YB, Iourov IY, Vorsanova SG, Liehr T, Kolotii AD, Kutsev SI, et al. Aneuploidy and confined chromosomal mosaicism in the developing human brain. PLoS One. 2007;2(6).

[24] Kaushal D, Contos JJ a, Treuner K, Yang AH, Kingsbury M a, Rehen SK, et al. Alteration of gene expression by chromosome loss in the postnatal mouse brain. J Neurosci. 2003;23(13):5599-606.

[25] Yurov YB, Vostrikov VM, Vorsanova SG, Monakhov VV, Iourov IY. Multicolor fluorescent in situ hybridization on post-mortem brain in schizophrenia as an approach for identification of low-level chromosomal aneuploidy in neuropsychiatric diseases. Brain and Development. 2001. p. S186–S190.

[26] Rehen SK, Yung YC, Mccreight MP, Kaushal D, Yang AH, Almeida BS V, et al. Constitutional aneuploidy in the normal human brain. J Neurosci. 2005;25(9): 2176-80.

[27] Pack SD, Weil RJ, Vortmeyer AO, Zeng W, Li J, Okamoto H, et al. Individual adult human neurons display aneuploidy: detection by fluorescence in situ hybridization and single neuron PCR. Cell Cycle. 2005 Oct 28;4(12):1758-60.

[28] Kingsbury M, Friedman B, McConnell M, Rehen S, Yang A, Kaushal D, et al. Aneuploid neurons are functionally active and integrated into brain circuitry. Proc Natl Acad Sci U S A. 2005;102(17):6143-7.

[29] Thomas P, Fenech M. Chromosome 17 and 21 aneuploidy in buccal cells is increased with ageing and in Alzheimer's disease. Mutagenesis. 2008 Jan;23(1):57-65.

[30] Fischer HG, Morawski M, Bruckner MK, Mittag A, Tarnok A, Arendt T. Changes in neuronal DNA content variation in the human brain during aging. Aging Cell. 2012 Aug;11(4):628-33.

[31] Pakkenberg B, Pelvig D, Marner L, Bundgaard MJ, Gundersen HJG, Nyengaard JR, et al. Aging and the human neocortex. Exp Gerontol. 2003. pp. 95-9.

[32] Muotri AR, Gage FH. Generation of neuronal variability and complexity. Nature. 2006;441(7097):1087-93.

[33] Singer T, McConnell MJ, Marchetto MCN, Coufal NG, Gage FH. LINE-1 retrotransposons: mediators of somatic variation in neuronal genomes? Trends Neurosci. 2010;33(8):345-54.

[34] Peterson SE, Yang AH, Bushman DM, Westra JW, Yung YC, Barral S, et al. Aneuploid cells are differentially susceptible to caspase-mediated death during embryonic cerebral cortical development. J Neurosci. 2012;32(46):16213-22.

[35] Devalle S, Sartore RC, Paulsen BS, Borges HL, Martins R a. P, Rehen SK. Implications of aneuploidy for stem cell biology and brain therapeutics. Front Cell Neurosci. 2012;6(September):1-13.

[36] Blaschke AJ, Staley K, Chun J. Widespread programmed cell death in proliferative and postmitotic regions of the fetal cerebral cortex. Development. 1996;122(4):1165-74.

[37] Yang AH, Kaushal D, Rehen SK, Kriedt K, Kingsbury MA, McConnell MJ, et al. Chromosome segregation defects contribute to aneuploidy in normal neural progenitor cells. J Neurosci. 2003;23(32):10454-62.

[38] McConnell MJ, Kaushal D, Yang AH, Kingsbury MA, Rehen SK, Treuner K, et al. Failed clearance of aneuploid embryonic neural progenitor cells leads to excess aneuploidy in the Atm-deficient but not the Trp53-deficient adult cerebral cortex. J Neurosci. 2004;24(37):8090-6.

[39] Sartore RC, Campos PB, Trujillo C a., Ramalho BL, Negraes PD, Paulsen BS, et al. Retinoic acid-treated pluripotent stem cells undergoing neurogenesis present increased aneuploidy and micronuclei formation. PLoS One. 2011;6(6):1-11.

[40] Yurov YB, Vorsanova SG, Iourov IY. The DNA replication stress hypothesis of Alzheimer's Disease. Sci World J. 2011;11(1537-744X (electronic)):2602-12.

[41] Mosch B, Morawski M, Mittag A, Lenz D, Tarnok A, Arendt T. Aneuploidy and DNA replication in the normal human brain and Alzheimer's disease. J Neurosci. 2007;27(26):6859-67.

[42] Arendt T. Cell cycle activation and aneuploid neurons in Alzheimer's disease. Mol Neurobiol. 2012;46(1):125-35.

[43] Herrup K, Yang Y. Cell cycle regulation in the postmitotic neuron: oxymoron or new biology? Nat Rev Neurosci. 2007;8(5):368-78.

[44] Busser J, Geldmacher DS, Herrup K. Ectopic cell cycle proteins predict the sites of neuronal cell death in Alzheimer's disease brain. J Neurosci. 1998;18(8):2801-7.

[45] Nagy Z, Esiri MM, Smith AD. Expression of cell division markers in the hippocampus in Alzheimer's disease and other neurodegenerative conditions. Acta Neuropathol. 1997;93(3):294-300.

[46] Smith MZ, Nagy Z, Esiri MM. Cell cycle-related protein expression in vascular dementia and Alzheimer's disease. Neurosci Lett. 1999;271(1):45-8.

[47] Yang Y, Mufson EJ, Herrup K. Neuronal cell death is preceded by cell cycle events at all stages of Alzheimer's disease. J Neurosci. 2003;23(7):2557-63.

[48] Hoozemans JJM, Brückner MK, Rozemuller AJM, Veerhuis R, Eikelenboom P, Arendt T. Cyclin D1 and cyclin E are co-localized with cyclo-oxygenase 2 (COX-2) in pyramidal neurons in Alzheimer disease temporal cortex. J Neuropathol Exp Neurol. 2002;61(8):678-88.

[49] Vincent I, Jicha G, Rosado M, Dickson DW. Aberrant expression of mitotic cdc2/cyclin B1 kinase in degenerating neurons of Alzheimer's disease brain. J Neurosci. 1997;17(10):3588-98.

[50] McShea A, Harris PL, Webster KR, Wahl AF, Smith MA. Abnormal expression of the cell cycle regulators P16 and CDK4 in Alzheimer's disease. Am J Pathol. 1997;150(6):1933-9.

[51] Yang Y, Geldmacher DS, Herrup K. DNA replication precedes neuronal cell death in Alzheimer's disease. J Neurosci. 2001;21(8):2661-8.

[52] Westra JW, Barral S, Chun J. A reevaluation of tetraploidy in the Alzheimer's disease brain. Neurodegener Dis. 2009;6(5-6):221-9.

[53] Spalding KL, Bergmann O, Alkass K, Bernard S, Salehpour M, Huttner HB, et al. Dynamics of hippocampal neurogenesis in adult humans. Cell. 2013;153(6):1219-27.

[54] Buckton KE, Whalley LJ, Lee M, Christie JE. Chromosome changes in Alzheimer's presenile dementia. J Med Genet. 1983;20(1):46-51.

[55] Buckton KE, Whalley LJ, Lee M, Christie JE. Chromosome aneuploidy in Alzheimer's disease. Exp Brain Res. 1982;(Suppl 5):58-63.

[56] Ward BE, Cook RH, Robinson A, Austin JH. Increased aneuploidy in Alzheimer disease. Am J Med Genet. 1979;3(2):137-44.

[57] Matsuyama SS, Bohman R. Variation in DNA content of mononuclear cells of patients with dementia of the Alzheimer type. Alzheimer Dis Assoc Disord. 1988;2(2):120-2.

[58] Geller LN, Potter H. Chromosome missegregation and trisomy 21 mosaicism in Alzheimer's disease. Neurobiol Dis. 1999;6(3):167-79.

[59] White BJ, Crandall C, Goudsmit J, Morrow CH, Alling DW, Gajdusek DC, et al. Cytogenetic studies of familial and sporadic Alzheimer disease. Am J Med Genet. 1981;10(1):77-89.

[60] Moorhead PS, Heyman A. Chromosome studies of patients with Alzheimer disease. AmJMedGenet. 1983;14(0148-7299):545-56.

[61] Migliore L, Testa a, Scarpato R, Pavese N, Petrozzi L, Bonuccelli U. Spontaneous and induced aneuploidy in peripheral blood lymphocytes of patients with Alzheimer's disease. Hum Genet. 1997;101:299-305.

[62] Migliore L, Botto N, Scarpato R, Petrozzi L, Cipriani G, Bonuccelli U. Preferential occurrence of chromosome 21 malsegregation in peripheral blood lymphocytes of Alzheimer disease patients. Cytogenet Cell Genet. 1999;87:41-6.

[63] Arendt T, Brückner MK, Mosch B, Lösche A. Selective cell death of hyperploid neurons in Alzheimer's disease. Am J Pathol. 2010;177(1):15-20.

[64] Iourov IY, Vorsanova SG, Liehr T, Yurov YB. Aneuploidy in the normal, Alzheimer's disease and ataxia-telangiectasia brain: differential expression and pathological meaning. Neurobiol Dis. 2009 May;34(2):212-20.

[65] Yurov YB, Vorsanova SG, Liehr T, Kolotii AD, Iourov IY. X chromosome aneuploidy in the Alzheimer's disease brain. Mol Cytogenet. 2014 Jan;7(1):20.

[66] van den Bos H, Spierings DCJ, Taudt AS, Bakker B, Porubský D, Falconer E, et al. Single-cell whole genome sequencing reveals no evidence for common aneuploidy in normal and Alzheimer's disease neurons. Genome Biol. 2016;17(1):116.

[67] Hamlett ED, Boger HA, Ledreux A, Kelley C, Mufson EJ, Falangola MF, et al. Cognitive impairment, neuroimaging, and Alzheimer neuropathology in mouse models of Down syndrome. Curr Alzheimer Res. 2016 Dec 7;13(1):35-52.

[68] Korenberg JR, Pulst SM, Neve RL, West R. The Alzheimer amyloid precursor protein maps to human chromosome 21 bands q21.105-q21.05. Genomics. 1989;5(1):124-7.

[69] Gardiner K, Herault Y, Lott IT, Antonarakis SE, Reeves RH, Dierssen M. Down syndrome: from understanding the neurobiology to therapy. J Neurosci. 2010;30(45):14943-5.

[70] Costa AC. Alzheimer disease: treatment of Alzheimer disease in Down syndrome. Nat Rev Neurol. 2012;8:1-18.

[71] Migliore L, Coppedè F, Fenech M, Thomas P. Association of micronucleus frequency with neurodegenerative diseases. Mutagenesis. 2011;26(1):85-92.

[72] Migliore L, Boni G, Bernardini R, Trippi F, Colognato R, Fontana I, et al. Susceptibility to chromosome malsegregation in lymphocytes of women who had a Down syndrome child in young age. Neurobiol Aging. 2006;27(5):710-6.

[73] Petersen MB, Schinzel AA, Binkert F, Tranebjaerg L, Mikkelsen M, Collins FA, et al. Use of short sequence repeat DNA polymorphisms after PCR amplification to detect the parental origin of the additional chromosome 21 in Down syndrome. Am J Hum Genet. 1991;48(1):65-71.

[74] Hassold T, Hunt PA, Sherman S. Trisomy in humans: incidence, origin and etiology. Curr Opin Genet Dev. 1993;3(3):398-403.

[75] Schupf N, Kapell D, Lee JH, Ottman R, Mayeux R. Increased risk of Alzheimer's disease in mothers of adults with Down's syndrome. Lancet. 1994;344(8919):353-6.

[76] Schupf N, Kapell D, Nightingale B, Lee JH, Mohlenhoff J, Bewley S, et al. Specificity of the fivefold increase in AD in mothers of adults with Down syndrome. Neurology. 2001;57(6):979-84.

[77] Hunter CL, Bimonte HA, Granholm ACE. Behavioral comparison of 4 and 6 month-old Ts65Dn mice: age-related impairments in working and reference memory. Behav Brain Res. 2003;138(2):121-31.

[78] Cataldo AM, Petanceska S, Peterhoff CM, Terio NB, Epstein CJ, Villar A, et al. App gene dosage modulates endosomal abnormalities of Alzheimer's disease in a segmental trisomy 16 mouse model of Down syndrome. J Neurosci. 2003;23(17):6788-92.

[79] Holtzman DM, Santucci D, Kilbridge J, Chua-Couzens J, Fontana DJ, Daniels SE, et al. Developmental abnormalities and age-related neurodegeneration in a mouse model of Down syndrome. Neurobiology. 1996;93:13333-8.

[80] Torres EM, Dephoure N, Panneerselvam A, Tucker CM, Whittaker CA, Gygi SP, et al. Identification of aneuploidy-tolerating mutations. Cell. 2010;143(1):71-83.

[81] Cai X, Evrony GD, Lehmann HS, Elhosary PC, Mehta BK, Poduri A, et al. Single-cell, genome-wide sequencing identifies clonal somatic copy-number variation in the human brain. Cell Rep. 2014 Aug;8(5):1280-9.

[82] McConnell M, Lindberg M, Brennand K, Piper J, Voet T, Cowing-Zitron C, et al. Mosaic copy number variation in human neurons. Science (80-). 2013 Nov 1;342(6158):632-3.

[83] Bakker B, van den Bos H, Lansdorp PM, Foijer F. How to count chromosomes in a cell: an overview of current and novel technologies. BioEssays. 2015;37(5):570-7.

[84] Imataka G, Arisaka O. Chromosome analysis using spectral karyotyping (SKY). Cell Biochem Biophys. 2012;62:13-7.

[85] Falconer E, Lansdorp PM. Strand-seq: a unifying tool for studies of chromosome segregation. Semin Cell Dev Biol. 2013;24(8-9):643-52.

[86] Hills M, O'Neill K, Falconer E, Brinkman R, Lansdorp PM. BAIT: organizing genomes and mapping rearrangements in single cells. Genome Med. 2013;5(9):82.

[87] Knouse KA, Wu J, Whittaker CA, Amon A. Single cell sequencing reveals low levels of aneuploidy across mammalian tissues. Proc Natl Acad Sci U S A. 2014 Sep 2;111(37): 13409-14.

[88] Westra JW, Peterson SE, Yung YC, Mutoh T, Barral S, Chun J. Aneuploid mosaicism in the developing and adult cerebellar cortex. J Comp Neurol. 2008 Apr 20;507(6):1944-51.

[89] Bakker B, Taudt A, Belderbos M, Porubsky D, Spierings D, De T, et al. Single cell sequencing reveals karyotype heterogeneity in murine and human tumours. Genome Biol. 2016;17: 1-15.

Chapter 6

Chromosomal Abnormalities and Menstrual Cycle Disorders

Ksenija Gersak and Ziva Miriam Gersak

Additional information is available at the end of the chapter

http://dx.doi.org/10.5772/67795

Abstract

Chromosomal abnormalities have long been recognized as a cause of menstrual cycle disorders, premature ovarian insufficiency, and recurrent pregnancy loss. In women with X chromosome abnormalities, premature ovarian insufficiency is mainly a consequence of ovarian follicle depletion, due to insufficient initial follicle number and/or spontaneous accelerated follicle loss. The level of X chromosome mosaicism and its reproductive significance is still under debate. In our study, we evaluated the contribution of X chromosome abnormalities in women with sporadic idiopathic premature ovarian insufficiency (POI) and in women with a history of recurrent pregnancy loss. The results show that X aneuploidy and low-level mosaicism have reproductive significance in the phenotypically normal women with recurrent pregnancy loss and/or fertility problems. These results have practical implications for genetic counseling and fertility treatment.

Keywords: X chromosome, X chromosome mosaicism, amenorrhea, premature ovarian insufficiency, recurrent pregnancy loss

1. Introduction

Chromosomal abnormalities have long been recognized as a cause of abnormal sexual development, recurrent pregnancy loss, infertility, menstrual cycle disorders, and premature ovarian insufficiency (POI). Regarding the genetic causes of menstrual cycle disorders and POI, they can either be chromosomal or caused by single genes, involving the X chromosome or autosomes. The X chromosome abnormalities represent 13% of the cases, followed by the FMR1 gene premutation that represents 6% of the cases [1].

In November 2010, the International Federation of Gynaecology and Obstetrics formally accepted a new classification system for causes of abnormal uterine bleeding and menstrual cycle disorders in the reproductive years. It was developed in response to concerns about the design and interpretation of basic science and clinical investigation that relates to the problem of abnormal uterine bleeding and is based on the acronym PALM-COEIN (polyps, adenomyosis, leiomyoma, malignancy and hyperplasia–coagulopathy, ovulatory disorders, endometrial causes, iatrogenic, not classified) [2]. Chromosomal abnormalities are usually involved in ovulatory disorders, which lead to POI and infertility.

2. Menstrual cycle disorders

Menstruation is the regular discharge of blood and mucosal tissue from the inner lining of the uterus through the vagina as a result of periodic hormonal changes. Bleeding that can be defined as a "period" is described according to the four parameters [2]:

- regularity of onset,
- frequency of onset,
- duration of menstrual flow, and
- heaviness (or volume) of menstrual flow (**Table 1**).

Clinical dimensions of menstruation and menstrual cycle	Descriptive term	Normal limits (5–95th percentiles)
	Frequent	<24 days
Frequency of menses	Normal	24–38 days
	Infrequent	>38 days
	Absent	No bleeding
Regularity of menses	Regular	Variation ± 2–20 days
Cycle-to-cycle variation over 12 months	Irregular	Variation > 20 days
	Prolonged	>8 days
Duration of flow	Normal	4,5–8 days
	Shortened	<4,5 days
	Heavy	>80 mL
Volume of monthly blood loss	Normal	5–80 mL
	Light	<5 mL

Adapted from Munro et al. [2].

Table 1. Normal/acceptable limit values for menstrual parameters.

http://dx.doi.org/10.5772/67795

Regular menstrual cycles are usually the outward manifestation of cyclical ovarian activity and ovulation. The establishment of regular ovulatory cycles at puberty depends on a complex series of interactions involving the hypothalamus, anterior pituitary, and the ovaries. With these series of complex interrelated events, it is hardly surprising that disorders of ovulation are relatively common causes of menstrual cycle disorders and POI.

Ovarian function in an ovulatory patients can be divided into three main groups [3]:

- hypergonadotrophic hypogonadism,
- hypogonadotrophic hypogonadism, and
- normogonadotrophic anovulation.

As per the World Health Organization, menstrual cycle disorders can also be classified either as a primary disorder of the ovaries or as a result of secondary causes:

- in primary ovarian insufficiency, the ovary fails to function normally in response to appropriate gonadotropin stimulation provided by the hypothalamus and pituitary (hypergonadotrophic hypogonadism),
- in secondary ovarian insufficiency, the hypothalamus and pituitary fail to provide appropriate gonadotropin stimulation (hypogonadotrophic hypogonadism) (**Figure 1**).

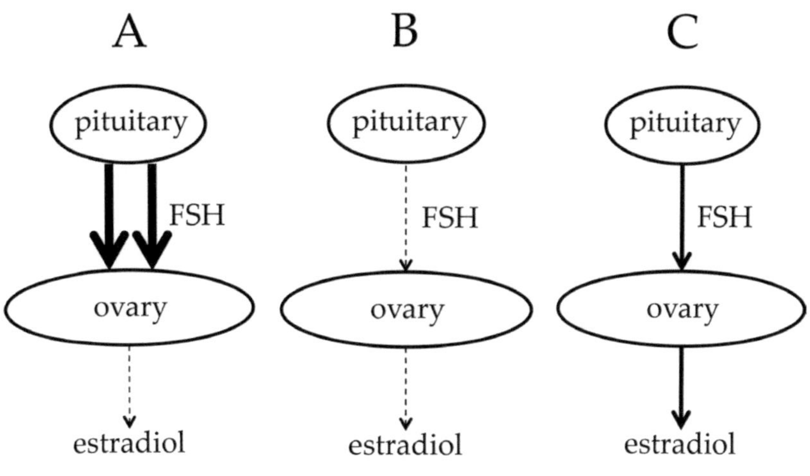

Figure 1. Gonadotrophic stimulation of the ovaries. A—hypergonadotrophic hypogonadism, B—hypogonadotrophic hypogonadism, C—normogonadotropic eugonadism. Adapted from Gersak [4].

3. Premature ovarian insufficiency

Premature ovarian insufficiency (POI) is a condition characterized by:

- amenorrhea (for at least 4 months),

- hypoestrogenism, and
- elevated serum gonadotropin levels two recordings of serum concentrations of follicle-stimulating hormone (FSH) of more than 40 IU/L at least 1 month apart in women younger than 40 years (>2 SD under the mean menopausal age).

Our current understanding of human ovarian reserve presumes that the ovary establishes several million nongrowing (primordial, intermediate and primary) follicles at around 5 months of gestational age. A steady decline of that number then follows, reaching the approximate value of 1000 at menopause, at the average age of 50–51 years [5–7]. With approximately 450 monthly ovulatory cycles that occur in the reproductive lifespan of a healthy human female, this progressive decline in nongrowing follicle count is chiefly attributed to follicle death by apoptosis. The peak of primordial follicle population, established at around 20-week postconception, determines the individual's age at menopause. Therefore, it is estimated that early or late menopause is related to low or high (respectively) peak follicle population at 18–22 weeks postconception. Women with around 295,000 nongrowing follicles per ovary at birth will reach menopause at the average age. In contrast, the ovaries of women, who are destined to have an earlier menopause, include around 35,000 nongrowing follicles at birth each, while those of women reaching a late menopause have over 2.5-million nongrowing follicles at birth each (**Figure 2**) [7].

Premature ovarian insufficiency can be caused by:

- ovarian follicle dysfunction,
- ovarian follicle depletion, or by
- mutations in genes associated with primary ovarian insufficiency.

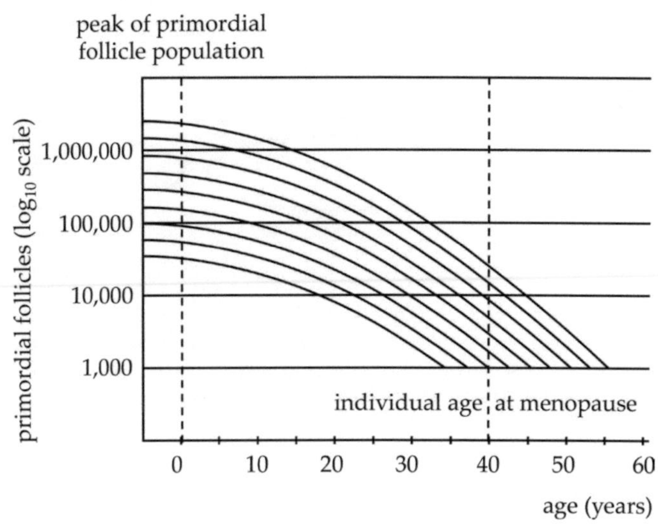

Figure 2. The correlation between ovarian reserve and age at menopause. This figure describes the hypothesis that the peak nongrowing follicle population established at around 20 weeks post-conception determines an individual's age at menopause. Adapted from Wallace and Kelsey [7].

They all result in a premature depletion of the primordial follicle pool [3, 5].

Acquired ovarian insufficiency can also occur because of a range of conditions that result in the destruction or loss of ovarian tissue (e.g., endometriosis, ovarian surgery, chemotherapy or radiotherapy).

4. Chromosomal abnormalities and premature ovarian insufficiency

Chromosome abnormalities have long been recognized as a main genetic cause of POI (**Figure 3**).

In women with numerical and structural abnormalities of the X chromosome, premature ovarian insufficiency is mainly a consequence of ovarian follicle depletion, due to an insufficient initial follicle number and/or spontaneous accelerated follicle loss.

Once they develop amenorrhea and are found to have elevated gonadotropin levels, ovarian failure is permanent except in a few extremely rare reported cases. These patients should not be given false hope; the term "primary ovarian insufficiency" instead of premature ovarian failure, premature menopause, or early menopause might be misleading for them unless its use is accompanied by honest, thorough, and compassionate counseling [8].

4.1. Monosomy X

Turner syndrome (monosomy X) occurs with an incidence of 1 in 2500 female births, which makes it the most common X chromosome abnormality leading to POI [9]. One fifth to one-third of affected girls is diagnosed as newborns because of puffy hands and feet or redundant nuchal skin. The second third of girls with 45,X are diagnosed in mid-childhood upon investigation of short stature. The rest are given their diagnosis at puberty due to primary or secondary amenorrhea.

Until the 18th week of gestation, the number of nongrowing follicles in the 45,X-fetus is normal. The presence of normal gonadotropin levels in the first 3–6 months of life suggests that residual ovarian function exists but does not ensure that the initiation and progression of puberty will be normal [9, 10].

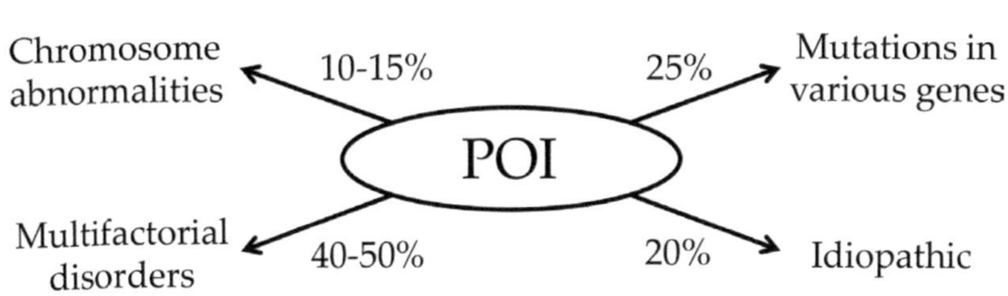

Figure 3. Causes of premature ovarian insufficiency (POI).

In many girls, pubic and axillary hair will develop spontaneously, because 45,X does not change the adrenarche. Some girls even possess enough residual ovarian function for breast budding and vaginal spotting to occur. Still, secondary amenorrhea will develop.

Although one X chromosome is sufficient to allow for ovarian differentiation, oocytes require two active X chromosomes. Therefore, haploinsufficiency of many genes located on the X chromosome in individuals with Turner's syndrome results in oocyte apoptosis and oocyte depletion within the first 10 years of life. The definite cause of the accelerated apoptosis is unknown. Two genes on the X chromosome are clearly implicated in premature ovarian insufficiency: bone morphogenetic protein 15 (BMP15) and fragile X mental retardation 1 (FMR1) [5, 11, 12]. Additional genes on the X chromosome have been implicated, however, but not proven, to have a role in ovarian failure specifically in females with 45,X.

The BMP15 gene is located on the short arm of the X chromosome (Xp11.2), within one of the "POF critical regions" (locus POF4; MIM number 300510) [12, 13]. Castronovo et al. performed a high-resolution comparative genome hybridization (CGH)-array analysis in a cohort of 45,X patients with or without spontaneous menarche [14]. They identified a tandem duplication of a single BMP15 gene in an 11-year-old patient with 45,X karyotype, who caught the pediatrician's attention because of a short stature but experienced a spontaneous menarche followed by regular menses for more than 4 years. Consistent with haploinsufficiency of the short stature homeobox gene (SHOX), this patient was short (145 cm at 34 years) despite growth hormone treatment. BMP15 duplication on the conserved X chromosome might have preserved a sufficient gene dosage in the developing ovary during the first meiotic phases, when a double dose of X-linked genes is required [12, 14]. BMP15 duplication led to the conservation of a certain amount of functional follicles at pubertal age and the ability to compensate, at least partially, for the loss of one copy of the other X-linked genes. BMP15 gene contributes to the ovarian phenotype of 45,X patients, supporting the hypothesis that BMP15 represents the first ovary-determining gene to have been identified on the X chromosome, which lends additional support to the idea that inactivating mutations in this gene can predispose to POI [12, 13].

4.2. Trisomy and polysomy X

Trisomy X or 47,XXX occurs in about 1 in 1000 newborn girls [15]. They generally have an unremarkable physical development, although there is a tendency toward tallness, usually presenting with an accelerated growth until puberty. Most of them have normal sexual development and are able to conceive children, but the occurrence of premature ovarian insufficiency probably exceeds the one in the general population. Recently, Stagi et al. reported that young 47,XXX girls show a premature activation of the GnRH pulse generator, which can occur even without puberty signs. In their study, basal and peak FSH levels in 47,XXX individuals were higher than in the control group, while E2 and inhibin levels, along with ovarian volume, were reduced, leading to a reduced gonadal function [16].

Trisomy X is associated with a very small amount of phenotypic abnormalities compared with autosomal trisomy states. The important factor is dosage compensation. Only one X chromosome in each cell needs to be fully active, whereas the other one is genetically inactivated. The inactivation occurs early in blastogenesis. The process originates at an X inactivation center within Xq13 and spreads in both directions. Certain parts of the X chromosome however are not subject to inactivation. The pseudoautosomal regions (PAR1 and PAR2) remain genetically active and function disomically [17]. Approximately 5–10% of additional genes outside the PAR regions on the X chromosome also escape X-inactivation.

In trisomy X, two of the three X chromosomes are inactivated. However, genes residing in the PAR regions along with other genes that escape X-inactivation are expressed from all three X chromosomes. The inactivation process is almost successful, resulting in an apparently normal in utero survival of 47,XXX fetuses. The fact that PARs are not subject to inactivation and may function in a trisomic or even polysomic state, it is hypothesized that the phenotypic abnormalities associated with trisomy X result from overexpression of these genes [18]. One exception is the SHOX gene, which escapes X-inactivation and is associated with the tall stature in polysomy X conditions.

Deficiency or overexpression of specific gene products on the X chromosome also influences oocyte quality.

Theoretically, it could be expected that three X chromosomes display 2:1 segregation during meiosis, with the production of an equal number of X and XX oocytes. However, no discernible increased risk for chromosomally abnormal offspring of 47,XXX women has been demonstrated [19]. This suggests that a "meiotic quality control" mechanism may exist to eliminate the errors. The spindle assembly checkpoint (SAC) monitors attachment to microtubules and tension on chromosomes. Usually, until all chromosomes are properly assembled at the spindle equator (chromosome congression) and under tension from spindle fibers, a complex between the anaphase promoting factor/cylosome (APC/C), its accessory protein Cdc20, and proteins of the SAC keep the APC/C in an inactive state [20].

4.3. X chromosome mosaicism

Mosaicism describes the presence of two or more populations of cells with different genotypes in one individual. If it occurs at the first cell division after conception, only two cell lines are possible. If nondisjunction occurs at a later cell division, two or more cell lines can persist [19].

When an abnormal number of sex chromosomes are seen in a low percentage of cells, the result could be interpreted either as a technical artifact, a genuine mosaicism, or being age related. The last option—loss of one X chromosome to give an occasional 45,X cell—is a normal characteristic of aging in 46,XX females. The rate of X chromosome loss in prepubertal females is around 1.5–2.5%, rising to 4.5–5% in women older than 75 years [21]. In contrast to sex chromosomes, the frequency of autosomal chromosome loss does not change during the course of aging.

The level of X chromosome mosaicism and its reproductive significance is still under debate. For clinical changes to occur, a minimum of 6% of X chromosome aneuploidy is required [22, 23]. "True" mosaicism represents the presence of more than 10% of aneuploid cells, whereas "low-level" mosaicism is defined as 6–10% of aneuploid cells. The frequency of X chromosome mosaicism in women with sporadic form of POI has been estimated to be between 3 and 21% [23]. Upon comparison between patients with X-chromosome mosaicism and those with a balanced structural autosomal rearrangement, patients with X-chromosome mosaicism have a significantly higher incidence of diminished ovarian reserve [24].

Additionally, X-chromosome mosaicism may be a manifestation of impaired genetic control of chromosome nondisjunction.

The diminished ovarian reserve and impaired genetic control of chromosome nondisjunction are probably also involved in the higher abortion rate and recurrent miscarriages in women with X-chromosome mosaicism.

4.4. X chromosome rearrangements

A variable degree of gonadal dysgenesis occurs in patients with X chromosome rearrangements. The majority of patients have oligomenorrhea, followed by secondary amenorrhea or POI [25].

Cytogenetically visible rearrangements occur in specific Xq regions. Two main critical regions have been located on the long arm of X chromosome, at Xq13-q21 and at Xq26-q27 [25, 26]. A few deletions in distal Xq have also been reported. Marozzi et al. described three POI cases with Xq chromosome deletions: two terminal, with breakpoints at Xq26.2 and Xq21.2, and one interstitial, with breakpoints at Xq23 and Xq28 [27]. In all three cases, the Xq deletion size and position did not correlate with age at POI occurrence. The smallest deleted region associated with POI was Xq26.2-q28. Rossetti et al. reported a distal interstitial deletion of the X chromosome in a fertile mother and her two affected daughters [28]. Also, Eggermann et al. presented a familial case of POI women with a small deletion from Xq27.2/Xq27.3 to Xqter [29]. In a population of 90 POI patients, Portnoi et al. identified three women bearing a large terminal Xq deletion involving Xq21-qter [30].

Mechanisms proposed for the explanation of the ovarian defect include the following: direct disruption of relevant loci and a position effect, caused by rearrangements on contiguous genes [1]. Position effect is a mechanism that involves the deletion or translocation of regulatory domains to a different position on the genome, which might be the cause of changes in gene transcription [12, 31].

The reason why women with similar X-chromosome rearrangements show a relatively great variability in the degree of ovarian failure is unclear. It may be related to natural cell selection, leading to X inactivation in germ cell precursors. In females with X-chromosome abnormalities, a nonrandom X inactivation is normally seen, resulting in a pattern that reflects the predominance of cells with the most functional gene imbalance.

http://dx.doi.org/10.5772/67795

Duplication located at the telomeric Xq region may alter pairing of X chromosomes during meiosis and therefore induce oocyte depletion [12].

5. Subjects and methods

Our study included 319 women with menstrual cycle disorders (sporadic idiopathic POI or secondary amenorrhea) referred to our Department of Obstetrics and Gynaecology in the period between 2000 and 2014. The diagnosis of POI was based on the criteria of either at least 6 months of amenorrhea or the age of menopause less than 40 years, combined with two consecutive values of serum follicle stimulating hormone (FSH) higher than 40 IU/l. Women with primary amenorrhea or gonadal dysgenesis, FRAXA permutation, mutations in the *FOXL2* or inhibin *INHα* genes were excluded.

During the same period, 424 women with a history of recurrent pregnancy loss and regular menstrual cycles were identified. A history of recurrent pregnancy loss was defined as two or more consecutive pregnancy losses before 22 weeks of gestation.

All women gave their informed consent.

Cytogenetic studies were carried out on peripheral blood samples, cultured for approximately 72 h. For each routine chromosomal analysis, 20–30 Giemsa-banded cells were analyzed, with three of those cells karyotyped. If the initial cytogenetic analysis revealed any cells with sex-chromosome hypoploidy or hyperploidy, 100 cells were counted and analyzed. The presence of more than 10% of aneuploid cells was characterized as true mosaicism, whereas low-level mosaicism was defined as 6–10% of aneuploid cells.

6. Results

Chromosome abnormalities were found in 62 (19.4%) women with POI. Twenty-six patients (26/319, 8.1%) had true X chromosome mosaicism; 28 patients (28/319, 8.7%) had low-level X mosaicism. Different types of sex-chromosome mosaicism present in our subject group (and their frequency) are shown in **Table 2**, while other abnormal karyotypes (8/319, 2.5%) are shown in **Table 3**.

Prevalence of chromosome abnormalities in patients with a history of recurrent pregnancy loss is represented in **Table 4**. Out of 424 women, X chromosome mosaicism was observed in 39 of them. Twenty-two (22/424, 5.2%) had true sex chromosome mosaicism; 17 had low-level X mosaicism.

Among those 39, 6 women had aneuploid offspring (**Table 5**). Moreover, one of those six, a woman with low-level X mosaicism, gave birth to a girl with true X mosaicism.

Number of patients	Type of sex chromosome mosaicism
18	45,X/46,XX
8	45,X/47,XXX
5	47,XXX/46,XX
19	45,X/47,XXX/46,XX
1	45,X/46,X,i(Xq10)
1	47,XXX/48,XXXX/46,XX
1	45,X/47,XXX/48,XXXX/49,XXXXX/46,XX
1	45,X/47,XXX/49,XXXX/47,XXY/46,XY/46,XX

Table 2. Sex chromosome mosaicism in women with POI ($n = 54$).

Patient	Age at karyotyping	Chromosome abnormalities [number of metaphases]
1	23	46,XX;t(X;16)dn [20]
2	36	46,XX;t(8;10)dn [20]
3	19	46,XX,t(4;12)(q21.1;p11.2)dn [20]
4	31	46,XX[30]/46,XX fra(2)(q13)[20]
5	32	46,X,del(X)(q21)dn [20]
6	25	46,X,i(X)(q10)dn [20]
7	35	45,X[44]/46,X,i(X)(q10)[2]/47,X,i(X)(q10),i,(X)(q10)[1]/46,XX[2]
8	33	46,X,del(X)(p11.2)[32]/45,X[27]/47,X,del(X)(p11.2,del(X)(p11.3)[3]

Table 3. Chromosome abnormalities (without X chromosome mosaicism) in women with POI ($n = 8$).

Number of pregnancy loss	Number of patients ($n = 424$)	Number of patients with X chromosome mosaicism ($n = 39$)	Number of patients with other chromosome abnormalities ($n = 64$)
2	134	16	21
3	201	19	34
4	33	3	6
≥5	13	1	3

Table 4. Prevalence of chromosome abnormalities in patients with a history of recurrent pregnancy loss.

http://dx.doi.org/10.5772/67795

Offspring with aneuploidy	Chromosome abnormalities (number of aneuploid cells, %)	Mother's chromosome abnormalities (number of aneuploid cells, %)
1	46,XX,+14,der(13;14)(q10;q10) dn; stillbirth	45,X/46,XX (>10%)
2	45,X/46/XX (>10%); live born	45,X/47,XXX/46,XX (<10%)
3	47,XXX/46,XX (<10%); live born	45,X/47,XXX/46,XX (>10%)
4	47,XY,+21; live born	45,X/47,XXX/46,XX (>10%)*
5	47,XXY/46,XX (>10%); live born	47,XXX/48,XXXX/46,XX (>10%)
6	46,X,i(Xq); live born	45,X/46,X,i(Xq) (100%)

* Patient No. 32 has also a brother with Down syndrome (47,XY,+21).

Table 5. Offspring with aneuploidy born to women with X chromosome abnormalities and recurrent pregnancy loss.

In 7 out of the aforementioned 39 patients (19%), pregnancies occurred with the assistance of ovulation induction.

7. Discussion

Our study has established an important role of X chromosome abnormalities in women with sporadic idiopathic POI or history of recurrent pregnancy loss. With routine G-banding, at least 50 cells have to be analyzed in order to exclude the presence of 6% mosaicism with a 0.95 level of confidence [32]. With an evaluation of 20 metaphases, only a mosaicism greater than 14% can be found with the same confidence.

If true and low-level mosaicisms are regarded as identical abnormal results, this study found mosaicism in 16.8% of patients. In our previous study, X chromosome mosaicism was found in 21.9% of patients [23].

Wu et al. [33]. reported 5 out of 61 (8.2%) POI cases with X chromosome mosaicism. In a Hong Kong group of 312 women with secondary amenorrhea, 11 cases with karyotype 45,X/46,XX and 3 cases with mosaic triple/poly X were found [34]. Lakhal et al. detected 34 (5.9%) patients with homogeneous or mosaic X-chromosome aneuploidy out of 568 with secondary amenorrhea. In contrast, Portnoi et al. identified no 45,X/46,XX or 46,XX/47,XXX chromosome mosaicisms in any of their POI patients or controls [30].

In our present study, true X chromosome mosaicism was found in 8.1% of women with sporadic idiopathic POI, whereas low-level mosaicism was found in 8.7%. Based on our present and previous results [23], we presume that at least two different subgroups of patients with X chromosome mosaicism exist. The mean age of women with true X mosaicism and low-level X mosaicism was significantly different in both studies; in our recent study, the values were

26.0 ± 5.65 years and 35.92 ± 3.87 years, respectively. Although peripheral blood does not reflect the situation in other tissues well, that is, in ovarian tissue, the onset of POI occurred earlier in women with true X mosaicism. In all patients, karyotyping was performed within a 12-month period after the last menses.

In couples with recurrent spontaneous abortion, X chromosome mosaicism was identified in 3–16% [33, 35–39]. In 50 cells counted, Düzcan et al. showed mosaicism of either structural rearrangements or aneuploidies of sex chromosomes in 7 cases out of 354 with reproductive failure [38]. In our present study, a significant number (≥6%) of X chromosome aneuploidy in lymphocyte cultures was found in 9.2% of women with history of reproductive failure. Five liveborn children and one stillborn with aneupoidy were identified. Unfortunately, we have no data about chromosomal aneuploidy in embryonic/fetal tissue recovered from the abortuses of the same women before they visited our department. Kaneko et al. reviewed 117 pregnancy outcomes in 49 cases of 45,X/46,XX, 45,X/47,XXX, 45,X/46,XX/47,XXX and 45,X/46,XX/47,XXX/48,XXXX mosaicism [40]. For cases with information available, miscarriage rate was 30%, stillbirth rate was 7%; 43% of babies were normal, and 20% were abnormal. Sex chromosome abnormalities were observed in 7% of the children of 45,X/46,XX women and in 23% of the children of 45,X/46,XX/47,XXX women; not one 45,X/47,XXX woman had a child with X aneuplody [19]. Kuo and Guo reported a 68.6% miscarriage rate in patients with X chromosome mosaicism and diminished ovarian reserve (FSH level of >11.0 mUI/ml), and as high as 44.1% for cases without diminished ovarian reserve [24].

Despite the lack of data about fetal karyotypes, an increased risk to have a child with aneuploidy may apply to our patients. Supporting this assumption, both the child and the brother of one of the previously mentioned 39 women with X chromosome mosaicism (**Table 5**) had Down syndrome (**Table 5**). This finding may reflect a genetic tendency toward mitotic and meiotic nondisjunction or errors in the "meiotic quality control" mechanism [20]. The fact that the meiotic segregation error of one chromosome may affect the segregation of other chromosomes was demonstrated also in XO female mice [41].

Information on meiotic and mitotic errors has become available with the advent of preimplatation genetic diagnosis—sequential testing of the first and second polar bodies [42]. In contrast to the traditional concept that aneuploidies mainly originate from female meiosis I, direct testing in patients of advanced reproductive age (average age 38.5 years) showed that chromosome abnormalities originate from both meiosis I and meiosis II in comparable proportions and are predominantly of chromatid origin. Although isolated errors in either meiosis I or meiosis II were observed, approximately one half of oocytes with meiosis I errors also had sequential meiosis II errors. The result of such sequential errors shows that ideally, almost one-third of these zygotes should be "euploid."

Balanced zygotes may represent a phenomenon of aneuploidy rescue in female meiosis [42]. The inherent predisposition for genomic instability in meiosis divisions can probably explain the nature of recurrent spontaneous abortions in women with X mosaicism [20, 40].

In a mosaic ovary, aberrant X chromosome pairing and impaired genetic control of chromosomal nondisjunction may cause premature germ cell death, thus decreasing the number of germ cells and accelerate follicle atresia [19, 24]. One obvious explanation could also lie in the haploinsufficiency of loci on the X chromosome [12, 14].

8. Conclusion

POI is a clinical syndrome defined by loss of ovarian activity before the age of 40 years. Although the prevalence is only 1%, POI is associated with numerous health problems preceded by menstrual cycle abnormalities and subfertility. The proper diagnostic criteria for POI are still lacking. In 2016, the ESHRE Guideline Group on POI published a less restrictive definition such as oligo/amenorrhea for at least 4 months and an elevated FSH level up to 25 IU/l on two occasions more than 4 weeks apart.

According to the results from several studies mentioned in this chapter, as well as ESHRE guidelines, cytogenetic analyses should be considered for all women with unexplained sporadic noniatrogenic POI. X chromosome abnormalities cause up to 20% of the cases, of which the contribution of "true" and "low-level" X chromosome mosaicism represents a significant proportion.

X aneuploidy and low-level mosaicism are reproductively significant also in phenotypically normal women with recurrent pregnancy loss.

In recent years, array-comparative genomic hybridization and next-generation sequencing are becoming important genetic tests in everyday practice, increasing the etiologic diagnosis rate up to 30%. However, they fail to detect chromosomal rearrangements if breakpoints are either located in introns or not associated with a gain or loss of genetic material [43]. On the other hand, FISH may be the most appropriate method for confirming a suspected numerical mosaicism. According to the ISCN, numerical and structural abnormalities still have to be excluded at a classical banding level.

We share the opinion that women with X mosaicism may be at increased risk of producing chromosomally abnormal offspring and should be offered prenatal diagnosis. These results have practical implications for genetic counseling and fertility treatment.

Author details

Ksenija Gersak[1,2]* and Ziva Miriam Gersak[2]

*Address all correspondence to: ksenija.gersak@mf.uni-lj.si

1 Department of Obstetrics and Gynaecology, University Medical Centre Ljubljana, Ljubljana, Slovenia

2 Faculty of Medicine, University of Ljubljana, Ljubljana, Slovenia

References

[1] Cordts EB, Christofolini DM, Dos Santos AA, Bianco B, Barbosa CP. Genetic aspects of premature ovarian failure: a literature review. Arch Gynecol Obstet. 2011;**283**:635-43. doi:10.1007/s00404-010-1815-4

[2] Munro MG, Critchley HO, Fraser IS. The FIGO systems for nomenclature and classification of causes of abnormal uterine bleeding in the reproductive years: who needs them? Am J Obstet Gynecol. 2012;**207**:259-65. doi:10.1016/j.ajog.2012.01.046

[3] ESHRE Capri Workshop Group. Health and fertility in World Health Organization group 2 anovulatory women. Hum Reprod Update. 2012;**18**:586-99. doi:10.1093/humupd/dms019

[4] Gersak K. Genetika zenske neplodnosti/Genetica dell'infertilità femminile. In: Peterlin B, (editor). Genetika v ginekologiji/La genetica in ginecologia. 1st ed. Ljubljana: Design studio; 2014. pp. 108-21. ISBN: 978-961-230-464-5

[5] De Vos M, Devroey P, Fauser BC. Primary ovarian insufficiency. Lancet. 2010;**376**:911-21. doi:10.1016/S0140-6736(10)60355-8

[6] Coulam C, Adamson S, Annegers J. Incidence of premature ovarian failure. Obstet Gynecol. 1986;**67**:604-06.

[7] Wallace WH, Kelsey TW. Human ovarian reserve from conception to the menopause. PLoS One. 2010;**5**:e8772. doi:10.1371/journal.pone.0008772

[8] Reindollar RH. Turner syndrome: contemporary thoughts and reproductive issues. Semin Reprod Med. 2011;**29**:342-52. doi:10.1055/s-0031-1280919

[9] Sybert VP, McCauley E. Turner's syndrome. N Engl J Med. 2004;**351**:1227-38.

[10] Heinrichs C, Bourdoux P, Saussez C, Vis HL, Bourguignon JP. Blood spot follicle-stimulating hormone during early postnatal life in normal girls and Turner's syndrome. J Clin Endocrinol Metab. 1994;**78**:978-81.

[11] Trolle C, Hjerrild B, Cleemann L, Mortensen KH, Gravholt CH. Sex hormone replacement in Turner syndrome. Endocrine. 2012;**41**:200-19. doi:10.1007/s12020-011-9569-8

[12] Persani L, Rossetti R, Di Pasquale E, Cacciatore C, Fabre S. The fundamental role of bone morphogenetic protein 15 in ovarian function and its involvement in female fertility disorders. Hum Reprod Update. 2014;**20**:869-83. doi:10.1093/humupd/dmu036

[13] Layman LC. Editorial: BMP15—the first true ovarian determinant gene on the X-chromosome?. J Clin Endocrinol Metab. 2006;**91**:1673-6.

[14] Castronovo C, Rossetti R, Rusconi D, Recalcati MP, Cacciatore C, Beccaria E, et al. Gene dosage as a relevant mechanism contributing to the determination of ovarian function in Turner syndrome. Hum Reprod. 2014;**29**:368-79. doi:10.1093/humrep/det436

[15] Otter M, Schrander-Stumpel CT, Curfs LM. Triple X syndrome: a review of the literature. Eur J Hum Genet. 2010;**18**:265-71. doi:10.1038/ejhg.2009.109

[16] Stagi S, di Tommaso M, Scalini P, Lapi E, Losi S, Bencini E, Masoni F, Dosa L, Becciani S, de Martino M. Triple X syndrome and puberty: focus on the hypothalamus-hypophysis-gonad axis. Fertil Steril. 2016;**105**:1547-53. doi:10.1016/j.fertnstert.2016.02.019

[17] Mangs HA, Morris BJ. The human pseudoautosomal region (PAR): origin, function and future. Curr Genomics. 2007;**8**:129-36.

[18] Tartaglia NR, Howell S, Sutherland A, Wilson R, Wilson L. Triple X syndrome with rare phenotypic presentation. Indian J Pediatr. 2008 Jun;**75**:629-31. doi:10.1007/s12098-008-0120-8

[19] Gardner RJM, Sutherland GR. Chromosome Abnormalities and Genetic Counseling. 2nd ed. New York: Oxford University Press; 1996. p. 478. ISBN 0-19-510615-6

[20] Vogt E, Kirsch-Volders M, Parry J, Eichenlaub-Ritter U. Spindle formation, chromosome segregation and the spindle checkpoint in mammalian oocytes and susceptibility to meiotic error. Mutat Res. 2008 Mar 12;**651**:14-29.

[21] Guttenbach M, Koschorz B, Bernthaler U, Grimm T, Schmid M. Sex chromosome loss and aging: in situ hybridization studies on human interphase nuclei. Am J Hum Genet. 1995;**57**:1143-50.

[22] Homer L, Le Martelot MT, Morel F, Amice V, Kerlan V, Collet M, De Braekeleer M. 45,X/46,XX mosaicism below 30% of aneuploidy: clinical implications in adult women from a reproductive medicine unit. Eur J Endocrinol. 2010;**162**:617-23. doi:10.1530/EJE-09-0750

[23] Gersak K, Veble A. Low-level X chromosome mosaicism in women with sporadic premature ovarian failure. Reprod Biomed Online. 2011;**22**:399-403. doi:10.1016/j.rbmo.2011.01.002

[24] Kuo PL, Guo HR. Mechanism of recurrent spontaneous abortions in women with mosaicism of X-chromosome aneuploidies. Fertil Steril. 2004;**82**:1594-601.

[25] Gersak K, Writzl K, Veble A, Liehr T. Primary amenorrhoea in a patient with mosaicism for monosomy X and a derivative X-chromosome. Genet Couns. 2010;**21**:335-42.

[26] Vásquez-Velásquez AI, Torres-Flores J, Leal CA, Rivera H. Apparent neotelomere in a 46,X,del(X)(qter→p11.2:)/46,X,rea(X)(qter→p11.2::q21.2→qter) novel mosaicism: review of 34 females with a recombinant-like dup(Xq) chromosome. Genet Test Mol Biomarkers. 2011;**15**:727-31. doi:10.1089/gtmb.2011.0017

[27] Marozzi A, Manfredini E, Tibiletti MG, Furlan D, Villa N, Vegetti W, et al. Molecular definition of Xq common-deleted region in patients affected by premature ovarian failure. Hum Genet. 2000;**107**:304-11.

[28] Rossetti F, Rizzolio F, Pramparo T, Sala C, Bione S, Bernardi F, et al. A susceptibility gene for premature ovarian failure (POF) maps to proximal Xq28. Eur J Hum Genet. 2004;**12**:829-34.

[29] Eggermann T, Meschede D, Schüler H, Palm S, Gläser D, Horsthemke B, et al. Premature ovarian failure associated with a small terminal Xq deletion: narrowing the POF1 region down to Xq27.2/Xq27.3-qter. Clin Genet. 2005;**67**:434-7.

[30] Portnoi MF, Aboura A, Tachdjian G, Bouchard P, Dewailly D, Bourcigaux N, et al. Molecular cytogenetic studies of Xq critical regions in premature ovarian failure patients. Hum Reprod. 2006;**21**:2329-34.

[31] Tachdjian G, Aboura A, Portnoï MF, Pasquier M, Bourcigaux N, Simon T, et al. Cryptic Xp duplication including the SHOX gene in a woman with 46,X, del(X)(q21.31) and premature ovarian failure. Hum Reprod. 2008;**23**:222-6.

[32] Hook EB. Exclusion of chromosomal mosaicism: tables of 90%, 95% and 99% confidence limits and comments on use. Am J Hum Genet. 1977;**29**:94-7.

[33] Wu RC, Kuo PL, Lin SJ, Liu CH, Tzeng CC. X chromosome mosaicism in patients with recurrent abortion or premature ovarian failure. J Formos Med Assoc. 1993;**92**:953-6.

[34] Wong MS, Lam ST. Cytogenetic analysis of patients with primary and secondary amenorrhea in HongKong: retrospective study. Hong Kong Med J. 2005;**11**:267-72.

[35] Horsman DE, Dill FJ, McGillivray BC, Kalousek DK. X chromosome aneuploidy in lymphocyte cultures from women with recurrent spontaneous abortion. Am J Med Genet. 1987;**28**:981-7.

[36] Radojcic Badovinac A, Buretic-Tomljanovic A, Starcevic N, Kapovic M, Vlastelic I, Randic L. Chromosome studies in patients with defective reproductive success. Am J Reprod Immunol. 2000;**44**:279-83.

[37] Morel F, Gallon F, Amice V, Le Bris MJ, Le Martelot MT, Roche S, et al. Sex chromosome mosaicism in couples undergoing intracytoplasmic sperm injection. Hum Reprod. 2002;**17**:2552-5.

[38] Duzcan F, Atmaca M, Cetin GO, Bagci H. Cytogenetic studies in patients with reproductive failure. Acta Obstet Gynecol Scand. 2003;**82**:53-6.

[39] Gonçalves RO, Santos WV, Sarno M, Cerqueira BA, Gonçalves MS, Costa OL. Chromosomal abnormalities in couples with recurrent first trimester abortions. Rev Bras Ginecol Obstet. 2014;**36**:113-7. doi:10.1590/S0100-720320140003000004

[40] Kaneko N, Kawagoe S, Hiroi M. Turner's syndrome-review of the literature with reference to a successful pregnancy outcome. Gynecol Obstet Invest. 1990;**29**:81-7.

[41] Hunt P, LeMaire R, Embury P, Sheean L, Mroz K. Analysis of chromosome behavior in intact mammalian oocytes: monitoring the segregation of a univalent chromosome during female meiosis. Hum Mol Genet. 1995;**4**:2007-12.

[42] Kuliev A, Verlinsky Y. Meiotic and mitotic nondisjunction: lessons from preimplantation genetic diagnosis. Hum Reprod Update. 2004;**10**:401-7.

[43] Pasquier L, Fradin M, Cherot E, Martin-Coignard D, Colin E, Journel H, et al. Karyotype is not dead (yet)! Eur J Med Genet. 2016;**59**:11-5.

Chapter 7

Chromosomal Abnormalities in Preimplantation Embryos and Detection Strategies in PGD and PGS

Pinar Tulay

Additional information is available at the end of the chapter

http://dx.doi.org/10.5772/67419

Abstract

Structural and numerical chromosomal abnormalities are common in early developing embryos, and these abnormalities may cause spontaneous abortions and implantation failure. The reproductive risk of carriers with structural chromosomal abnormalities depends on the breakpoint positions, the segregation patterns and the sex of the carrier. These carriers have a lower chance of producing normal or balanced gametes due to abnormal segregation of chromosomes at meiosis leading to repeated spontaneous abortions and infertility. Preimplantation genetic diagnosis (PGD) is offered to couples who have already been diagnosed with a single gene disorder or a chromosome imbalance to select an embryo free from the mutation or an embryo with a balanced karyotype prior to implantation and pregnancy. PGS is applied to patients experiencing repeated implantation failures or spontaneous abortions with normal karyotypes. Translocations are the most common type of structural chromosome rearrangement. Both reciprocal and Robertsonian translocations are phenotypically normal. PGD for translocations was initially performed by fluorescence in situ hybridization (FISH) at cleavage stage embryos. However, with the recent developments, many centers have opted for the use of array comparative genomic hybridization (aCGH), single-nucleotide polymorphism (SNP) arrays and next generation sequencing (NGS).

Keywords: chromosomal abnormalities, PGD, FISH, aCGH

1. Introduction

Preimplantation embryo development follows a series of critical events. These events start at gametogenesis and lasts until parturition. Gametogenesis is a process of gamete formation. Male and female gametes are derived from primordial germ cells (PGCs) by the processes of spermatogenesis and oogenesis, respectively. PGCs have unique properties of gene expression, epigenetics, morphology and behavior. Once the PGCs undergo mitosis, spermatogenesis and oogenesis progress differently. In spermatogenesis, spermatogonia undergo mitosis starting at puberty until death, and each primary spermatocyte produces four spermatids at the end of meiosis. In oogenesis, PGCs differentiate into oogenia, and they enter meiosis and arrest until puberty. Unlike meiosis II in spermatogenesis, secondary oocyte and first polar body do not undergo meiosis II until fertilization. After fertilization, meiosis II starts and each oogenia produce a single viable oocyte [1].

At fertilization, the oocyte completes meiosis, and the fertilized oocyte is called the zygote. Oocyte and sperm nuclei fuse resulting in syngamy. The zygote undergoes series of cleavage divisions, forming 2-cell, 4-cell, 8-cell, morula and blastocyst stages [2]. During cleavage stage divisions programming of maternal and paternal chromosomes takes place to create the embryonic genome (embryonic genome activation, EGA) and to start the preimplantation embryo development. If the EGA fails, the development does not continue because of the inability of the embryo to have cellular functions [3]. This activation is initiated by degradation of maternal nucleic acids, specific RNAs stored in oocytes, proteins and other macromolecules [4]. Upon EGA, which starts at the 2-cell stage in mouse and 4–8-cell stage in human [5], remarkable reprogramming of expression occurs in the preimplantation embryo. These reprogramming events are controlled by DNA methylation, histone acetylation, transcription, translation and miRNA regulation [6].

Both conception and embryonic developments during pregnancy are vulnerable processes since a large number of the conceptions are chromosomally abnormal. Chromosomal imbalances, gains or losses of segments/whole chromosomes, are common in human, and they are observed in 1/380 live births [7]. Chromosomal imbalances have been observed in preimplantation embryos mostly in the form of aneuploidies and translocations, and they may lead to embryo death or development of an affected embryo [8, 9]. The incidence of chromosomally abnormal embryos increases vividly with advanced maternal age [10–12]. The main causes of spontaneous abortions and repeated implantation failure are these numerical and structural chromosomal abnormalities [13–17]. Therefore, in the last decades, a great focus has been put on detecting these chromosomal aberrations in preimplantation embryos. Preimplantation genetic diagnosis has been applied to patients with known structural chromosomal abnormalities as well as single gene disorders, whereas preimplantation genetic screening has aimed to detect aneuploid embryos and lower the risk of implantation failures and spontaneous abortions following in assisted reproductive technology treatments [18–20].

In this chapter, the applications of preimplantation genetic diagnosis for translocations and preimplantation genetic screening for aneuploidy testing will be discussed. Translocations are the most common type of rearrangements that we come across in fertility clinics. Different techniques that are being used currently will be thoroughly evaluated. Finally, different aspects of preimplantation genetic screening will be evaluated.

2. Structural chromosomal abnormalities in human embryos

Majority of conceptus with chromosomal abnormality aborts spontaneously with <1% of abnormal conceptus resulting in term pregnancy. Chromosomal abnormalities can arise at three stages during human development, gametogenesis, fertilization and embryogenesis. Analysis of chromosomes in human gametes and embryos has become available with the development of artificial reproductive (ART) technologies developed to treat infertility.

Balanced structural chromosome rearrangements are common in human. Approximately 1/500 to 1/1000 live births carry a balanced translocation [21]. Translocations are formed due to rearrangements of nonhomologous chromosome segments. They can be caused by abnormal DNA repair, chromosome breakage, centric fission followed by malsegregation of that chromosome or through the formation of isochromosomes or terminal deletion accompanied by a duplication of the rest of the chromosome [22]. Translocations are grouped in two categories: reciprocal, the most common form, and Robertsonian. Reciprocal translocations occur due to an exchange of two ends of nonhomologous chromosomes. Robertsonian translocations involve rearrangement of two acrocentric chromosomes (chromosomes 13, 14, 15, 21 and 22) with the loss of the short arms occurring in 1/900 live births [7]. The most common Robertsonian translocation involves chromosomes 13 and 14 [23].

Although the carriers of both reciprocal and Robertsonian translocations are phenotypically normal, the reproductive risk of balanced carriers varies depending on the chromosomes involved, breakpoint positions, the segregation patterns and the sex of the translocation carrier [24]. However, they generally have a lower chance to produce normal or balanced gametes due to abnormal segregation of chromosomes at meiosis leading to repeated spontaneous abortions and infertility [21, 25]. At pachytene stage of meiosis I, chromosomes with reciprocal translocation rearrangements form quadrivalent. At the end of meiosis I, these chromosomes can segregate in four different ways: alternate (2:2), adjacent (2:2), 3:1 and 4:0 (**Figure 1a**). Alternate segregation either leads to a normal or a balanced rearrangement, and therefore, it results in a viable birth. Studies suggest that the most common segregation pattern of gametes produced by the carriers of reciprocal translocations is alternate (balanced) segregation [26]. In the case of an adjacent segregation, homologous chromosomes cause a monosomy for one centric center and trisomy for the other centric center. Studies suggest that adjacent two segregation pattern is rather uncommon [26] and may rise in cases of maternal meiotic errors [21]. Three to one segregation leads to a tertiary trisomy/monosomy or interchange trisomy/monosomy. This type of segregation can be viable. If the chromosomes fail to segregate, it leads to 4:0 segregation resulting in double trisomy or double monosomy. In case of a Robertsonian translocation, one normal with one derivative chromosome or single chromosomes of derivative or the single chromosomes of the normal chromosome can segregate resulting in an abnormal gamete (**Figure 1b**). The only way of a Robertsonian carrier can produce a normal gamete is if the two normal chromosomes segregate together at meiosis I [27].

Insertions can be classified as a type of translocations, and these are uncommon rearrangements. The simple insertion involves three breaks where the first two removes the part of the chromosome, and the segment is reinserted within the third break. The conceptus with a smaller insertional segment has a potential to be viable [28]. The insertions, especially the small ones, may be passed on from generations to generations without being detected. However, with the use of newer technologies, such as microarrays, more patients with insertions are likely to be detected [29]. Insertions are one the rearrangements with the highest reproductive risk, in such approximately 32% of male and 36% of female carriers are having a chromosomally abnormal child [30].

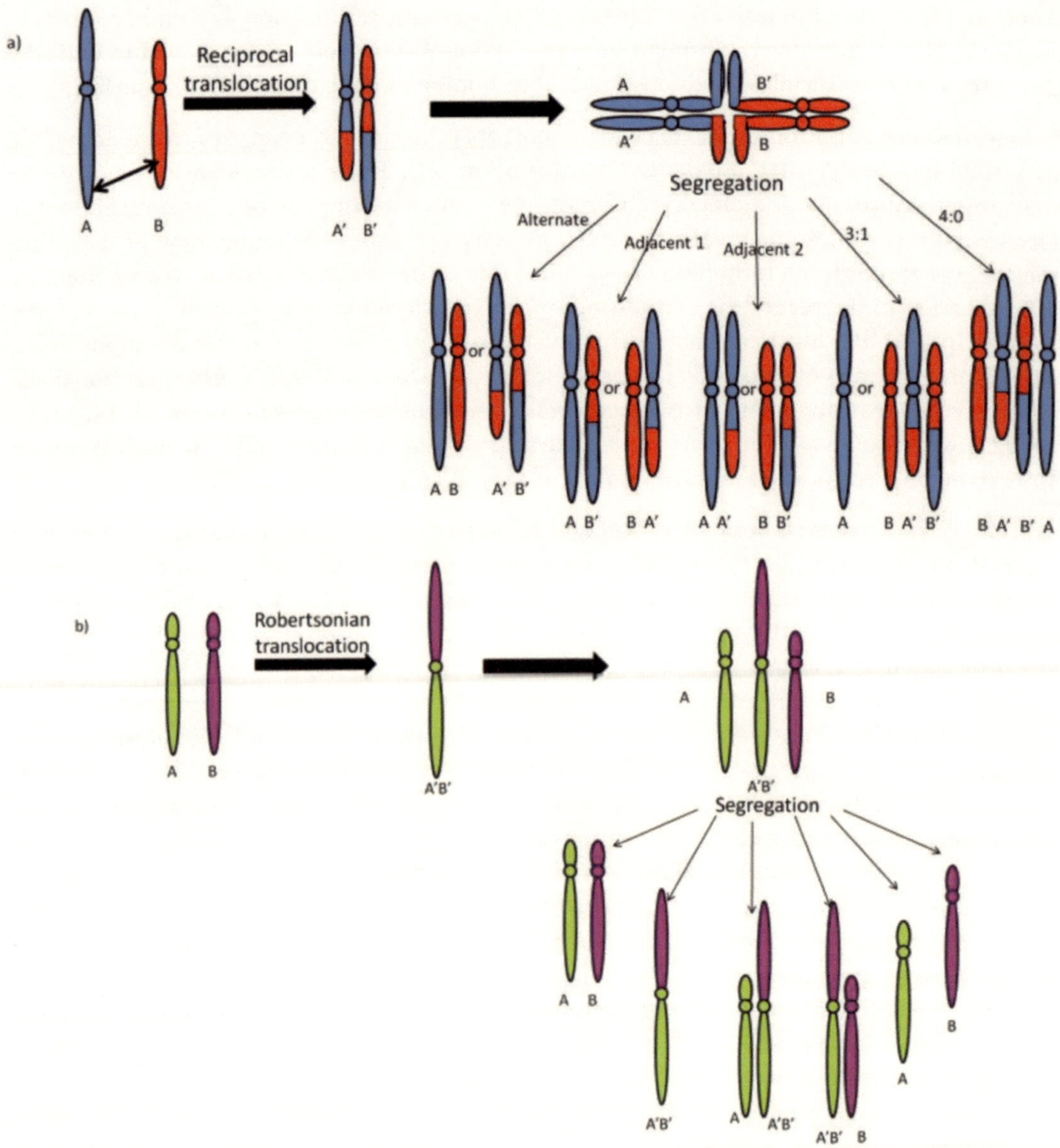

Figure 1. Segregation patterns of translocation carriers (a. Reciprocal and b. Robertsonian translocation carriers) during meiosis.

Another example of chromosomal rearrangements is inversions. These are intrachromosomal structural rearrangements. The simple inversion involves two break points within the same chromosome where the intercalcary segment gets rotated and reinserted. The inversions can be subcharacterized as pericentric, where the inverted segment involves the centromere, and paracentric, where the inverted segment is reinserted on the same chromosome arm. It is very rare that an inversion, especially pericentric inversions, would cause infertility [31]. However, abnormal synapsis of a chromosome pair may cause the development of an abnormal embryo due to malsegregation of chromosomes during gametogenesis. Depending on the break point, whether it involves genes or not, the size of the inversion could result in detrimental effects. Therefore, the risk of an inversion carrier varies among couples, and each has their own risk. The risk estimate can be performed by family studies, literature with similar inversion break points and gamete (sperm) analysis. Sperm studies have shown that during spermatogenesis, inversions with larger segments could result in spermatogenic arrest [32].

The carriers with a chromosomal rearrangements have the option to pursue pregnancy without seeking for any medical help and wish for a chromosomally normal child. Some of these carriers may have had an abnormal child due to the chromosomal abnormalities, and some of these carriers, especially translocation carriers, may have experienced repeated spontaneous abortions. Therefore, these patients may choose to seek for different options to avoid such experiences. These couples may opt for donor gametes, prenatal diagnosis or preimplantation genetic diagnosis.

3. Preimplantation genetic diagnosis

Preimplantation genetic diagnosis (PGD) is offered to couples who have already been diagnosed with a single gene disorder or a chromosome imbalance to select an embryo free from the mutation or an embryo with a balanced karyotype prior to implantation and pregnancy [9]. The first application of PGD was performed for a couple with X-linked recessive disorder almost a quarter century ago by Handyside and colleagues [33].

PGD is a highly invasive technique that requires IVF and biopsy of the polar body of the mature oocyte or the developing embryo (cleavage stage or blastocyst stage). Polar body biopsy involves biopsying the first only or the first and the second polar bodies. Neither the first polar body nor the second polar body is required for fertilization or a normal embryonic development [34]. Polar body biopsy is advantageous since it provides sufficient time for analysis. First polar body biopsy alone only allows analysis of meiotic errors (maternal origin only), and it does not give any information on the mitotic errors. Although the biopsy of both polar bodies provides information on both the meiotic and mitotic errors, it is still limited to detect the maternal errors only [35].

Biopsy at the cleavage stage on day 3 postfertilization provides more complete diagnosis than polar body biopsy and with enough time to finish the diagnosis before the embryo transfer [36, 37]. However, mosaicism (presence of at least two cell lines) at this stage is a major issue for PGS. In mosaic embryos, one or two cells may not represent the rest of the embryo due to different cell types in every cell [38–43].

Blastocyst biopsy has been applied more frequently in PGS in the last years. Biopsy of trophectoderm cells provides more number of cells for diagnosis and therefore overcomes the trouble of the single cell diagnosis [44]. Even though some studies report mosaicism at the blastocyst stage [45–47], due to the activation of cell cycle control points by the 8-cell stage embryo, many mosaic embryos are arrested or are repaired [48]. The lower rates of mosaicism in addition to analysis of several cells instead of just one provide less diagnostic errors. Conversely, blastocyst stage biopsy is limited before the procedure can even begin as it depends on the development of the embryo into a blastocyst [49].

4. Numerical chromosomal abnormalities in embryos and preimplantation genetic screening

Since the initial applications of PGD for sex-linked disorders and monogenic diseases, the indications have been expanded to aneuploidy screening by preimplantation genetic screening (PGS). PGS is applied to patients with advanced maternal age, recurrent miscarriages, repeated in vitro fertilization (IVF) failures or male infertility. Unlike PGD, patients undergoing PGS do not carry a genetic disorder and they have a normal karyotype. The main goal of PGS is to test embryos for aneuploidies that arise spontaneously in human gametogenesis, more prevalent in female meiosis, or early embryonic development [50, 51]. Aneuploidy is a common feature in preimplantation embryos causing the low success rates and high miscarriage rates in assisted reproductive technology (ART) treatments [52, 53]. Although embryos with autosomal monosomies are mainly lethal; embryos with some trisomies (13, 18 and 21) have higher chances of survival with the risk of developing genetic disorders [54], and some trisomies (15, 16 and 22) can cause embryonic developmental arrest or implantation failures [55, 56]. Therefore, selecting an embryo with a normal chromosomal complement helps to improve the implantation rates and increases the chances of birth of a healthy child.

The first PGS was performed by fluorescence in situ hybridization (FISH) in polar bodies and cleavage stage embryos in 1995 [57–59]. Up until recently, FISH was the preferred method of analysis in cleavage stage embryos [60]. As discussed earlier, although at cleavage stage, both maternal and paternal errors can be analyzed, it is complicated by high levels of mosaicsism. Mosaicsism is rare for monogenic diseases; however, it is very common for aneuploidies in the embryos at cleavage stage. There are more than ten randomized control trials showing that cleavage stage biopsy and FISH analysis does not improve the delivery rates [61–71]. In 2010, European Society of Human Reproduction and Embryology (ESHRE) reported that cleavage stage biopsy using FISH is not recommended for PGS [72]. The majority of the aneuploidies in the embryos affecting the pregnancy rates are believed to occur in the oocyte, and therefore, polar body (PB) biopsy may have an added advantage in PGS, especially since PBs are not affected by mosaicim arising in mitosis [73]. However, biopsy of the first PB does not provide a complete aneuploidy screening since biopsy of first PB only gives errors occurring in meiosis I, and it does not reveal any information about meiosis II. Therefore, performing both PB I and PB II biopsies are recommended for better analysis. Biopsy of PBs is considered less invasive than biopsy of a blastomere or trophectoderm, and the use of aCGH in PB biopsy was shown to have improved implantation rates [74]. Furthermore, the multicenter randomized control trial set by the ESHRE Task force reported that PGS using the first and the second PB by aCGH increases the delivery rates significantly in patients with advanced maternal age [75]. One of the pitfalls of polar body biopsy is that oocytes diagnosed as aneuploid may actually form a euploid embryo due to a chromatid predivision error in MI with a balanced segregation at MII [75, 76]. Moreover, Geraedts and colleagues (2011) reported that at least 1 in 10 oocytes biopsied do not provide a diagnostic result [75]. Therefore, embryos with no diagnostic results and developed normally are either discarded or biopsied at a later stage. This increases the labor for both embryology and genetics teams, and it causes an added economical burden to the patients.

With the recent improvements in IVF laboratories, blastocyst biopsy has become the preferred method for PGS. In the past, one of the main problems of performing blastocyst biopsy was the limited time allowed for the diagnosis since the embryonic cells are either biopsied on day 5 or on day 6 for the slow developing embryos. With the use of vitrification, high embryo survival rates were reported [77–80], and many centers have opted performing PGS at blastocyst stage [81]. Furthermore, vitrifying embryos provide chance of an embryo transfer during an unstimulated cycle that was shown to result in high pregnancy rates [82–84]. In good prognosis patients, a pilot randomized clinical trial showed that trophectoderm biopsy and use of aCGH for PGS increases the implantation and ongoing pregnancy rates [85]. The pitfall of trophectoderm biopsy is that some embryos may not reach to the blastocyst stage in vitro that may be viable in utero [86]. As an added evaluation of aneuploidy screening, mitochondrial DNA (mtDNA) copy number has been investigated in euploid embryos showing that high mtDNA copy number indicates lower embryo viability and implantation [87, 88].

In addition to the array comparative genomic hybridization (aCGH) platforms, validation and the initial applications of single-nucleotide polymorphism (SNP) arrays [22, 76, 89–91] and next generation sequencing (NGS) platforms [92–96] showed promising results for their use in PGS. With the use of SNP arrays, the aneuploidies including monosomies or partial deletions as well as parental origin of any chromosomal abnormality can be identified [97].

Although PGD is widely accepted and applied throughout the world, there is still an ongoing debate on whether PGS is beneficial to infertile couples due to variable success rates depending on the maternal age, the technique used and the time of biopsy. Therefore, more and more studies are being developed for indirect aneuploidy assessment of the embryos.

5. PGD for translocations

Up until recently, the most common technique used to detect translocations in PGD was FISH. Polymerase chain reaction (PCR), which has been widely used to detect monogenic disorders, has also been used to detect translocations in PGD [98]. Other techniques that have been introduced to detect translocations in PGD are aCGH and more recently SNP arrays and NGS platforms.

5.1. PGD for translocations by FISH

FISH is a cytogenetic technique that had been used to detect structural chromosome analysis for patients with translocations and X-linked disorders. FISH is based on the hybridization of interphase chromosomes on specific DNA probes [99]. Although FISH is a rapid and accurate technique, it is limited as only a few chromosomes can be examined in a single cell. Moreover, it is restricted to analyze only the regions known to have imbalances. Signal interpretation is very important for correct diagnosis since the hybridization efficiency with each successive round could be lowered due to signal splitting and signal overlap. Additionally, loss of micronuclei during fixation of the blastomere causes difficulties in diagnosis [100].

5.2. PGD for translocations by PCR

PCR, a technique to amplify DNA by in vitro enzymatic replication, is mainly used to detect monogenic disorders [37] and recently, to detect translocations [98]. PCR is a technically demanding procedure, especially single cell PCR for PGD. The most important issues with PCR are the high risk of contamination, allele dropout (ADO) and amplification failure. ADO, which occurs when one of the alleles fails to amplify in a heterozygote cell for that particular region and is usually caused by a low amount of DNA in single cell PCR procedures, incomplete lysis or imperfect denaturation temperature [101], could lead to a misdiagnosis [101]. Fluorescent-PCR and multiplex PCR, which are more sensitive than conventional PCR, can be used to lower the ADO risk and amplification failure [102]. Although PCR has its limitations, it has the potential to conquer the drawbacks of FISH in detecting translocations.

Quantitative fluorescent PCR (QF-PCR) has been incorporated to the analysis of chromosomal imbalances. Studies have shown that QF-PCR is a sensitive, rapid and accurate technique that has been applied to study chromosomal abnormalities in spontaneous miscarriages [103] and in prenatal diagnosis [104]. Not only the parental and meiotic origin of aneuploidy can be detected by QF-PCR by using semi/fully informative short tandem repeat (STR) markers, but also the possible recombination events can be analyzed using informative STR markers. QF-PCR results of this study are preliminary, and more studies must be carried out.

5.3. PGD for translocations by array comparative genomic hybridization

aCGH, which is a similar technique to metaphase CGH, is used to determine total or partial aneuploidy by detecting chromosomal gains and losses of the entire genome [105]. Manual identification of chromosomes is not required with aCGH, and this technique has higher sensitivity and specificity for small genomic changes [106]. aCGH not only is used in prenatal diagnoses for identification of translocations [107, 108] and being reported as a rapid technique to detect de novo chromosome imbalances [109] but also is used to detect translocations in PGD clinically [110–112].

The comprehensive chromosome screening using aCGH has an added advantage to FISH in detecting aneuploidies and interchromosomal effect. Interchromosomal effect is the phenomenon known as the interference of chromosomes involved in rearrangement with the segregation of the structurally normal chromosomes [113–115]. Twenty-four chromosome aneuploidy screening revealed that segregation errors occur at high frequency even for the chromosomes not tested by FISH [8, 9, 20, 100, 116–120]. Furthermore, aCGH can detect copy number differences more precisely compared to FISH and PCR analyses since these methods are at much lower resolution than aCGH [121]. However, one of the limitations of aCGH is its inability to detect ploidy [122].

The methodology of aCGH is similar to metaphase-CGH, such that the only difference is that aCGH does not require metaphase chromosomes, and it can use target DNA for hybridization from cloned DNA segments, such as PCR-generated sequences, bacterial artificial chromosome (BAC) and cDNA clones [49]. More importantly, aCGH is much faster technique compared to metaphase CGH in detecting chromosomal abnormalities within less than 1 day [123]. The test and reference DNA are labeled with green and red fluorochromes, respectively. After hybridizing the labeled test and reference DNA on the array covered with BAC/cDNA clones or PCR-generated sequences, an array scanner captures the scanned image and computer systems are used to analyze the ratio of green to red fluorescence. If the test DNA is normal, the ratio of green to red signal should be 1:1. If the test DNA is monosomic, the green labeled chromosome will be less compared to the red labeled, and therefore, the ratio of green to red ratio is decreased and vice versa [124].

One of the most important advantages of aCGH is that it requires a small amount of genomic DNA for hybridization, as low as 2–4 μg [44]. However, in PGD/PGS, WGA, a technique used to amplify the whole genome for molecular analysis using small amounts of DNA [125], is fundamental. This technique can abolish DNA as being a limiting factor for genetic analysis by generating large quantities of DNA from starting material as small as 6pg, such as from a single blastomere [126]. Multiple WGA techniques have been used in the past, such as primer extension preamplification [127], linker-adaptor PCR [128], degenerate oligonucleotide primed-PCR [9, 129–131] and multiple displacement amplification [132–134].

5.4. PGD for translocations by single nucleotide polymorphism arrays

SNP arrays consist of oligonucleotide probes and most of them examine between 10,000–500,000 SNPs with high accuracy and reproducibility. SNP arrays utilize an approach similar to metaphase-CGH, such that the labeled test sample is hybridized separately on a different area of the array than the reference sample that is analyzed in parallel. The alleles detected at each SNP locus for the embryo are compared with the SNPs detected for the parents, and then, fluorescence intensities obtained for the test (embryo) and reference samples are analyzed by the brightness of the signals obtained. Brighter signals of the test sample indicate excess of that chromosome and *vice versa* [135].

The main advantage of SNP arrays is that they can determine the inheritance of genes that can allow simultaneous analysis of monogenic diseases and chromosome rearrangements, such as translocations including the balanced translocations unlike aCGH or FISH [100]. The drawback of SNP arrays is their high susceptibility to noise and bias, especially with the amplified single cell samples. SNP arrays cannot detect duplications. When SNP arrays are used in PGD/PGS, vitrification of embryos is necessary to enable enough time to complete the procedure [135].

SNP arrays have been applied in research to detect total aneuploidy and structural chromosomal imbalances to identify disease risks such as for type-2 diabetes, prostate cancer, glaucoma and some cardiovascular conditions [136]. SNP arrays were shown to analyze the copy number differences and chromosomal instability in studies following WGA of cells from cell lines [100] and amplified blastomeres from human cleavage-stage embryos [22, 137, 138]. Clinical applications of SNP arrays have been reported for several cancers [139] and for Gaucher disease and Marfan syndrome following blastomere biopsy [140]. SNP arrays have also been clinically applied in PGD and PGS [141–143].

5.5. PGD for translocations by next-generation sequencing

NGS is a technology that is used to sequence the nucleotides in a massively parallel manner. With the use of NGS, higher throughput data with lower cost can be obtained in a faster way compared to Sanger sequencing. Furthermore, for NGS platforms, bacterial cloning procedures are not required. On the other hand, NGS technologies require complex alignment algorithms in order to assemble and map the genome using short reads [144]. Up until this year, three main NGS platforms have been introduced, Roche (454), Life technologies and Illumina. Roche (454) generates 700 base pair fragments of approximately 1 million reads [145]. With the Life Technologies platform, semiconductor-sequencing technology has been used with solid-state pH meter. In this platform, proton generates up to 200 bp fragments of about 60–80 million reads. This technology generates up to 10 Gb of sequence in every run [145]. Illumina's platform generates up to 150 bp fragments of about 6 billion reads with approximately 1.8 Tb of sequence in each run over a period of 3 days [145]. Since NGS has become cost-effective, this comprehensive analysis has been applied in assessment of numerical and structural chromosomal abnormalities in PGS and PGD [96, 141, 146–149].

6. Conclusion

One of the most important reasons of the development of PGD was to avoid termination of pregnancy or avoid a severe congenital abnormality. Soon after the PGD implications have developed; PGS has been introduced aiming to select a euploid embryo to improve the implantation rates and avoid spontaneous abortions. However, PGD is not an easy reproductive option especially since there is no guarantee of pregnancy or even an embryo transfer in cases where all the embryos have the mutation or chromosomal imbalance [72]. Complex and multidisciplinary approaches are required for a successful PGD cycle combining the expertise of geneticists, embryologists and fertility doctors. Each PGD cycle starts with genetic counseling, fertility assessment, hormonal ovarian stimulation, development of embryos in vitro, biopsy of these embryos and preimplantation genetic testing of the embryonic samples. Initial studies were performed by a molecular cytogenetic technique, FISH, with some limitations including problems with fixation of the nucleus, hybridization problems and intensity of the fluorescence of the probes. As the newer technologies have been introduced, the fields of PGD and PGS have also improved. In the last past few years, with the development of aCGH, SNP arrays and NGS technologies, precise and reliable results have obtained from embryo biopsies with improvements in the implantation and take home baby rates.

Author details

Pinar Tulay

Address all correspondence to: pinar.tulay@neu.edu.tr

Near East University, Department of Medical Genetics, Faculty of Medicine, Nicosia, North Cyprus

References

[1] Jaroudi, S. and S. SenGupta, DNA repair in mammalian embryos. Mutat Res, 2007. **635**(1): pp. 53-77.

[2] William, L., Human Embryology. Vol. 2nd edition. Churchill Livingstone, New York. 1997.

[3] Schultz, R.M., The molecular foundations of the maternal to zygotic transition in the preimplantation embryo. Hum Reprod Update, 2002. **8**(4): pp. 323-331.

[4] Moore, K. and T.V.N. Persaud, The Developing Human. Saunders Company, Philadelphia. Vol. 6. 1998.

[5] Telford, N.A., A.J. Watson, and G.A. Schultz, Transition from maternal to embryonic control in early mammalian development: a comparison of several species. Mol Reprod Dev, 1990. **26**(1): pp. 90-100.

[6] Bell, C.E., M.D. Calder, and A.J. Watson, Genomic RNA profiling and the programme controlling preimplantation mammalian development. Mol Hum Reprod, 2008. **14**(12): pp. 691-701.

[7] Traversa, M.V., L. Carey, and D. Leigh, A molecular strategy for routine preimplantation genetic diagnosis in both reciprocal and Robertsonian translocation carriers. Mol Hum Reprod, 2010. **16**(5): pp. 329-337.

[8] Voullaire, L., et al., Chromosome analysis of blastomeres from human embryos by using comparative genomic hybridization. Hum Genet, 2000. **106**: pp. 210-217.

[9] Wells, D. and J.D. Delhanty, Comprehensive chromosomal analysis of human preimplantation embryos using whole genome amplification and single cell comparative genomic hybridization. Mol Hum Reprod, 2000. **6**: pp. 1055-1062.

[10] Kuliev, A., et al., Chromosomal abnormalities in a series of 6,733 human oocytes in preimplantation diagnosis for age-related aneuploidies. Reprod Biomed Online, 2003. **6**(1): pp. 54-59.

[11] Pellestor, F., et al., Maternal aging and chromosomal abnormalities: new data drawn from in vitro unfertilized human oocytes. Hum Genet, 2003. **112**(2): pp. 195-203.

[12] Fragouli, E., et al., Increased susceptibility to maternal aneuploidy demonstrated by comparative genomic hybridization analysis of human MII oocytes and first polar bodies. Cytogenet Genome Res, 2006. **114**(1): pp. 30-38.

[13] Kim, J.W., et al., Chromosomal abnormalities in spontaneous abortion after assisted reproductive treatment. BMC Med Genet, 2010. **11**(153). pp. 1-6

[14] Hodes-Wertz, B., et al., Idiopathic recurrent miscarriage is caused mostly by aneuploid embryos. Fertil Steril, 2012. **98**(3): pp. 675-680.

[15] Raziel, A., et al., Increased frequency of female partner chromosomal abnormalities in patients with high-order implantation failure after in vitro fertilization. Fertil Steril, 2002. **78**(3): pp. 515-519.

[16] Munne, S., et al., Outcome of preimplantation genetic diagnosis of translocations. Fertil Steril, 2000. **73**(6): pp. 1209-1218.

[17] Verlinsky, Y., et al., Preimplantation testing for chromosomal disorders improves reproductive outcome of poor-prognosis patients. Reprod Biomed Online, 2005. **11**(2): pp. 219-225.

[18] Munne, S., et al., Preimplantation genetic diagnosis reduces pregnancy loss in women aged 35 years and older with a history of recurrent miscarriages. Fertil Steril, 2005. **84**(2): pp. 331-335.

[19] Liang, L., et al., Identification of chromosomal errors in human preimplantation embryos with oligonucleotide DNA microarray. PLoS One, 2013. **8**(4): pp. e61838–e61838.

[20] Fiorentino, F., et al., PGD for reciprocal and Robertsonian translocations using array comparative genomic hybridization. Hum Reprod, 2011. **26**: pp. 1925-1935.

[21] Simopoulou, M., et al., Preimplantation genetic diagnosis of chromosome abnormalities: implications from the outcome for couples with chromosomal rearrangements. Prenat Diagn, 2003. **23**(8): pp. 652-662.

[22] Vanneste, E., et al., Chromosome instability is common in human cleavage-stage embryos. Nat Med, 2009. **15**(5): pp. 577-583.

[23] Anton, E., et al., Sperm FISH studies in seven male carriers of Robertsonian translocation t(13;14)(q10;q10). Hum Reprod, 2004. **19**(6): pp. 1345-1351.

[24] Faraut, T., et al., Cooperation of selection and meiotic mechanisms in the production of imbalances in reciprocal translocations. Cytogenet Cell Genet, 2000. **88**: pp. 15-21.

[25] Scriven, P.N., A.H. Handyside, and C.M. Ogilvie, Chromosome translocations: segregation modes and strategies for preimplantation genetic diagnosis. Prenat Diagn, 1998. **18**(13): pp. 1437-1449.

[26] Estop, A.M., V. Van Kirk, and K. Cieply, Segregation analysis of four translocations, t(2;18), t(3;15), t(5;7), and t(10;12), by sperm chromosome studies and a review of the literature. Cytogenet Cell Genet, 1995. **70**(1-2): pp. 80-87.

[27] Gardner, R.J.M. and G.R. Sutherland, Chromosome Abnormalities and Genetic Counselling. 2nd ed. Oxford University Press, New York. 1996.

[28] Doheny, K.F., et al., Segregation of a familial balanced (12;10) insertion resulting in Dup(10)(q21.2q22.1) and Del(10)(q21.2q22.1) in first cousins. Am J Med Genet, 1997. **69**(2): pp. 188-193.

[29] Kang, S.H., et al., Insertional translocation detected using FISH confirmation of array-comparative genomic hybridization (aCGH) results. Am J Med Genet A, 2010. **152A**(5): pp. 1111-1126.

[30] Van Hemel, J.O. and H.J. Eussen, Interchromosomal insertions. Identification of five cases and a review. Hum Genet, 2000. **107**: pp. 415-432.

[31] De Braekeleer, M. and T.N. Dao, Cytogenetic studies in male infertility: a review. Hum Reprod, 1991. **6**: pp. 245-250.

[32] Gabriel-Robez, O. and Y. Rumpler, The meiotic pairing behaviour in human spermatocytes carrier of chromosome anomalies and their repercussions on reproductive fitness I: Inversions and insertions. Ann Génét, 1994. **37**: pp. 3-10.

[33] Handyside, A.H., et al., Pregnancies from biopsied human preimplantation embryos sexed by Y-specific DNA amplification. Nature, 1990. **344**: pp. 768-770.

[34] Kaplan, B., et al., Viability of embryos following second polar body removal in a mouse model. J Assist Reprod Genet, 1995. **12**(10): pp. 747-749.

[35] Dreesen, J.C., et al., RS46(DXS548) genotyping of reproductive cells: approaching preimplantation testing of the fragile-X syndrome. Hum Genet, 1995. **96**(3): pp. 323-329.

[36] Goossens, V., et al., Diagnostic efficiency, embryonic development and clinical outcome after the biopsy of one or two blastomeres for preimplantation genetic diagnosis. Hum Reprod, 2008. **23**(3): pp. 481-492.

[37] Goossens, V., et al., ESHRE PGD Consortium data collection IX: cycles from January to December 2006 with pregnancy follow-up to October 2007. Hum Reprod, 2009. **24**(8): pp. 1786-1810.

[38] Munne, S., et al., Diagnosis of major chromosome aneuploidies in human preimplantation embryos. Hum Reprod, 1993. **8**(12): pp. 2185-2191.

[39] Delhanty, J.D., et al., Detection of aneuploidy and chromosomal mosaicism in human embryos during preimplantation sex determination by fluorescent in situ hybridisation, (FISH). Hum Mol Genet, 1993. **2**(8): pp. 1183-1185.

[40] Harper, J.C., et al., Mosaicism of autosomes and sex chromosomes in morphologically normal, monospermic preimplantation human embryos. Prenat Diagn, 1995. **15**(1): pp. 41-49.

[41] Delhanty, J.D., et al., Multicolour FISH detects frequent chromosomal mosaicism and chaotic division in normal preimplantation embryos from fertile patients. Hum Genet, 1997. **99**(6): pp. 755-760.

[42] Munne, S., et al., Preimplantation diagnosis of the aneuploidies most commonly found in spontaneous abortions and live births: XY, 13, 14, 15, 16, 18, 21, 22. Prenat Diagn, 1998. **18**(13): pp. 1459-1466.

[43] Los, F.J., D. Van Opstal, and C. van den Berg, The development of cytogenetically normal, abnormal and mosaic embryos: a theoretical model. Hum Reprod Update, 2004. **10**(1): pp. 79-94.

[44] Basille, C., et al., Preimplantation genetic diagnosis: state of the art. Eur J Obstet Gynecol Reprod Biol, 2009. **145**(1): pp. 9-13.

[45] McArthur, S.J., et al., Blastocyst trophectoderm biopsy and preimplantation genetic diagnosis for familial monogenic disorders and chromosomal translocations. Prenat Diagn, 2008. **28**(5): pp. 434-442.

[46] Sandalinas, M., et al., Developmental ability of chromosomally abnormal human embryos to develop to the blastocyst stage. Hum Reprod, 2001. **16**(9): pp. 1954-1958.

[47] Bielanska, M., et al., Diploid-aneuploid mosaicism in human embryos cultured to the blastocyst stage. Fertil Steril, 2005. **84**(2): pp. 336-342.

[48] Richeldi, L., et al., T cell-based tracking of multidrug resistant tuberculosis infection after brief exposure. Am J Respir Crit Care Med, 2004. **170**(3): pp. 288-295.

[49] Wells, D. and B. Levy, Cytogenetics in reproductive medicine: the contribution of comparative genomic hybridization (CGH). Bioessays, 2003. **25**(3): pp. 289-300.

[50] Wells, D. and J.D. Delhanty, Preimplantation genetic diagnosis: applications for molecular medicine. Trends Mol Med, 2001. **7**(1): pp. 23-30.

[51] Hassold, T., H. Hall, and P. Hunt, The origin of human aneuploidy: where we have been, where we are going. Hum Mol Genet, 2007. **16 Spec No. 2**: pp. R203–R208.

[52] Spandorfer, S.D., et al., Relationship between maternal age and aneuploidy in in vitro fertilization pregnancy loss. Fertil Steril, 2004. **81**(5): pp. 1265-1269.

[53] Menasha, J., et al., Incidence and spectrum of chromosome abnormalities in spontaneous abortions: new insights from a 12-year study. Genet Med, 2005. **7**(4): pp. 251-263.

[54] Munne, S., et al., Improved implantation after preimplantation genetic diagnosis of aneuploidy. Reprod Biomed Online, 2003. **7**(1): pp. 91-97.

[55] Macklon, N.S., J.P. Geraedts, and B.C. Fauser, Conception to ongoing pregnancy: the 'black box' of early pregnancy loss. Hum Reprod Update, 2002. **8**(4): pp. 333-343.

[56] Iwarsson, E., et al., A high degree of aneuploidy in frozen-thawed human preimplantation embryos. Hum Genet, 1999. **104**(5): pp. 376-382.

[57] Munne, S., et al., The use of first polar bodies for preimpantation diagnosis of aneuploidy. Hum Reprod, 1995. **10**: pp. 1015-1021.

[58] Munne, S., et al., Assessment of numeric abnormalities of X, Y, 18, and 16 chromosomes in preimplantation human embryos before transfer. Am J Obstet Gynecol, 1995. **172**(4 Pt 1): pp. 1191-9; discussion 1199-201.

[59] Verlinsky, Y., et al., Pregnancies following pre-conception diagnosis of common aneuploidies by fluorescent in-situ hybridization. Hum Reprod, 1995. **10**(7): pp. 1923-1927.

[60] Goossens, V., et al., ESHRE PGD Consortium data collection XI: cycles from January to December 2008 with pregnancy follow-up to October 2009. Hum Reprod, 2012. **27**(7): pp. 1887-1911.

[61] Hardarson, T., et al., Preimplantation genetic screening in women of advanced maternal age caused a decrease in clinical pregnancy rate: a randomized controlled trial. Hum Reprod, 2008. **23**(12): pp. 2806-2812.

[62] Staessen, C., et al., Comparison of blastocyst transfer with or without preimplantation genetic diagnosis for aneuploidy screening in couples with advanced maternal age: a prospective randomized controlled trial. Hum Reprod, 2004. **19**(12): pp. 2849-2858.

[63] Staessen, C., et al., Preimplantation genetic screening does not improve delivery rate in women under the age of 36 following single-embryo transfer. Hum Reprod, 2008. **23**(12): pp. 2818-2825.

[64] Mastenbroek, S., et al., What next for preimplantation genetic screening? More randomized controlled trials needed? Hum Reprod, 2008. **23**(12): pp. 2626-2628.

[65] Mastenbroek, S., et al., Preimplantation genetic screening: a systematic review and meta-analysis of RCTs. Hum Reprod Update, 2011. **17**(4): pp. 454-466.

[66] Mastenbroek, S., et al., In vitro fertilization with preimplantation genetic screening. N Engl J Med, 2007. **357**(1): pp. 9-17.

[67] Debrock, S., et al., Preimplantation genetic screening for aneuploidy of embryos after in vitro fertilization in women aged at least 35 years: a prospective randomized trial. Fertil Steril, 2010. **93**(2): pp. 364-373.

[68] Schoolcraft, W.B., et al., Preimplantation aneuploidy testing for infertile patients of advanced maternal age: a randomized prospective trial. Fertil Steril, 2009. **92**(1): pp. 157-162.

[69] Blockeel, C., et al., Prospectively randomized controlled trial of PGS in IVF/ICSI patients with poor implantation. Reprod Biomed Online, 2008. **17**(6): pp. 848-854.

[70] Mersereau, J.E., et al., Preimplantation genetic screening to improve in vitro fertilization pregnancy rates: a prospective randomized controlled trial. Fertil Steril, 2008. **90**(4): pp. 1287-1289.

[71] Meyer, L.R., et al., A prospective randomized controlled trial of preimplantation genetic screening in the "good prognosis" patient. Fertil Steril, 2009. **91**(5): pp. 1731-1738.

[72] Harper, J.C., et al., ESHRE PGD Consortium data collection X: cycles from January to December 2007 with pregnancy follow-up to October 2008. Hum Reprod, 2010. **25**(11): pp. 2685-2707.

[73] Hens, K., et al., Dynamics and ethics of comprehensive preimplantation genetic testing: a review of the challenges. Hum Reprod Update, 2013. **19**(4): pp. 366-375.

[74] Magli, M.C., et al., Polar body array CGH for prediction of the status of the corresponding oocyte. Part II: technical aspects. Hum Reprod, 2011. **26**(11): pp. 3181-3185.

[75] Geraedts, J., et al., Polar body array CGH for prediction of the status of the corresponding oocyte. Part I: clinical results. Hum Reprod, 2011. **26**(11): pp. 3173-3180.

[76] Scott, R.T., Jr., et al., Comprehensive chromosome screening is highly predictive of the reproductive potential of human embryos: a prospective, blinded, nonselection study. Fertil Steril, 2012. **97**(4): pp. 870-875.

[77] Kokkali, G., et al., Birth of a healthy infant following trophectoderm biopsy from blastocysts for PGD of beta-thalassaemia major. Hum Reprod, 2005. **20**(7): pp. 1855-1859.

[78] McArthur, S.J., et al., Pregnancies and live births after trophectoderm biopsy and preimplantation genetic testing of human blastocysts. Fertil Steril, 2005. **84**(6): pp. 1628-1636.

[79] Youssry, M., et al., Current aspects of blastocyst cryopreservation. Reprod Biomed Online, 2008. **16**(2): pp. 311-320.

[80] Tulay, P., et al., Number of embryos biopsied as a predictive indicator for the outcome of preimplantation genetic diagnosis by fluorescence in situ hybridisation in translocation cases. Zygote, 2014. **24**(1):107-14.

[81] Van Landuyt, L., et al., Influence of cell loss after vitrification or slow-freezing on further in vitro development and implantation of human Day 3 embryos. Hum Reprod, 2013. **28**(11):2943-9.

[82] Chang, E.M., et al., Use of the natural cycle and vitrification thawed blastocyst transfer results in better in-vitro fertilization outcomes: cycle regimens of vitrification thawed blastocyst transfer. J Assist Reprod Genet, 2011. **28**(4): pp. 369-374.

[83] Zhu, D., et al., Vitrified-warmed blastocyst transfer cycles yield higher pregnancy and implantation rates compared with fresh blastocyst transfer cycles—time for a new embryo transfer strategy? Fertil Steril, 2011. **95**(5): pp. 1691-1695.

[84] Ku, P.Y., et al., Comparison of the clinical outcomes between fresh blastocyst and vitrified-thawed blastocyst transfer. J Assist Reprod Genet, 2012. **29**(12): pp. 1353-1356.

[85] Yang, Z., et al., Selection of single blastocysts for fresh transfer via standard morphology assessment alone and with array CGH for good prognosis IVF patients: results from a randomized pilot study. Mol Cytogenet, 2012. **5**(1): pp. 24.

[86] Parriego, M., F. Vidal, and A. Veiga, Blastocyst Biopsy, in Preimplantation Genetic Diagnosis, J. Harper, Editor. 2009, Cambridge University Press: Cambridge.

[87] Diez-Juan, A., et al., Mitochondrial DNA content as a viability score in human euploid embryos: less is better. Fertil Steril, 2015. **104**(3): pp. 534-541.

[88] Fragouli, E., et al., Altered levels of mitochondrial DNA are associated with female age, aneuploidy, and provide an independent measure of embryonic implantation potential. PLoS Genet, 2015. **11**(6): pp. e1005241.

[89] Treff, N.R., et al., Single nucleotide polymorphism microarray-based concurrent screening of 24-chromosome aneuploidy and unbalanced translocations in preimplantation human embryos. Fertil Steril, 2011. **95**: pp. 1606-1612.

[90] Forman, E.J., et al., Single embryo transfer with comprehensive chromosome screening results in improved ongoing pregnancy rates and decreased miscarriage rates. Hum Reprod, 2012. **27**: pp. 1217-1222.

[91] Treff, N.R., et al., Accurate 23 chromosome aneuploidy screening in human blastomeres using single nucleotide polymorphism (SNP) microarrays. Fertil Steril, 2007. **86**(S217): pp. S1.

[92] Fiorentino, F., et al., Development and validation of a next-generation sequencing-based protocol for 24-chromosome aneuploidy screening of embryos. Fertil Steril, 2014. **101**(5): pp. 1375-1382.

[93] Fiorentino, F., et al., Application of next-generation sequencing technology for comprehensive aneuploidy screening of blastocysts in clinical preimplantation genetic screening cycles. Hum Reprod, 2014. **29**(12):2802-13.

[94] Wells, D., et al., Clinical utilisation of a rapid low-pass whole genome sequencing technique for the diagnosis of aneuploidy in human embryos prior to implantation. J Med Genet, 2014. **51**(8): pp. 553-562.

[95] Wang, L., et al., Detection of chromosomal aneuploidy in human preimplantation embryos by next-generation sequencing. Biol Reprod, 2014. **90**(5): p. 95.

[96] Yin, X., et al., Massively parallel sequencing for chromosomal abnormality testing in trophectoderm cells of human blastocysts. Biol Reprod, 2013. **88**(3): p. 69.

[97] Brezina, P.R., et al., Single-gene testing combined with single nucleotide polymorphism microarray preimplantation genetic diagnosis for aneuploidy: a novel approach in optimizing pregnancy outcome. Fertil Steril, 2011. **95**(5): pp. 1786 e5–e8.

[98] Fiorentino, F., et al., Polymerase chain reaction-based detection of chromosomal imbalances on embryos: the evolution of preimplantation genetic diagnosis for chromosomal translocations. Fertil Steril, 2010. **94**(6):2001-11.

[99] Griffin, D.K., et al., Dual fluorescent in situ hybridisation for simultaneous detection of X and Y chromosome-specific probes for the sexing of human preimplantation embryonic nuclei. Hum Genet, 1992. **89**(1): pp. 18-22.

[100] Treff, N.R., et al., Accurate single cell 24 chromosome aneuploidy screening using whole genome amplification and single nucleotide polymorphism microarrays. Fertil Steril, 2010. **94**: pp. 2017-2021.

[101] Spits, C. and K. Sermon, PGD for monogenic disorders: aspects of molecular biology. Prenat Diagn, 2009. **29**(1): pp. 50-56.

[102] Dreesen, J.C., et al., Multiplex PCR of polymorphic markers flanking the CFTR gene; a general approach for preimplantation genetic diagnosis of cystic fibrosis. Mol Hum Reprod, 2000. **6**(5): pp. 391-396.

[103] Ban, Z., et al., Rapid diagnosis of triploidy of maternal origin using fluorescent PCR and DNA fragment analysis in the third trimester of pregnancy. Prenat Diagn, 2002. **22**(11): pp. 984-987.

[104] Hulten, M.A., S. Dhanjal, and B. Pertl, Rapid and simple prenatal diagnosis of common chromosome disorders: advantages and disadvantages of the molecular methods FISH and QF-PCR. Reproduction, 2003. **126**(3): pp. 279-297.

[105] Weiss, M.M., et al., Comparative genomic hybridisation. Mol Pathol, 1999. **52**(5): pp. 243-251.

[106] Solinas-Toldo, S., et al., Matrix-based comparative genomic hybridization: biochips to screen for genomic imbalances. Genes Chromosomes Cancer, 1997. **20**(4): pp. 399-407.

[107] Callier, P., et al., Contribution of array CGH in prognosis and genetic counselling of prenatally diagnosed supernumerary ring chromosome 20. Prenat Diagn, 2009. **29**(10): pp. 1002-1005.

[108] Colmant, C., et al., Interstitial deletion 6p22.3-p24.3 characterized by CGH array in a foetus with multiple malformations. Prenat Diagn, 2009. **29**(9): pp. 908-910.

[109] Vialard, F., et al., Array comparative genomic hybridization in prenatal diagnosis: another experience. Fetal Diagn Ther, 2009. **25**(2): pp. 277-284.

[110] PGDIS, 10th international congress on preimplantation genetic diagnosis, in Trophectoderm biopsy and array CGH to detect unbalanced forms of t(9;15)(q22.2;q11.1) R. Edwards, et al., Editors. 2010, Reproductive BioMedicine online: Montpellier.

[111] Christodoulou, C., et al., Preimplantation genetic diagnosis for chromosomal rearrangements with the use of array comparative genomic hybridization at the blastocyst stage. Fertil Steril, 2017. **107**(1):212-219.e3.

[112] Garcia-Herrero, S., et al., Genetic analysis of human preimplantation embryos. Curr Top Dev Biol., 2016. **120**: pp. 421-447.

[113] Alfarawati, S., et al., Embryos of robertsonian translocation carriers exhibit a mitotic interchromosomal effect that enhances genetic instability during early development. PLoS Genet, 2012. **8**(10): p. e1003025.

[114] Estop, A.M., et al., Is there an interchromosomal effect in reciprocal translocation carriers? Sperm FISH studies. Hum Genet, 2000. **106**(5): pp. 517-524.

[115] Munne, S., et al., Negligible interchromosomal effect in embryos of Robertsonian translocation carriers. Reprod Biomed Online, 2005. **10**(3): pp. 363-369.

[116] Fishel, S., et al., Live birth after polar body array comparative genomic hybridization prediction of embryo ploidy the future of IVF? Fertil Steril, 2010. **3**: pp. 1006.e7-1006.e10.

[117] Treff, N.R., et al., SNP microarray-based 24 chromosome aneuploidy screening is significantly more consistent than FISH. Mol Hum Reprod 2010. **8**: pp. 583-589.

[118] Schoolcraft, W.B., et al., Clinical application of comprehensive chromosomal screening at the blastocyst stage. Fertil Steril, 2010. **94**: pp. 1700-1706.

[119] Fiorentino, F., Array comparative genomic hybridization: its role in preimplantation genetic diagnosis. Curr Opin Obstet Gynecol, 2012. **4**: pp. 203-209.

[120] Gutierrez-Mateo, C., et al., Validation of microarray comparative genomic hybridization for comprehensive chromosome analysis of embryos. Fertil Steril, 2011. **3**: pp. 953-958.

[121] Shaffer, L.G. and B.A. Bejjani, A cytogeneticist's perspective on genomic microarrays. Hum Reprod Update, 2004. **10**(3): pp. 221-226.

[122] Harper, J.C. and G. Harton, The use of arrays in preimplantation genetic diagnosis and screening. Fertil Steril, 2010. **94**(4): pp. 1173-1177.

[123] Le Caignec, C., et al., Single-cell chromosomal imbalances detection by array CGH. Nucleic Acids Res, 2006. **34**(9): p. e68.

[124] Daphnis, D.D., et al., Analysis of the evolution of chromosome abnormalities in human embryos from Day 3 to 5 using CGH and FISH. Mol Hum Reprod, 2008. **14**(2): pp. 117-125.

[125] Luthra, R. and L.J. Medeiros, Isothermal multiple displacement amplification: a highly reliable approach for generating unlimited high molecular weight genomic DNA from clinical specimens. J Mol Diagn, 2004. **6**(3): pp. 236-242.

[126] Pinard, R., et al., Assessment of whole genome amplification-induced bias through high-throughput, massively parallel whole genome sequencing. BMC Genomics, 2006. **7**: p. 216.

[127] Zhang, L., et al., Whole genome amplification from a single cell: implications for genetic analysis. Proc Natl Acad Sci U S A, 1992. **89**(13): pp. 5847-5851.

[128] Peng, W., H. Takabayashi, and K. Ikawa, Whole genome amplification from single cells in preimplantation genetic diagnosis and prenatal diagnosis. Eur J Obstet Gynecol Reprod Biol, 2007. **131**(1): pp. 13-20.

[129] Barbaux, S., O. Poirier, and F. Cambien, Use of degenerate oligonucleotide primed PCR (DOP-PCR) for the genotyping of low-concentration DNA samples. J Mol Med, 2001. **79**(5-6): pp. 329-332.

[130] Voullaire, L., et al., Detection of aneuploidy in single cells using comparative genomic hybridization. Prenat Diagn, 1999. **19**(9): pp. 846-851.

[131] Little, E.S., et al., Array CGH using whole genome amplification of fresh-frozen and formalin-fixed, paraffin-embedded tumor DNA. Genomics, 2005. **87**(2): pp. 298-306.

[132] Lasken, R.S. and M. Egholm, Whole genome amplification: abundant supplies of DNA from precious samples or clinical specimens. Trends Biotechnol, 2003. **21**(12): pp. 531-535.

[133] O'Geen, H., et al., Comparison of sample preparation methods for ChIP-chip assays. Biotechniques, 2006. **41**(5): pp. 577-580.

[134] Talseth-Palmer, B.A., et al., Whole genome amplification and its impact on CGH array profiles. BMC Res Notes, 2008. **1**(56): pp. 1-8.

[135] Wells, D., S. Alfarawati, and E. Fragouli, Use of comprehensive chromosomal screening for embryo assessment: microarrays and CGH. Mol Hum Reprod, 2008. **14**(12): pp. 703-710.

[136] Kittai, A., E. Widra, and R. Leach, SNP PGD microarray analysis from single embryonic cell. in ASHG. 2008.

[137] Handyside, A.H., et al., Karyomapping: a universal method for genome wide analysis of genetic disease based on mapping crossovers between parental haplotypes. J Med Genet, 2010. **47**(10): pp. 651-658.

[138] Kearns, W.G., et al. Comprehensive Preimplantation Genetin Diagnosis(PGD) by single cell SNP microarrays. in ASHG. 2009.

[139] PGDIS, 10th international congress on preimplantation genetic diagnosis, in Comprehensive microarray genetic analyses on single cell(s) from polar bodies or embryos to determine 23-chromosome aneuploidy, structural chromosome aberrations and genome-wide scans using single nucleotide polymorphisms (SNPs); to identify what partner provided the extra chromosome in aneuploid embryos; and to determine what embryo implanted following an in vitro fertilisation (IVF) cycle. R. Edwards, et al., Editors. 2010, Reproductive BioMedicine online: Montpellier.

[140] PGDIS, 10th international congress on preimplantation genetic diagnosis, in First clinical application of karyomapping for PGD of Gaucher disease combined with 24 chromosome screening. R. Edwards, et al., Editors. 2010, Reproductive BioMedicine online: Montpellier.

[141] Tan, Y., et al., Clinical outcome of preimplantation genetic diagnosis and screening using next generation sequencing. Gigascience, 2014. **3**(1): pp. 30.

[142] Xu, J., et al., Comparative study of single-nucleotide polymorphism array and next generation sequencing based strategies on triploid identification in preimplantation genetic diagnosis and screen. Oncotarget, 2016. **7**(49): 81839-81848.

[143] Ottolini, C.S., et al., Karyomapping identifies second polar body DNA persisting to the blastocyst stage: implications for embryo biopsy. Reprod Biomed Online, 2015. **31**(6): pp. 776-782.

[144] Miller, J.R., S. Koren, and G. Sutton, Assembly algorithms for next-generation sequencing data. Genomics 2010. **95**: pp. 315-327.

[145] Park, S.T. and J. Kim, Trends in next-generation sequencing and a new era for whole genome sequencing. Int Neurourol J, 2016. **20** (Suppl 2): pp. S76–S83.

[146] Zhang, W., et al., Clinical application of next-generation sequencing in preimplantation genetic diagnosis cycles for Robertsonian and reciprocal translocations. J Assist Reprod Genet, 2016. **33**(7): pp. 899-906.

[147] Lukaszuk, K., et al., Healthy baby born to a robertsonian translocation carrier following next-generation sequencing-based preimplantation genetic diagnosis: a case report. AJP Rep, 2015. **5**(2): pp. e172–e175.

[148] Zhang, C., et al., A single cell level based method for copy number variation analysis by low coverage massively parallel sequencing. PLoS One., 2013. **8**(1): pp. e54236.

[149] Aleksandrova, N., et al., Comparison of the results of preimplantation genetic screening obtained by a-CGH and NGS methods from the same embryos. Gynecol Endocrinol., 2016. **32**(suppl. 2): pp. 1-4.

Chapter 8

The Effect of *TBP-Related Factor 2* on Chromocenter Formation and Chromosome Segregation in *Drosophila Melanogaster*

Julia Vorontsova, Roman Cherezov and
Olga Simonova

Additional information is available at the end of the chapter

http://dx.doi.org/10.5772/67314

Abstract

Chromosome nondisjunction in meiosis causes the gene disbalance and a number of anomalies in development and fertility. Otherwise, genetically programmed sex-ratio meiotic drive occurs in a number of species. One of the forms of eukaryotic genome organization is a chromocenter evolutionally involved in the regulation of chromosome behavior in dividing cells among insects, plants, mammals, mollusks, and even yeast. In *Drosophila, TBP related factor 2 (Trf2)* belongs to a conservative *Tbp (TATA box-binding protein)* gene family and encodes a basic transcription factor. Recent data demonstrates that a decrease in TRF2 expression can result in the abnormalities of chromatin condensation; however, no details of this process have been studied. We demonstrated that a decrease in the TRF2 expression damaged proper chromocenter structure and abolished chromatin condensation and it was a reason for the chromosome nondisjunction. We found that compact chromocenter and correct homologue pairing were abolished in flies with a lower *Trf2* expression in germline and in somatic cells. We conclude that TRF2 can not only be involved in transcription activation, but also may perform structural function in pericentromeric heterochromatin organization. The possibility of TRF2 to regulate the evolutionary genetically programmed sex-ratio meiotic drive is discussed.

Keywords: chromocenter, chromosome nondisjunction, asinapsis, *TBP-related factor 2*, *Drosophila*

1. Introduction

Chromosome nondisjunction during meiosis causes the gene disbalance and, consequently, a number of anomalies in development and fertility. On the other hand, genetically programmed sex-ratio meiotic drive occurs in a number of animal species when mainly males or females are born, which is normal within the given species [1]. The genetic regulation of these processes is actively being studied. There are many factors that can result in the incorrect chromosome segregation. The correct segregation of sister chromatids between daughter cells depends on the coordinated interaction of centrosomes, centromeres, kinetochores, spindle fibrils, topoisomerases, proteolytic processes, and motor proteins [2]. On the other hand, chromosomes must be "prepared" (or structurally organized) when they enter meiosis (or mitosis). Structural disorganization of chromosome or same their regions that control the correct pairing of homologs during meiosis frequently results in the incorrect chromosome segregation. The one way of eukaryotic genome organization is chromocenter, which is evolutionally involved in the regulation of chromosome behavior in dividing cells not only among insects but also among plants, mammals, mollusks, and even yeast [3–7]. This nuclear structure arises in differentiated somatic and germ cells during interphase and meiotic prophase. The chromocenter is generated by the association of pericentromeric regions of all or separate groups of chromosomes and plays an important role in spatial organization of chromosomes [8]. Studies on *Drosophila* have clearly demonstrated that its disorganization leads to genomic disbalance [9, 10]. The screening for genes that control the formation and reorganization of chromocenter is performed [11, 12]. The high frequency of chromosome nondisjunction in the progeny of mutant parents is a main characteristic of mutations in these genes.

In *Drosophila, TBP-related factor 2* (*Trf2*) encodes an alternative basic transcription factor that is homologous to vertebrate *Trf2* protein and belongs to a conservative *TATA box-binding protein* (*Tbp*) gene family [13]. It was shown that previously discovered $lawc^{p1}$ (*leg-arista-wing complex*) mutation [14] appeared to be the only viable mutation that decreases *Trf2* gene expression [15]. The high conservatism of the *Trf2* protein allows us to study its functions on *Drosophila*.

In the previous studies, we demonstrated that the $lawc^{p1}$ mutation suppresses the phenotype of mutations in genes that encode polycomb group (PcG) proteins, which are negative epigenetic regulators of transcription via chromatin modification [16]. At the same time, we have found that $lawc^{p1}$ increased the effect of transvection (or allelic complementation [17]) caused by disruptions of the homologous chromosome pairing at a number of loci.

Recent data demonstrated that a decrease in *Trf2* gene expression could result in the disruption of chromatin condensation [18]; however, almost no details of this process have been studied. At the same time, we have noted frequent cases of chromosome nondisjunction during genetic experiments with hypomorphic *Trf2* mutations in *Drosophila melanogaster*. The question is whether a decrease in the *Trf2* gene expression really increases the frequency of chromosome nondisjunction in the female meiosis and if it is so, is this anomaly associated with an abnormal chromatin packaging (and particularly with the disruption in the chromocenter structure)?

Data of genetic experiments for the analysis of the frequency of X-chromosome nondisjunction in mutant lines and of cytogenetic experiments studding the structure of chromosomes in germ and somatic cells are presented below.

2. Analysis of frequency of X-chromosome nondisjunction in lines with lethal *Trf2* mutations

We calculated frequencies of X-chromosome nondisjunction in two groups of lines that contain lethal *Trf2* mutations. The lines of first group were obtained from Bloomington Drosophila Stock Centre: *l(1)G0039/FM7a*; *l(1)G0356/FM7a*; *l(1)G0424/FM7a*; *l(1)G0376/FM7a*; *l(1)G0425/FM7a*; *l(1)G0332/FM7a*; *l(1)G0152/FM7a*; *l(1)G0166/FM7a*; and *l(1)G0178/FM7a* [19]. Subsequently, we will call these lines "museum" lines. In museum lines, the lethality is caused by the integration of the *p{lacW}* transposon in the regulatory noncoding *Trf2* region (**Figure 1A**). Previously, we demonstrated that these lethal mutations did not complement *lawc*^{p1} mutation suggesting that they are in the same gene region [15].

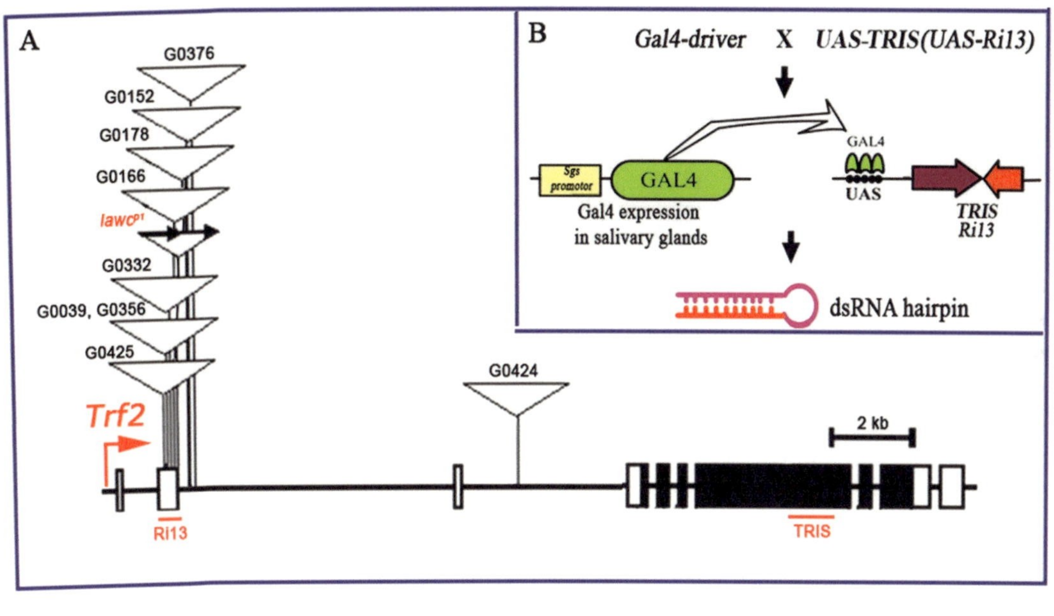

Figure 1. (A) Organization of the *Trf2* gene. Coding regions are shown as filled boxes, and noncoding ones are indicated with open boxes. Lethal insertions are marked with triangles. Double arrows mark the insertion of a double copy of the P element in the *lawc*^{p1} mutation. Red lines indicate the regions for *UAS-Ri13* and *UAS-TRIS* constructs which express RNA hairpins under the control of inducible *UAS* yeast promoter. (B) The scheme of two component *GAL4-UAS* system. The system is composed of two independent parent transgenic lines, the *Gal4* driver line in which the yeast transcription activator *Gal4* gene is expressed in a tissue-specific manner and the *Upstream Activating Sequence* (*UAS*) responder line in which the gene of interest is under *UAS* control. Mating of the *UAS*-containing responder flies with the *Gal4* driver-containing flies results in progeny bearing the two components, in which the *UAS*-transgene expresses dsRNA hairpins in a transcriptional pattern that reflects that of the *Gal4* driver. In our experiment the *Gal4* driver is *Sgs3* which express in larvae salivary glands.

The lines of second group were obtained in our laboratory: *l(1)lawc*^{4}*/FM4, l(1)lawc*^{16}*/FM4, l(1) lawc*^{18}*/FM4, l(1)lawc*^{53}*/FM4, l(1)lawc*^{60}*/FM4, l(1)lawc*^{67}*/FM4, l(1)lawc*^{73}*/FM4, l(1)lawc*^{75}*/FM4*, and *l(1) lawc*^{90}*/FM4* [20]. We will further call these lines "laboratory" lines. They carry lethal *Trf2* mutations obtained after the destabilization of the mobile *P* element in the initial *lawc*^{P1} allele [20].

In lines with lethal mutation, the X chromosome is maintained on the *In(1)FM* balancer chromosome. This chromosome carries a dominant *Bar* (*B*) marker mutation (narrow eyes) and recessive allele of the *yellow* (*y*) gene (yellow body). We crossed *y*$^{+}$*l(1)/In(1)FM, yB* females with males that carried the X chromosome marked by the y^1 mutation (y^1/Y) in order to identify exceptional classes of descendants and estimate the frequency of X-chromosome nondisjunction in these lines. Males and females of normal classes (the phenotype of which is easily identified) appeared in descendants of this crossing, including *In(1)FM, yB/Y* males with narrow eyes and yellow body and two classes of females including (1) *In(1)FM, yB/yB*$^{+}$ (yellow body and kidney-shaped eyes) and (2) *y*$^{+}$*l(1)/yB*$^{+}$ (grey body and normal oval eyes).

When X-chromosome nondisjunction occurred, males and females of exceptional classes (that always differ phenotypically) were detected in descendants. These were X/0 males with normal oval eyes and yellow bodies and XX/Y females with grey bodies and kidney-shaped eyes. Males of the normal class hemizygous for the X chromosome with a lethal allele—*l(1)/Y*—die. Exceptional classes of Y/0 males and XX/X super-females also die. Therefore, the frequency of X-chromosome nondisjunction (*Q*) was calculated according to the formula, $Q = 100\% \cdot \frac{2(X0 + XXY)}{XX + 2XY + 2X0 + 2XXY}$, where X0 and XXY are the number of flies of exceptional classes; XX and XY are the number of flies of normal classes. The sum of exceptional classes in the numerator was multiplied by two in order to take into account lethal classes with the XX/X and Y/0 genotype. The number of XY males in denominator was multiplied by two in order to take into account the class of lethal *l(1)/Y* males [21].

To estimate the influence of the *In(1)FM* balancer chromosome on the frequency of X-chromosome nondisjunction and compare it with the frequency of *Q* nondisjunction calculated for our lines, a control experiment was performed. For this, we crossed *In(1)FM, B/In(1) FM*, and *B* females with y^1/Y males. Females of normal class *In(1)FM* and *B/y*^{1} must have kidney-shaped eyes in the progeny of this crossing caused by a combination of one copy of the *Bar* mutant allele with one copy of the wild-type allele of this locus while *In(1)FM* and *B/Y* males must have narrow eyes caused by the presence of one copy of the *Bar* mutant allele. Exceptional females—*In(1)FM, B/In(1)FM, B/Y*—must have narrow eyes caused by two copies of the *Bar* mutant allele, while $y^1/0$ exceptional males must have normal oval eyes and yellow bodies.

To determine the influence of *p{lacW}* transposon on X-chromosome nondisjunction in museum lines and to take into account the genetic background of laboratory lines, additional control experiments were performed. As a control for museum lines, we calculated the frequency of X-chromosome nondisjunction in *l(1)G0071* line with lethal mutation caused by the insertion of *p{lacW}* transposon not to *Trf2* gene region. As a control for laboratory line, we used line with *lawc*$^{P1+}$ reversion and unknown lethal mutation (complemented to *Trf2*), which we obtained after the destabilization of a mobile *P* element in the initial *lawc*^{P1} allele.

All experiments were repeated three times, and the average frequency of X-chromosome nondisjunction Δ*Q* was calculated for each line. As a result of the experiment, it was found that the frequency of X-chromosome nondisjunction was increased in *lawc* mutants with decreased expression of the *Trf2* protein. The maximal frequency of X-chromosome nondisjunction was in the line *l(1)G0166* (31.2%), which increases the frequency of nondisjunction in the control line (1.4%) by approximately 22 times (**Table 1**).

Alleles	**Normal classes**		**Exceptional classes**		***Q* (%)**
	♀♀ X/X	**♂♂ X/Yx2**	**♂♂ X/0**	**♀♀ XX/Y**	
Museum lines					
l(1)G0039	379	328	13	44	13.9
l(1)G0178	296	240	14	15	9.8
l(1)G0332	345	328	13	38	13.2
l(1)G0152	454	348	28	16	9.9
l(1)G0166	306	262	57	72	31.2
l(1)G0356	377	342	46	47	20.6
l(1)G0424	324	258	14	19	10.2
l(1)G0376	345	298	4	15	5.6
l(1)G0425	183	218	6	6	5.6
Laboratory lines					
l(1)1awc^{4}	450	402	10	52	12.7
l(1)1awc^{16}	478	530	32	6	7.0
l(1)1awc^{18}	290	268	8	14	7.3
l(1)1awc^{53}	220	224	26	54	26.5
l(1)1awc^{60}	361	292	6	8	4.1
l(1)1awc^{67}	450	306	20	14	8.3
l(1)1awc^{73}	427	304	34	34	15.7
l(1)1awc^{75}	439	334	12	8	4.9
l(1)1awc^{90}	466	360	6	20	5.9
Control lines					
In(1)FM	1242	1186	6	11	1.4
l(1)G0071	363	282	1	4	1.5
lawc^{p1+}*l(1)*	356	320	1	3	1.2

First column indicates *Trf2* alleles. Next two columns indicate the amount of viewed males and females of normal classes. X/X—total amount of females with $y^{+}l(1)B^{+}/yB^{+}$ and yB/yB^{+} genotypes; X/Yx2—doubled amount of males with *yB/Y* genotype. Next two columns indicate the amount of detected males and females of exceptional classes: X/0, males with $yB^{+}/0$; XX/Y, females with $y^{+}l(1)B^{+}/yB/yB^{+}$ genotype. *Q*—frequency of X-chromosome nondisjunction.

Table 1. The frequency of X-chromosome nondisjunction in females with lethal *Trf2* mutations.

3. Study of the origin of chromosome nondisjunction in *lawc* mutants

To identify the source of chromosome nondisjunction, we decided to study the meiosis of mutant females. We performed the cytological analysis of the oocyte nucleus in mutant *lawc^{p1}/l(1)EF520* females (the frequency of X-chromosome nondisjunction is 5.2%) with low *Trf2* expression. Squash preparations of ovaries were prepared by modified Puro and Nokkala method [10, 22].

In germarium, the oocyte passes through the premeiotic DNA replication, meiosis prophase I, prometaphase I, and metaphase I. In mature oocyte of stage 14, division arrest usually occurs at the stage of metaphase I; chromosomes are collected in karyosome; and only achiasmatic chromosomes (IV and rarely X chromosome) are already oriented to opposite poles (**Figure 2A**).

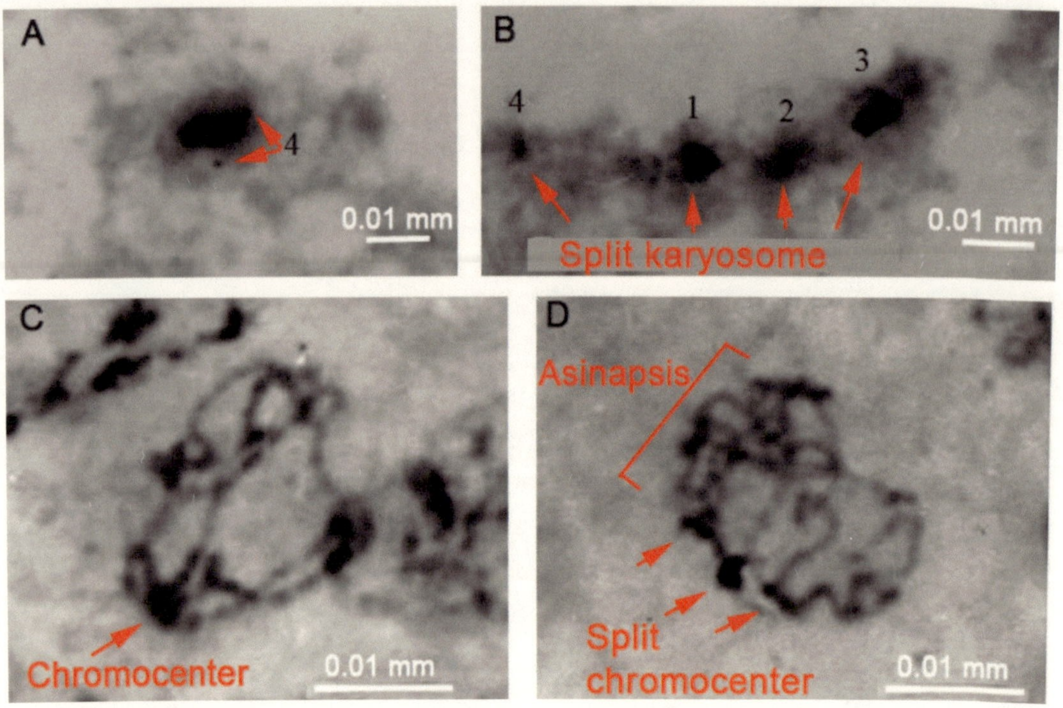

Figure 2. *Trf2* is necessary for chromatin condensation and chromocenter formation. (A–B) Late meiosis, the beginning of anaphase I, the oocyte nuclei of 13–14 stage. (A) Wild type; chromosomes of oocyte nucleus are assembled to karyosome with compact structure, while fourth chromosomes are oriented to opposite poles (arrows). (B) Mutant females; karyosome splitting. (C–D) Early meiosis, prophase I, the oocyte nuclei of 3rd stage. (C) Wild type; all chromosomes are attached by pericentromeric heterochromatin regions and thereby compact chromocenter is formed (arrow) following a correct pairing of homologous chromosomes. (D) Mutant females; chromocenter splitting occurs; chromosome compaction and homolog pairing are disturbed. Split chromocenter is indicated by arrows; failure of chromosome compaction is indicated by bracket.

We found that in anaphase I the chromocenter in mutant oocyte was often split and the compact karyosome structure was often broken (**Figure 2B**). The split karyosome assumes the disruption of the chromocenter; therefore, we performed an analysis of the early oocyte at the stage of meiosis prophase I when oocyte chromosomes were held together by pericentromeric heterochromatin, and the compact chromocenter was easy to distinguish. As a result, we found that chromosome compaction and homolog pairing were disturbed in mutant females, and the splitting of the chromocenter was proved to exist (**Figure 2C** and **D**).

Thus, a decreasing of *Trf2* gene expression leads to failure of chromocenter formation and chromatin condensation required for proper homolog paring at premeiotic stages, and it is evidently a reason for the chromosome nondisjunction that we observe in genetic experiments.

4. *Trf2* participates in pericentromeric heterochromatin formation

Chromocenter splitting assumes the disruption of interchromosomal ectopic contacts in the pericentromeric heterochromatin region. We decided to examine *Trf2* influence the pericentromeric heterochromatin formation. We used the line with paracentric inversion on X chromosome *In(1)*w^{m4} [23]. This inversion transfers the white locus next to the pericentromeric region, and as a result, w^{m4} mutants get a red-white mosaic colored eyes due to the position-effect variegation. To determine the ability of the $lawc^{p1}$ mutation to modify the position-effect variegation, we performed a genetic experiment using w^{m4} mutation as a sensitive test system. The combination of w^{m4} with the hypomorphic $lawc^{p1}$ mutation resulted the restoring of eye coloration in compound $w^{m4}lawc^{p1}$ flies (**Figure 3A**). This suggests that decrease in the concentration of *Trf2* protein causes the decompaction of normally tightly packed pericentromeric heterochromatin that results in *white* gene derepression. Thus, the *Trf2* is normally required for the formation of pericentromeric heterochromatin, which in turn participates in the chromocenter organization.

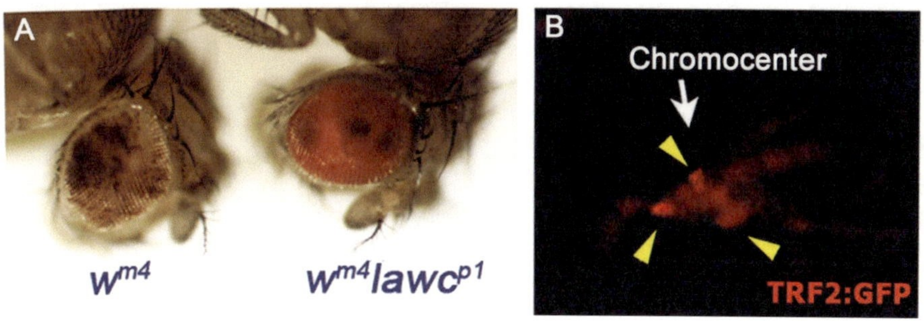

Figure 3. *Trf2* participates in pericentromeric heterochromatin formation. (A) The $lawc^{p1}$ mutation suppresses the position-effect variegation. Left: w^{m4} mutant with mosaic eye coloration. Right: double $w^{m4}lawc^{p1}$ mutant, the eye color of which is restored almost to wild type. (B) Localization of fusion *Trf2*:GFP protein in pericentromeric heterochromatin. Immunofluorescence staining of y^1w^1; *P{*w^+*, [GFP~Trf2-1]}* larvae salivary gland polytene chromosomes by antibodies to GFP. Arrows indicate *Trf2* localization in the chromocenter region.

As the *Trf2* protein is a transcription factor and can indirectly influence the chromatin structure (through the activation of genes responsible for chromatin compaction), the question arises: whether *Trf2* protein can directly participate in chromocenter formation? To answer this question, we used the y^1w^1; *P{*w^+*, [GFP~Trf2-1]}* flies express the hybrid GFP:*Trf2* protein (short *Trf2* isoform fused with green fluorescent protein [GFP]) under the control of the constitutive *Hairy wing* (*Hw*) gene promoter. We performed the immunofluorescence staining of *y^1w^1; P{w^+, [GFP~Trf2-1]}* larvae salivary gland polytene chromosomes by antibodies to GFP and analyzed the distribution of fusion GFP:*Trf2* in chromocenter. As a result, we found sites of *Trf2* localization in pericentromeric heterochromatin regions (**Figure 3B**). These data allow us to confirm the direct participation of the *Trf2* in the chromocenter formation.

5. The effect of *Trf2* knockdown on salivary glands polytene chromosome morphology

We demonstrated in the above described experiments that the decrease in *Trf2* concentration influences proper chromatin compaction and chromocenter structure in germ cells. However, *Trf2* localization found in pericentromeric salivary glands heterochromatin region assumes the involvement of this protein in the compaction of chromosomes also in somatic cells.

As considered, polytene chromosomes are very favor objects for the analysis of numerous features of interphase chromosome organization and the genome as a whole [24]. To confirm our hypothesis, we decided to use *UAS-GAL4* two-component system [25] for specific RNA interference (RNAi)–mediated *Trf2* depletion in salivary gland. We obtained two *Drosophila* UAS-containing transgenic lines using P-element–mediated transformation. These lines contain constructs that express double-stranded RNA hairpins that are complementary to either 5′UTR *Trf2* regulatory (*P{w^+; UAS-Ri}13*) or encoding (*P{w^+; UAS-TRIS}*) *Trf2* gene region (**Figure 1A**). Both *UAS-Ri13* and *UAS-TRIS* constructs are able to express RNA hairpins under the control of inducible *UAS* yeast promoter element (**Figure 1B**).

For specific *Trf2* depletion in somatic cells, we used the *Sgs3-GAL4* driver (the line *w^{1118}; P{Sgs3-GAL4.PD}TP1*) that expresses yeast GAL4 activator in larvae salivary glands. After crossing *UAS*-containing flies with *Sgs3-GAL4* driver flies, the morphology of polytene chromosomes in descendant larvae *Sgs3>Ri13* and *Sgs3>TRIS* was analyzed. Larvae from *UAS*/+ lines and larvae from *Sgs3-GAL4*/+ line were used as the controls.

Normally, polytene chromosomes are present in salivary glands in singular due to the somatic synapsis occurs when two homologous chromosomes remain consistently conjugated. Polytene nonhomologous chromosomes in the nucleus are joined by their centromeres to form the most compact common region—chromocenter (**Figure 4A, C**, and **E**). Studies of *Trf2*-depleted salivary gland polytene chromosomes show a number of structural aberrations in the polytene chromosomes morphology. Its banding patterns are changed, the pairing is significantly disturbed, and asynapsis frequently involves very extensive regions (almost the entire chromosome; **Figure 4B, D**, and **F**). These defects were found approximately in 95% of analyzed nuclei (N = 100) in the experimental sample and approximately in 5% (N = 50) of analyzed nuclei in the control sample.

http://dx.doi.org/10.5772/67314

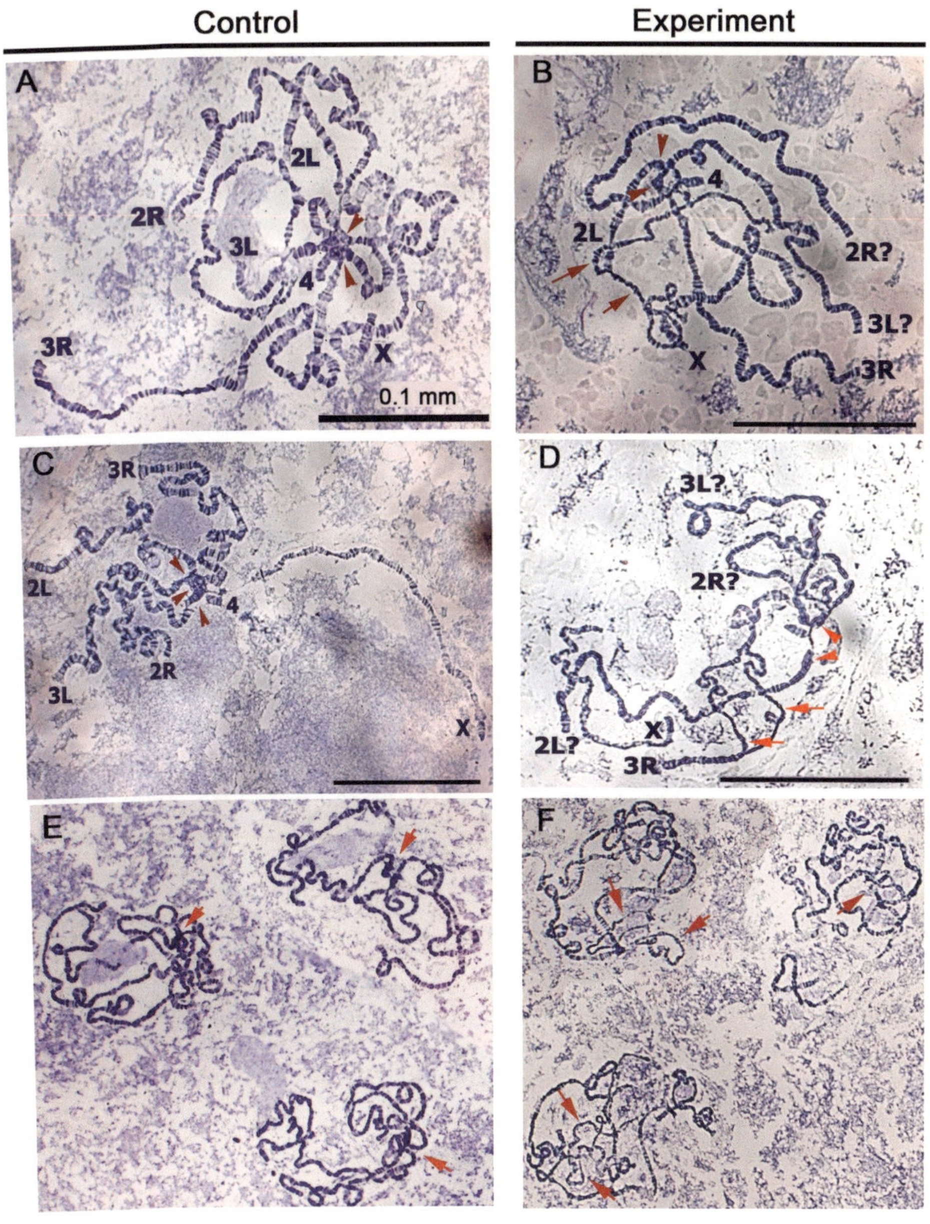

Figure 4. The effect of *Trf2* depletion on salivary glands polytene chromosomes morphology. Polytene chromosomes before and after *Trf2* depletion in salivary glands. Control—polytene chromosomes of larvae from *Sgs3-GAL4* driver (A) and from line with *UAS* transgene (C). Experiment—polytene chromosomes of *Sgs3>TRIS* (B) and *Sgs3>Ri13* (D) larvae containing activated constructions. Marks: X chromosome (X), left (2L) and right (2R) arms of the second autosome, left (3L) and right (3R) arms of the third autosome, and fourth (4) chromosome. Chromocenters and asynapses are indicated by arrowheads and arrows correspondently. Total view of polytene chromosomes in control (E) and experiment (F). Chromocenters are indicated by arrows on (E); homolog chromosome asynapses are indicated on (F). The regions of chromocenter on (F) are difficult to identify. Question marks mean that same chromosomes are hard to identify due to their abnormal morphology.

It is known that partial asynapsis is not a consequence of squashing of nuclei and variations in methods used to make preparations do not affect the frequencies of asynapsis [26]. So, we concluded that high frequency of chromosome asynapsis was induced by *Trf2* depletion. However, the main trait of nuclei in lines with depleted *Trf2* was the failure of chromocenter formation. Thus, the suppression of the *Trf2* expression in salivary glands reveals the involvement of *Trf2* gene in a chromocenter organization and in the correct pairing of homologous chromosomes not only in meiosis but also in somatic cells.

It is known that the chromocenter is responsible for the chromosome co-orientation during cell division and facilitates the paring of homologs [9, 27]. The disturbance of paring affects the transvection (or allelic complementation)—the phenomenon in which gene regulatory elements located in one of the homologs control a promoter of the same gene but located in another homolog [28, 29]. It is interesting to note that hypomorphic *lawc* mutations suppress transvection effect induced by *zeste* mutations [16]. This fact confirms the existence of abnormal homolog paring in lines with lower *Trf2* expression.

The study a set of mutations that cause chromosome nondisjunction allowed to conclude that the chromocenter is a genetically programmed structure, that is, there are genes that control its formation and reorganization [11]. For example, it was demonstrated that the recessive mutation of *crossover suppressor on 3 of Gowen* (*c(3)G*) gene influences the structure of the lateral element and the length of meiotic chromosomes [30–32].

The *Syntaxin 13* (*Syx13*) gene mutation (*ff16*) causes sterility and chromosome nondisjunction in males and females meiosis. Oocytes of mutant *ff16* females demonstrate a split karyosome and the disruption in the chromocenter formation. The product of this gene is homologous to the receptor of synaptosomal-associated protein of 25 kDa (SNAP-25) and is involved in cytokinesis [32, 33].

Another gene—*no distributive disjunction* (*nod*)—is involved in the organization and orientation of the spindle during mitosis and meiosis and is required for its binding to chromosomes in the *Drosophila* oocyte nucleus. This gene encodes the protein that contains DNA-binding domain and the conservative motor domain homologous to the Kinesin. *nod* mutations disrupt chromocenter formation in germ and somatic cells and cause achiasmatic chromosome nondisjunction in *Drosophila* females meiosis [30, 34]. All these proteins have distinct functions; however, a decrease in their activity leads to a similar result, that is, the disruption of chromocenter formation and chromosome nondisjunction.

It was shown that *Trf2* may be the part of the macromolecular chromatin-remodeling complex NUcleosome Remodeling Factor (NURF) which is correlated with transcriptional activation [35]. Nevertheless, the data we obtained have demonstrated that *Trf2* could not only be involved in transcription activation but also could perform structural functions in chromatin organization. This idea is supported by the observation that there is no proper chromatin condensation in early spermatids of mice with null *Trf2* mutation and, in particular, the chromocenter formation is disturbed [36]. Thus, we may conclude that the role of *Trf2* in the organization of chromocenter structure and chromatin condensation is evolutionarily conservative.

In yeast, it was demonstrated that kinetochores—large protein complexes assembled on the centromeric region of the chromosomes, to which spindle microtubule is attached during cell division—are formed by the epigenetic mechanism. This mechanism involves the generation of specialized nucleosomes in which a canonical histone H3 is replaced by its centromere-specific homologs—centromere protein A (CENP-A). This protein served as a landmark for kinetochore assembly to define the identity of centromeres [37, 38]. The high frequency of chromosome nondisjunction induced by decondensation of pericentric heterochromatin in *lawc* mutants allows us to assume that *Trf2* may be involved in the epigenetic regulation of kinetochores formation in *Drosophila*.

As it was mentioned above, the correct distribution of chromatids between daughter cells depends on the coordinated interaction of centrosomes, centromeres, kinetochores, spindle fibrils, topoisomerase, proteolytic processes, and motor proteins. The error of accurate spatiotemporal interactions between any of these factors results in a genomic disbalance. We cannot completely exclude the probability that *Trf2*, being transcription factor, can indirectly influence the process of cellular division through the regulation of genes that control mitosis and meiosis. In previous experiments, while looking for interactions between the *Trf2* and other genes, we performed genetic screening to detect cytological regions that are sensitive to a decreased level of *Trf2* expression [39]. **Table 2** shows genes of meiosis and mitosis localized in these regions. The genes involved in chromatin compaction are the largest group.

Process	**Genes**	
Chromatin compaction	*Top2 (topoisomerase 2)* *Top3alpha (topoisomerase 3alpha)* *Mcm7 (minichromosome maintenance 7)* *eIF-4E (eukaryotic initiation factor 4E)* *cid (centromere identifier)*	*kis (kismet)* *vls (valois)* *barr* *Bj1* *Df31 (decondensation factor 31)*
Assembly of division spindle	*mad2* *cnn (centrosomin)*	*αTub67C*
Chromosome disjunction	*Sse (Separase)* *Gap1 (GTPase-activating protein 1)*	*Dub (double or nothing)* *cdc23 (cell-division-cycle 23)*
Organization of actin components of cytoskeleton	*spir (spire)* *dia (diaphanous)*	
Checkpoint	*mus304 (mutagen-sensitive 304)* *Cdk8 (Cyclin-dependent kinase 8)* *Myt1*	*hay (haywire)* *lok (loki)*
?	*Hs2st (heparan sulfate 2-O-sulfotransferase)* *I-2 (Inhibitor-2)*	

Table 2. The classification of mitosis and meiosis genes that may interact with *Trf2*.

This does not mean that *Trf2* interacts with each of them; nevertheless, we cannot exclude the probability that decompaction of pericentric heterochromatin and defects in chromosome segregation in mitosis and meiosis in *lawc* mutant are induced by low expression of some of these genes. However, the localization of *Trf2* in the chromocenter supports the idea that this factor can be independently involved in the organization of chromatin structure.

6. Conclusion

We demonstrated that a decrease in the *Trf2* expression damages proper chromocenter structure and abolishes chromatin condensation required for correct homologs pairing at premeiotic stages and is evidently a reason for the chromosome nondisjunction that we observed in genetic experiments. Moreover, we found that compact chromocenter and correct homolog pairing were abolished in flies with a lower *Trf2* expression not only in germline but also in somatic cells. As *Trf2* is localized in pericentromeric regions, we conclude that *Trf2* can not only be involved in transcription activation but also may perform structural function in pericentromeric heterochromatin organization that is responsible for a chromocenter formation.

In conclusion, we would like to note that in the recent screening for genes that control the sex-ratio meiotic drive in *Drosophila simulans* (closely related species to *D. melanogaster*), the *Trf2* was suggested as the candidate for the factor responsible for this natural phenomenon typical for some animal species [40, 41]. It is interesting that in studied *D. simulans* population *Trf2* locus underwent the tandem duplication [41]. Thus, the function to control the specific X-chromosome nondisjunction may be adapted during the evolution by one of *Trf2* copies.

Author details

Julia Vorontsova, Roman Cherezov and Olga Simonova*

*Address all correspondence to: osimonova@hotmail.com

Koltsov Institute of Developmental Biology, Russian Academy of Sciences, Moscow, Russian Federation

References

[1] Jaenike J. Sex chromosome meiotic drive. Annu. Rev. Ecol. Syst. 2001; 32: 25-49. DOI: 10.1146/annurev.ecolsys.32.081501.113958

[2] Kirsch-Volders M, Cundari E, Verdoodt B. Towards a unifying model for the metaphase/anaphase transition. Mutagenesis. 1998; 13: 321-335. DOI: 10.1093/mutage/13.4.321

[3] Simon L, Voisin M, Tatout C, Probst A. Structure and function of centromeric and pericentromeric heterochromatin in *Arabidopsis thaliana*. Front. Plant Sci. 2015; 6: 1049. DOI: 10.3389/fpls.2015.010

[4] Zowalaty A, Baumann C, Li R, Chen W, De La Fuente R, Ye X. Seipin deficiency increases chromocenter fragmentation and disrupts acrosome formation leading to male infertility. Cell Death Dis. 2015; 6: e1817. DOI: 10.1038/cddis.2015.188

[5] Belli M, Vigone G, Merico V, Redi C, Garagna S, Zuccotti M. Time-lapsed of the mouse oocyte chromatin organization during meiotic resumption. Biomed. Res. Int. 2014; 2014: Article ID 207357, 10 pages. DOI: 10.1155/2014/207357

[6] Zalenskaya A, Zalensky O. Non-random positioning of chromosomes in human sperm nuclei. Chromosome Res. 2004; 12(2): 163-173. DOI: 10.1023/B:CHRO.0000013166.04629.97

[7] Funabiki H, Hagan I, Uzawa S, Yanagida M. Cell cycle dependent specific positioning and clustering of centromeres and telomeres in fission yeast. J. Cell Biol. 1993; 121(5): 961-976. DOI: 10.1083/jcb.121.5.961

[8] Stegnii V. The problem of systemic mutation. Russ. J. Genet. 1996; 32(1): 9-16.

[9] Chubykin V. The structure of the chromocenter in the oocytes, the initiation of homologous pairing and the regulation of the formation of crossing over in *Drosophila*. Tsitologiya. 1995; 37(5-6): 481-490.

[10] Chubykin V. Role of the chromocenter in nonrandom meiotic segregation of nonhomologous chromosomes in *Drosophila melanogaster* females. Russ. J. Genet. 2001; 37(3): 205-212. DOI: 10.1023/A:1009058323327

[11] Chubykin V. Genetic control of formation and reorganization of the chromocenter in Drosophila. Russ. J. Genet. 2001; 37(8): 888-893. DOI: 10.1023/A:1016721531557

[12] Berkovits B, Wolgemuth D. The first bromodomain of the testis-specific double bromodomain protein Brdt is required for chromocenter organization that is modulated by genetic background. Dev. Biol. 2011; 360(2): 358-368. DOI: 10.1016/j.ydbio.2011.10.005

[13] Rabenstein M, Zhou S, Lis J, Tjian R. TATA box-binding protein (TBP)-related factor 2 (TRF2), a third member of the TBP family. Proc. Natl. Acad. Sci. U.S.A. 1999; 96(9): 4791-4796. DOI: 10.1073/pnas.96.9.4791

[14] Simonova O, Kuzin B, Georgiev P, Gerasimova T. Novel regulatory mutation in *Drosophila melanogaster*. Russ. J. Genet. 1992; 28(2): 164-167.

[15] Vorontsova Yu, Modestova E, Burdina N, Korochkin L, Simonova O. Restoring viability of lethal mutants for the *leg-arista-wing complex* gene in rescue experiments with transgenic constructs that express the *trf2* gene domains in *Drosophila melanogaster*. Dokl. Akad. Nauk. 2007; 417(1-6): 429-431. DOI: 10.1134/S0012496607060051

[16] Simonova O, Petruk S, Dzhagaeva I, Korochkin L. Role of the *lawc*^{p1} mutation in the regulation of the *white* locus expression in *Drosophila*. Russ. J. Genet. 1998; 34(3): 267-272.

[17] Wu C. Transvection, nuclear structure and chromatin proteins. J. Cell Biol. 1993; 120(3): 587-590. DOI: 10.1083/jcb.120.3.587

[18] Kopytova D, Krasnov A, Kopantceva M, Nabirochkina E, Nikolenko J, Maksimenko O, Kurshakova M, Lebedeva L, Yerokhin M, Simonova O, Korochkin L, Tora L, Georgiev P, Georgieva S. Two isoforms of *Drosophila* TRF2 are involved in embryonic development, premeiotic chromatin condensation and proper differentiation of germ cells of both sexes. Mol. Cell. Biol. 2006; 26(20): 7492-7505. DOI: 10.1128/MCB.00349-06.

[19] Peter A, Schottler P, Werner M, et al. Mapping and identification of essential gene functions on the X chromosome of Drosophila. EMBO Rep. 2002; 3(1): 34-38. DOI: 10.1093/embo-reports/kvf012.

[20] Modestova E, Vorontsova Yu, Korochkin L, Simonova O. Induction of lethal mutations of the *leg-arista-wing complex* gene of *Drosophila melanogaster*. Dokl. Akad. Nauk. 2005; 403(1-6): 282-283. DOI: 10.1134/S1022795413050128.

[21] Zitron A, Hawley R. The genetic analysis of distributive segregation in *Drosophila melanogaster*: 1. Isolation and characterization of aberrant X segregation (Axs), a mutation defective in chromosome partner choice. Genetics. 1989; 122(4): 801-821.

[22] Puro J, Nokkala S. Meiotic segregation of chromosomes in *Drosophila melanogaster* oocytes: a cytological approach. Chromosoma. 1977; 63: 273-286. DOI: 10.1007/BF00327454

[23] Muller H. Types of visible variations induced by X-rays in *Drosophila*. J. Genet. 1930; 22: 299-334. DOI: 10.1007/BF02984195

[24] Zhimulev I, Koryakov D. Polytene chromosomes. eLS. 2009; DOI: 10.1002/9780470015902.a0001183.pub2.

[25] Brand AH, Perrimon N. Targeted gene expression as a means of altering cell fates and generating dominant phenotypes. Development. 1993; 118: 401-415.

[26] Zhimulev I. Morphology and structure of polytene chromosomes. Adv. Genet. 1996; 34: 1-497. DOI: 10.1016/S0065-2660(08)60533-7.

[27] Chubykin V. Homologue pairing: initiation sites and effects on crossing over and chromosome segregation in *Drosophila melanogaster*. Russ. J. Genet. 1996; 32(1): 1-8. DOI: 10.1134/S1022795409090026.

[28] Pirrotta V. Transvection and chromosomal trans-interaction effects. Biochim. Biophys. Acta. 1999; 1424(1): 1-8. DOI: 10.1016/S0304-419X(99)00019-0.

[29] Qian S, Varjavand B, Pirrotta V. Molecular analysis of the *zeste-white* interaction reveals a promoter_proximal element essential for distant enhancer-promoter communication. Genetics. 1992; 131(1): 79-90.

[30] Chubykin V. Structural characteristics of the chromocenter in ovary cells of *c(3)G* and *NOD* mutants of *Drosophila melanogaster*. Russ. J. Genet. 2001; 37(9): 1032-1040. DOI: 10.1023/A:1011909530640

[31] Bogdanov Yu, Grishaeva T, Dadashev S. Gene *CG17604* of *Drosophila melanogaster* may be a functional homolog of yeast gene *Zip1* and mammal gene *SCP1 (SYCP1)* encoding proteins of the synaptonemal complex. Russ. J. Genet. 2002; 38(1): 90-94. DOI: 10.1023/A:1013728214562.

[32] Fedorova S, Nokkala S, Chubykin V, Omelyanchuk L. The isolation of a mutation causing abnormal cytokinesis in male and split chromocenter in female meiosis in *Drosophila melanogaster*. Hereditas. 2001; 134: 125-134. DOI: 10.1111/j.1601-5223.2001.00125.x

[33] Nokkala S, Fedorova S, Tuohimaa J, et al. The syntaxin gene *Syx13* participates in mitotic and male meiotic cytokinesis and chromocenter formation in female meiosis. In: Program and Abstracts. 43rd Annual Drosophila Research Conference. San Diego. 2002. p. 158.

[34] Cui W, Hawley R. The HhH(2)/NDD domain of the *Drosophila* Nod chromokinesin-like protein is required for binding to chromosomes in the oocyte nucleus. Genetics. 2005; 171(4): 1823-1835. DOI: 10.1534/genetics.105.047464

[35] Hochheimer A, Zhou S, Zheng S, Holmes M, Tjian R. TRF2 associates with DREF and directs promoter-selective gene expression in *Drosophila*. Nature. 2002; 420: 439-445. DOI: 10.1038/nature01167

[36] Martianov I, Brancorsini S, Gansmuller A, et al. Distinct functions of TBP and TLF/TRF2 during spermatogenesis: requirement of TLF for heterochromatic chromocenter formation in haploid round spermatids. Development. 2002; 129(4): 945-955.

[37] Pidoux A, Allshire R. The role of heterochromatin in centromere function. Philos. Trans. R. Soc. Lond. B Biol. Sci. 2005; 360(1455): 569-579. DOI: 10.1098/rstb.2004.1611.

[38] Yamagishi Y, Sakuno T, Goto Y, Watanabe Y. Kinetochore composition and its function: lessons from yeasts. FEMS Microbiol. Rev. 2014; 38(2): 185-200. DOI: 10.1111/1574-6976.12049.

[39] Simonova O, Modestova E, Vorontsova Yu, Cherezov R. Screening of genomic regions affecting *lawc/Trf2* gene expression during *Drosophila melanogaster* development. Russ. J. Dev. Biol. 2012; 43(5): 301-317. DOI: 10.1134/S1062360412050086

[40] Montchamp-Moreau C. Sex-ratio meiotic drive in *Drosophila simulans*: cellular mechanism, candidate genes and evolution. Biochem. Soc. Trans. 2006; 34(4): 562-565. DOI: 10.1042/BST0340562

[41] Fouvry L, Ogereau D, Berger A, Gavory F, Montchamp-Moreau C. Sequence analysis of the segmental duplication responsible for Paris sex-ratio drive in *Drosophila simulans*. G3 (Bethesda). 2011; 1(5): 401-410. DOI: 10.1534/g3.111.000315

Chapter 9

Reference Karyotypes and Chromosomal Variability: A Journey with Fruit Flies and the Key to Survival

Alicia Leonor Basso Abraham

Additional information is available at the end of the chapter

http://dx.doi.org/10.5772/intechopen.69835

Abstract

My goal is to present the analysis of concepts on the "normal" karyotype and chromosomal abnormalities through comprehension of chromosomal variation within fruit flies populations, advantages of these insects as models to study genetic polymorphisms and the methodology from field to strains. Cytological preparations were obtained from cerebral ganglion. Staining methods include routine and fluorescent bandings as well as *in situ* hybridization using DNA probes. We define a more frequent karyotype of each one species and take them as the reference karyotype. The reference as well as the chromosomal variants studied within each species were isolated in different strains. The techniques applied revealed differences among individuals belonging to different strains, thus documenting the mutations into the DNAr cluster, variation in the patterns of heterochromatin, mosaic specimens carrying nuclei with different chromosomal numbers. Hoecht revealed double-minute chromosomes and CG- rich banding marked somatic crossing over between sister chromatids. The most frequent karyotype is the reference karyotype, namely, the normal karyotype. Chromosomal mutations produce variability. In man, a number of these mutants are considered chromosomal abnormalities. We learnt that variation is the key to survival and that many individuals could be in the right place in the wrong moment.

Keywords: *Anastrepha fraterculus*, chromosomal abnormalities, somatic crossing over, sister chromatids interchange, chromosomal rearrangements, evolutive advantage, hybridization, rDNA cluster, genetic disorders, chromosomal mutations, aneuploidies, mosaic specimens, double-minute chromosomes

1. Introduction

When we talk about chromosomal abnormalities, we are referring to a particular group of karyotypes which differ from the most frequent one known as the "species karyotype." The "species karyotype" is known as "normal" karyotype.

The denomination "chromosomal abnormalities" refers to human mutations involving entire chromosomes or large segments of them which are missing, duplicated, and rearranged, showing that the relevant cellular processes are prone to a high level of error.

The consequences of such changes are physiogenetic disorders which are more evident in diploid species such as human beings and flies. The reason why fruit flies are a good model to study the inheritance of chromosomal mutations is because of their short life cycle, the possibility of their artificial rearing, and their large progenies.

Most genetic abnormalities appear spontaneously. Physical or chemical agents in the environment are capable of causing mutations in genes, and these mutations will be passed from parents to offsprings.

The purpose of this chapter is to clarify the concepts of normal karyotype or chromosomal composition throughout my prolonged research on populations of fruit flies, the materials and methods I used in my research, the lessons I learnt on this subject, and the conclusions I drew concerning chromosomal abnormalities on human beings.

I organized the main subject into different sections: (i) the South American fruit fly and the laboratory rearing technique for genetic studies; (ii) some concepts when studying karyotypes in men and flies; (iii) working with fruit flies; and (iv) original research findings in fruit flies.

1.1. The South American fruit fly *Anastrepha fraterculus* (Wied.)

A. fraterculus and *C. capitata* belong to the Tephritidae family which groups the true fruit flies. Both are agricultural pests with complete metamorphosis. The complete life cycle begins when females oviposit their eggs inside fruits where eclosion takes place and the larvae feed and develop passing through three instars. Immobilization of larva III marks the beginning of metamorphosis along with chitinization of the larval cuticle. Inside the puparium, histolysis of many larval tissues is followed by a *de novo* synthesis to reconstruct the adult fly. Ecdysis takes place at approximately 45 days from egg eclosion.

Their life cycles last between 35 and 45 days, while human beings produce one generation each in 20–25 years.

1.1.1. A laboratory rearing technique adjusted for genetic studies

An artificial rearing technique of the species for genetic studies begins with a representative sampling of a particular population and ensures abundant offspring. A genetic study looks for understanding chromosomal variation; thus, it is based in the study of families [1] founded by one male and one female. Reference works for the laboratory rearing techniques of *C. capitata* are Refs. [2–4] and for *A. fraterculus* is Ref. [5].

These techniques allow us to establish colonies and to study families of flies in order to isolate chromosomal variants and to understand their behavior and significance within a population [6].

1.2. Some concepts when studying karyotypes in man and flies

The karyotype is the full set of chromosomes in a person's cells or in a fly's cell.

A very particular feature of flies is somatic pairing, an unusual event that makes the recognition of chromosomal pairs and their changes during mitosis easier.

A chromosome contains hundreds to thousands of genes. A gene is a segment of DNA containing the code used to synthesize a protein, an enzyme, an RNAt, or RNAr, so a gene can code for different polypeptides at different moments of life and in different organs.

Sexual reproduction of these organisms occurs in cycles of alternated phases and delineate times between two generations, and it is represented as:

Female 2n---MEIOSIS----n

FERTILIZATION produces a new zygote 2n

Male 2n------MEIOSIS-----n

where "n" is a gamete and "2n" is a zygote. We use a slightly different nomenclature to clearly distinguish between the zygote and the number of chromosome sets or ploidy level.

Almost every human cell is diploid (2x), since it contains two sets of 23 chromosomes inherited or received from each parent, for a total of 46 chromosomes/cell.

The human karyotype is composed of 23 chromosomal pairs, so almost every cell carries 46 chromosomes. Sperm cells and egg cells are gametes (n) which are haploid (x) since they carry only one set of 23 chromosomes ($n = x = 23$), and during fertilization ($n + n$), the new fertilized egg called zygote (2n) will be diploid $2n = 2x = 46$ chromosomes (two sets of chromosomes). So almost all of the persons' cells are diploid $2n = 2x = 46$ except for their gametes, either sperm or oocytes, which are haploid $n = x = 23$.

The fruit flies *C. capitata* and *A. fraterculus* are also diploid species with six pairs of chromosomes for a total of 12 chromosomes ($2n = 2x = 12$). Sperm cells and egg cells carry six chromosomes, so gametes are $n = x = 6$.

Karyotypes are obtained from good mitotic metaphases by cutting each chromosome and its homolog and ordering pairs from the largest to the shortest: a normal human karyotype will show 46 chromosomes, and a normal *Anastrepha's* or *Ceratitis'* karyotype will show 12 chromosomes.

We define a more frequent karyotype of each one species and take it as the reference karyotype, ordinarily known as the "normal karyotype." The reference karyotype as well as the chromosomal variants studied within each species were isolated in different laboratory strains and maintained throughout the generations in order to understand their significance. Chromosomal variants arise by mutations which are changes affecting chromosomal structure and/or chromosomal number. The rearing methodology allowed to associate each chromosomal mutation to particular physiological or morphological mutations or types of behaviors.

When chromosomal variants are found to be associated to physiological or morphological disorders, they are called chromosomal abnormalities. In human beings, they produce disorders known as syndromes and cancers. They are chromosomal mutations detected through cytological techniques. Chromosomal mutations are changes in chromosome structure which involve at least one chromosome breakage. Changes in chromosome number mostly arise as a consequence of failures during cell division, although they can also be produced by breakage of a chromosome segment. Sometimes, a change in chromosome structure causes a change in chromosome number.

1.3. Chromosomal mutations affecting chromosome number

1.3.1. Polyploids

Duplication of complete sets of chromosomes will modify ploidy levels and consequently chromosome number. For instance, we could use triploid flies carrying $2n = 3x = 18$ chromosomes in their somatic cells to study sex determination in *Ceratitis capitata*. Triploidy is caused because of nondisjunction of chromosomes during meiosis I of one of the parents. Although this phenomenon could be an extremely rare event in living babies, a triploid bearing $2n = 3x = 69$ was reported to live 9 months (Conference: La Española Hospital, 2013).

1.3.2. Aneuploids: nondisjunction of homologous chromosomes

Trisomy 21 in humans $2n = 2x + 1 = 47$ is known as Down syndrome. Most affected persons have an extra copy of chromosome 21 due to nondisjunction of chromosome 21 in a parent with normal karyotype. This syndrome can eventually be produced by a translocation which occurs when the long arm of chromosome 21 breaks off and attaches to another chromosome at the centromere.

Monosomy: One chromosome of a pair is missing ($2n = 2x - 1$). A nulisomic is $2n = 2x - 2$ because a complete pair is absent, which could be detected in triploid individuals or others with higher levels of ploidy.

1.4. Chromosomal mutations altering chromosome morphology

One chromosome breakage causes deletion of a chromosome segment in one chromosome of a pair.

Two chromosome breakages involving two chromosomes of a pair "o" from different pairs, cause translocations, inversions, and duplications of chromosomal segments

1.5. Original research findings in fruit flies

The main topics of this subsection are the comprehension of chromosomal variation within populations of fruit flies and the advantages of these insects as models to study genetic polymorphisms. We define a more frequent karyotype of the species and considered it as the reference karyotype, ordinarily known as the "normal karyotype." The reference as well as the chromosomal variants studied in the species were isolated in different laboratory strains and maintained throughout the generations in order to understand their significance.

http://dx.doi.org/10.5772/intechopen.69835

2. Methodologies

A very particular feature of flies is somatic pairing, an unusual event that makes the recognition of chromosomal changes easier.

A genetic study is based on the transmission of traits from one generation to the next. A long time between generations as well as a reduced progeny, greatly delays the comprehension on how mutations transmission is carried out.

An artificial rearing technique of the species for genetic studies begins with a representative sampling of a particular population and ensures abundant offspring (**Image 1**). A genetic study looks for understanding chromosomal variation; thus, it is based in the study of families [1] founded by one male and one female (**Image 1**). A good rearing technique ensures a good oviposition rate.

Reference works for the laboratory rearing techniques of *C. capitata* are Refs. [2–4] and for *A. fraterculus* see Ref. [5].

Cytological preparations were obtained from cerebral ganglion of third instars. The preparation of ganglia was as described in Ref. [7].

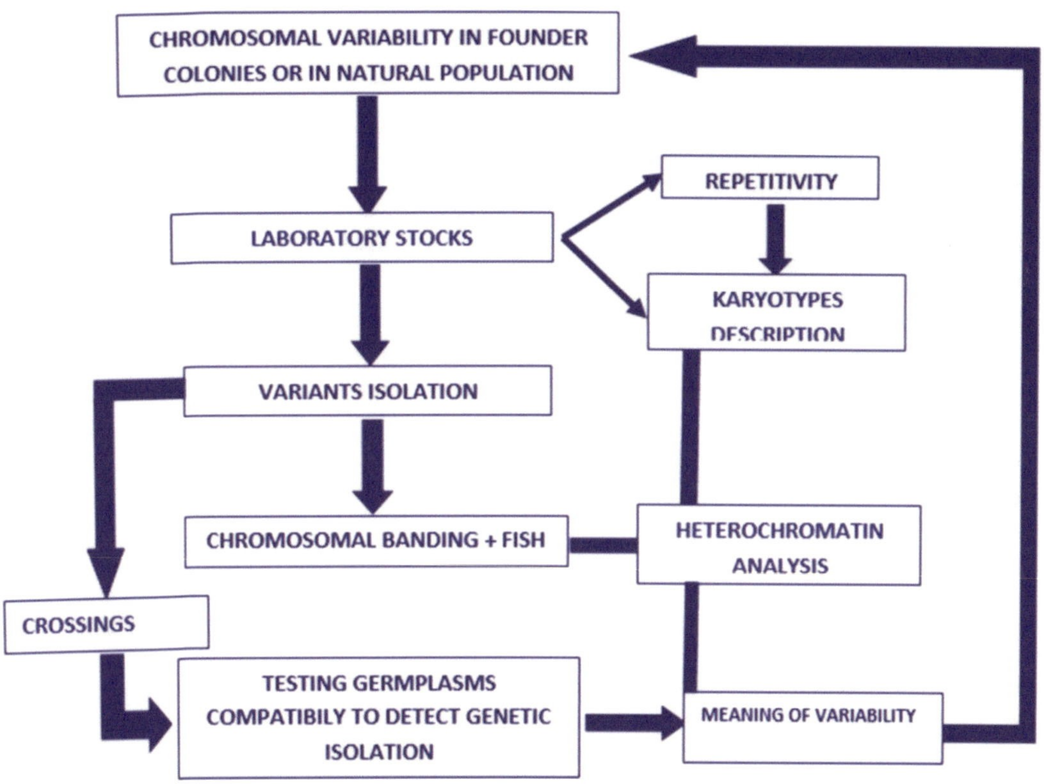

Image 1. Genetic methodology: work design scheme.

Chromosome banding and ideograms were from mitotic chromosome spreads from cerebral ganglia. C-banded preparations were obtained using the technique of Ref. [8]. H-banding was as described in Ref. [9]. GC-rich banding using $CMA_3$was as described in Ref. [10]. Mounting was performed in McIlvaine buffer with pH = 7 (0.16 M dibasic sodium phosphate, 0.04 M sodium citrate). Preparations were kept in the dark during 24 hours before examination under a Zeiss Axioplan fluorescence microscope. N-banding was obtained as described in Ref. [11]. At least 10 metaphase plates per chromosome spread were analyzed. Approximately 5000 larvae were dissected to obtain 1654 cytological preparations of *A. fraterculus* with good quality metaphases.

The fluorescent *in situ* hybridization (*FISH*) technique described by Willhoeft and Franz [7] was carried out using three different probes. (1) The *Drosophila hydei* probe pDh2-H8 corresponds to a cloned genomic fragment of 310 bp containing a 28S rRNA coding region interrupted by an intron [12]. (2) The *C. capitata* probe pCc-18S corresponds to an AT-rich cloned fragment of 720 bp derived from the 18S gene [13, 14]. (3) The *A. fraterculus* probe pK18 corresponds to a genomic fragment of 300 bp originated from a differential sex band [13]. All three probes were labeled by random priming with Digoxigenin-11-dUTP and revealed with anti-Digoxigenin-Fluorescein using propidium iodide as counter staining. The preparations were kept in the dark during 24 hours before examination under a Zeiss Axioplan fluorescence microscope. Images were recorded with an Olympus DP72 digital camera, time exposure being manually adjusted.

3. Results

Key results change two paradigms: *C. capitata* is a species considered to have karyotypic uniformity, and *A. fraterculus* was considered a complex of cryptic species. The possibility of rearing these species under laboratory conditions made possible the isolation of strains with complexities previously detected in natural populations of these flies (**Image 1**). Throughout 30 years, we could study polyploids, sexual aneuploids, and chromosomal rearrangements like translocations, inversions, deletions, duplications, ring chromosomes, jumping elements, cell mosaic specimens, B-chromosomes, and double-minute chromosomes. The rearing technique gave as the possibility of repeating a technique and/or applying different chromosomal markers on the same genetic material as well as to perform compatibility tests to understand the significance of chromosomal variation (**Image 1**).

Comprehension of populations' structures is an unavoidable task for geneticists.

3.1. *Ceratitis capitata*

The analysis of genetic variation within and between natural populations of *C. capitata* [15] explains the history of our reference laboratory strain *Arg 17* as well as all the morphological, chromosomal, and physiological variants along with the study of Mendoza polymorphisms colonies used in control strategies [15, 16]. We now summarize the chromosomal mutations found in the species throughout the years: reciprocal translocations, multiple translocations, and translocations between a sex chromosome and an autosome. The X-chromosome polymorphism due to attachment of a B-chromosome producing the X_L [16] could be understood through the analysis of 64 families involving reciprocal crosses of one male and one female. The transmission of the $Y + B = Y_L$ was analyzed in Ref. [15]. The deletions affecting the long arm of the sexual Y chromosome produces a mutant Y named Y_B [15]. The polymorphism Ya-Yb is analyzed in Ref. [15]. Other chromosomal mutations were also isolated in different families such as inversions involving the autosomes, sexual aneuploidies: sexual trisomics $2n = 2x + 1 = 13$ XXX, XXY, and sexual tetrasomics $2n = 2x + 2 = 14$ XXYY. Finally, we studied triploids: $2n = 3x = 18$ XXY and tetraploids: $2n = 4x = 24$.

3.2. *Anastrepha fraterculus*

The taxonomic status of *A. fraterculus* has been a controversial subject, mainly because of misinterpretation of the observed chromosomal variation. In an 11 years work, the different karyotypes and DNA polymorphism of geographically defined populations from Argentina were studied, using derived stocks maintained in the laboratory during 25 generations.

This fruit fly is the main native tephritid pest and only second to the invading Mediterranean fruit fly *C. capitata*. Previous to this work, almost 38 species have been written after or are synonymies of *A. fraterculus*. Our studies have been performed utilizing wild flies as well as laboratory stocks. This was the first time that *A. fraterculus* stocks were successfully isolated and maintained. The emphasis of this work was in the analysis of chromosomal characteristics since misinterpretation of genetic variation has been the origin of the current taxonomic confusion. More than 2500 specimens from 24 habitats (host-fruit/locality) were cytologically analyzed using specific cytological techniques. The different approaches (cytological, biochemical, and molecular) including *in situ hybridization*, on the same genetic material (stocks) made it possible the rigorous karyotypic and molecular analysis of the stocks and population samples [13].

The main results obtained are:

That—contrary to what many specialists have postulated—the chromosomal polymorphisms in *A. fraterculus* described and analyzed throughout this work are not a barrier for intercrossings (in the wild and in laboratory conditions) and represent a single species.

The basic knowledge of the species' chromosomal variability was widened for different populations of South America: Argentina, Brazil, and Uruguay.

This was the first time the rDNA cluster is localized and the autosomes of the species are described and identified.

This was the first time that cytological ploidy mosaicism in natural populations of *A. fraterculus* is described, assigning a role in the regulation of differential gene expression during insect development.

For the first time, double-minute chromosomes are described in natural populations of an invertebrate, a physiological adaptive role is proposed.

It was determined that the different chromosomal variants can be associated to particular host fruits or particular geographic localities.

It was demonstrated that habitat heterogeneity maintains the coexistence of different karyotypes and rearrangements present as polymorphisms whose frequencies vary from one population to the other.

We demonstrated that no correlation exists between data from traps and those obtained from samples of infested fruits, strengthening that *A. fraterculus* mating system is not based in larval feeding resources. This is highly significant since host registering must be unavoidably done on the base of effectively infested fruits. Pest status must depend on registration of hosts.

The reference karyotype *fraterculus Arg 1*, from now on *fArg1*, carries a 2n = 2x = 12 chromosome complement composed—as revealed by C-banding by an acrocentric X-chromosome, a quasi-metacentric Y-chromosome and 4 autosomal pairs not easy to distinguish except for chromosomal pair II which is the largest of the complement [13, 17, 18].

We found variants for all the chromosomal pairs in comparing them with *fArg1*. We studied and documented 1654 specimens of good cytological quality, applying different techniques on the same material. We maintained stocks of flies and founded 85 families as described previously. We had to confine our study to the sexual chromosome variants.

C-banding of the most frequent karyotype named *fArg 1* shows two telomeric bands on the X-chromosomes and one on the Y-chromosome [13, 17]. N-banding was a valuable marker of chromosome 3 which otherwise is difficult to distinguish from chromosome 4: a negative N-band resulted as a strong marker of pair 3 (**Figure 1A**). In the same family, we could detect the presence of triploid individuals (**Figure 1B**).

We described four variants of the X-chromosome and six variants of the Y-chromosome [13].

C-banding of the X_1, X_2, X_3, X_4, Y_1, Y_2, Y_3, Y_4, and Y_5 variants can be found in Refs. [13, 17, 18].

H-banding along with somatic pairing revealed the heterozygous autosomal rearrangements which are clearly seen and indicated by arrows (**Figure 2**).

The combination of banding techniques provided profiles to characterize the 10 sex chromosomal variants isolated in laboratory stocks (**Images 2–5**).

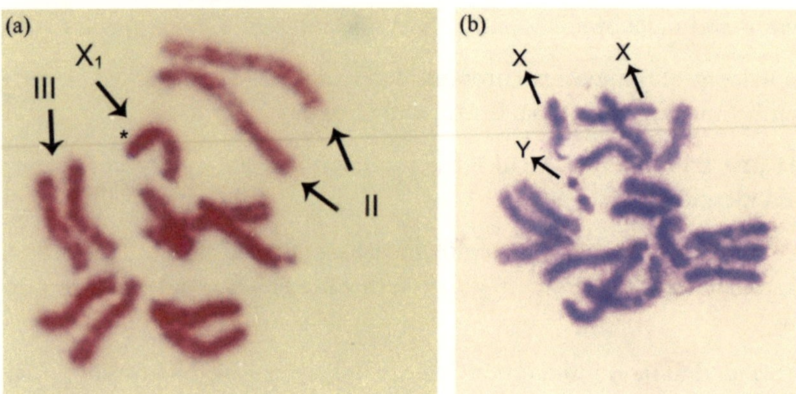

Figure 1. *N-banding* of neuroblast metaphases in *fArg1*. (A) Diploide X_1 Y_1 where asterisk indicates differential staining between positive banding and negative banding. 2800×. (B) Metaphase plate from a triploid male XXY. 2200×

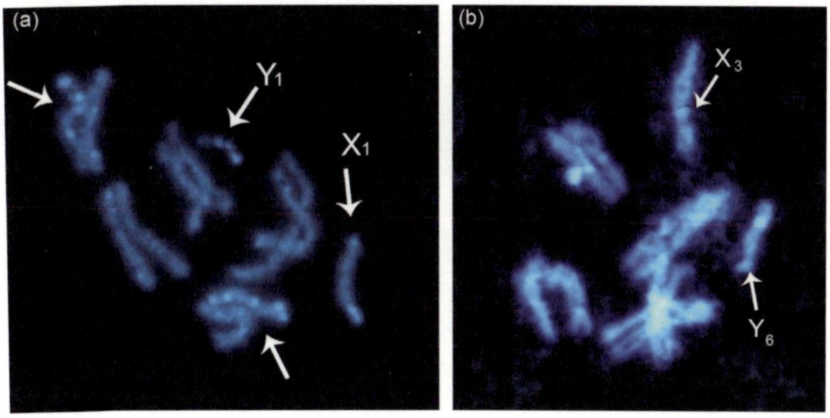

Figure 2. H-banding of metaphase plates. (A) X_1Y_1 specimen, arrows show heterozygous rearrangements. 2800×. (B) X_3Y_6 specimen. 2600×.

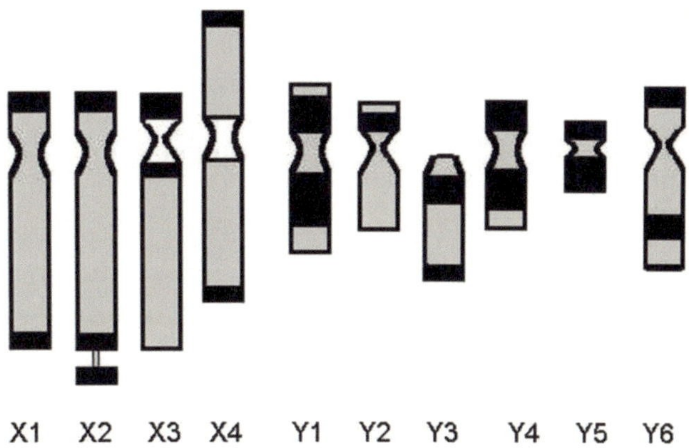

Image 2. Idiograms of the main variants of sex chromosomes for *Anastrepha fraterculus:* C-banding.

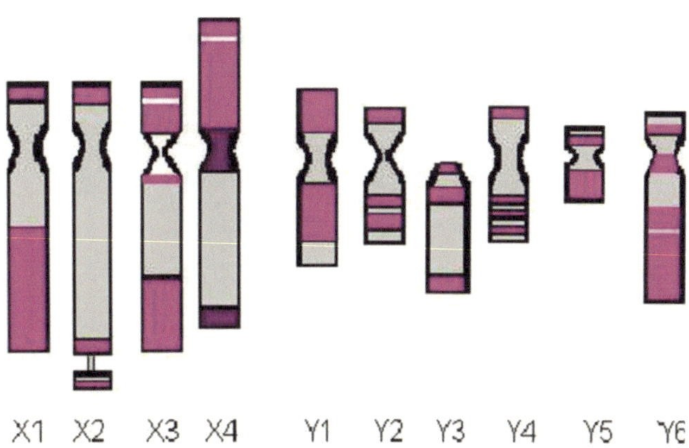

Image 3. Idiograms of the main variants of sex chromosomes for *Anastrepha fraterculus:* N-banding.

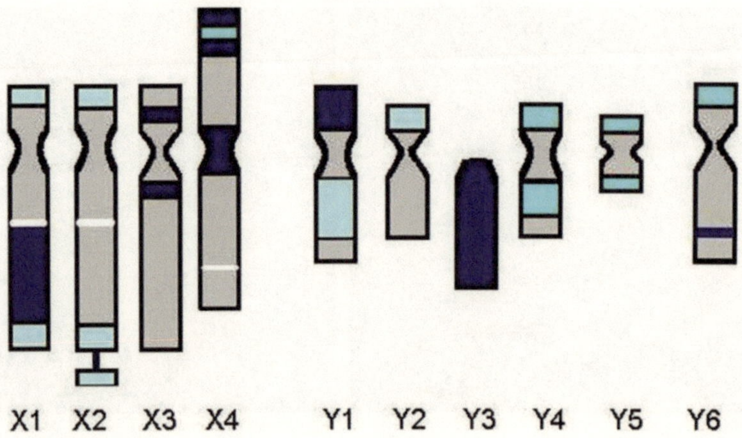

Image 4. Idiograms of the main variants of sex chromosomes for *Anastrepha fraterculus:* H-banding.

Ring chromosomes such as the X in (**Figure 3**) and the X-w (**Figure 4**) are evidence for duplication events. The X-w is shown in a prometaphase plate, as well as in an anaphase plate with bridge. This chromosomal rearrangement is a noticeable system during the evolution of *A. fraterculus*.

Ploidy mosaics (**Figures 5–7**) and double-minute chromosomes are also evidences for duplication events (**Figure 8**).

Mosaic individuals carrying diploid nuclei along with sexual tetrasomic nuclei X1X1Y5Y5 were found within some families of flies (**Figure 7**).

We also detected aneuploids such as monosomics (**Figure 9**) and sexual trisomics (**Figure 11**). Chromomicin A3 evidenced chromosomes with unequal sister chromatids (**Figure 10**) as a result of the somatic crossing over with interchange between sister chromatids (**Figure 11**) [19, 20].

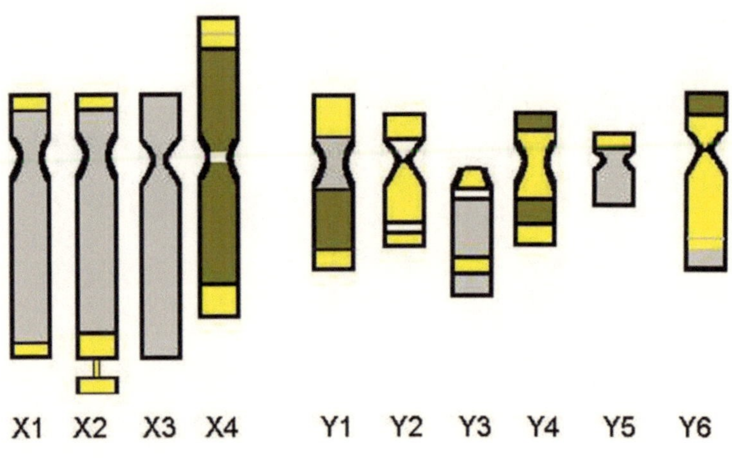

Image 5. Idiograms of the main variants of sex chromosomes for *Anastrepha fraterculus:* CMA_3-banding.

http://dx.doi.org/10.5772/intechopen.69835

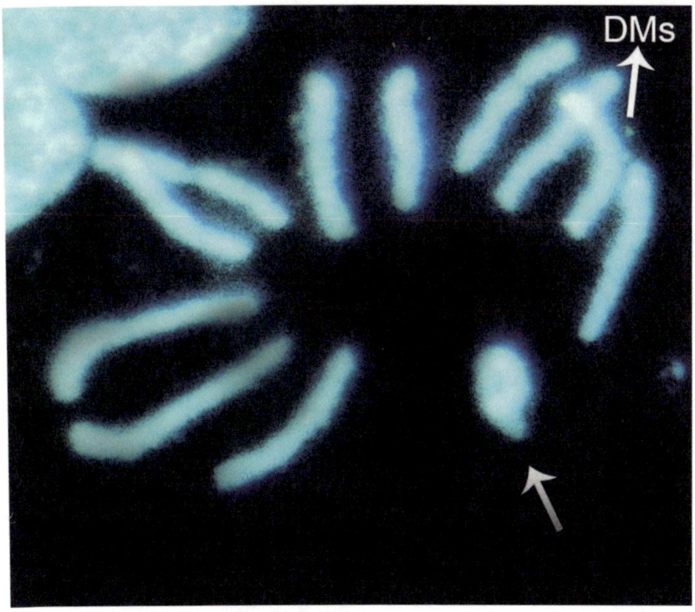

Figure 3. Metaphase carrying an X_2 ring chromosome. See arrow. 3200×.

The ribosomal DNA cluster was first located in *A. fraterculus* and in *C. capitata* using the 720 bp probe of the 18S gene of *C. capitata* [13]. This probe tested on the reference stock of *A. fraterculus* hybridized the short-arm telomere of X1 chromosome and the centromere and pericentromeric region of the short arm of Y1 chromosome in *fArg1* (**Figure 12**). In different strains of *A. fraterculus,* the localization of the ribosomal cluster was observed on the variants of sexual chromosomes such as Y_2 and Y_5 (**Figures 13–14**).

Except for the sexual karyotypes X_3X_3 and X_3X_4, we found all the combinations among the X chromosomes and among the X and Y chromosomes (**Image 6**).

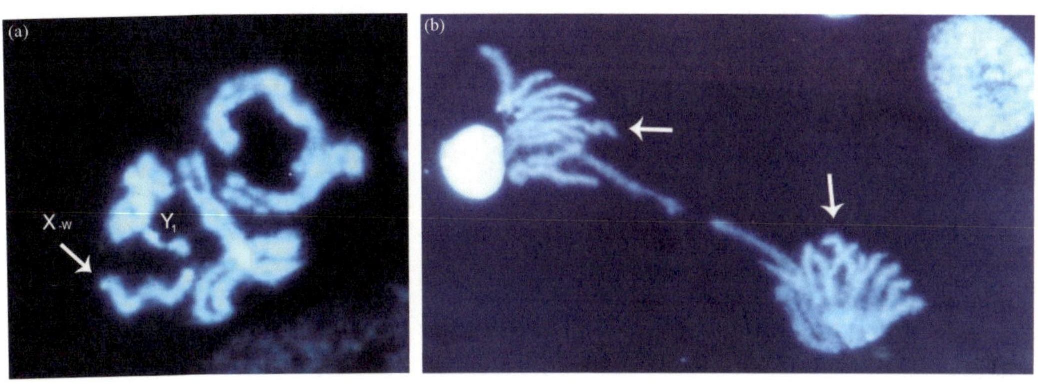

Figure 4. The X-w chromosome. (A) Prometaphase carrying X-w Y_1 and translocations. 2600×. (B) Anaphase with bridge, arrows show the X-w chromosome in each pole. 2600×.

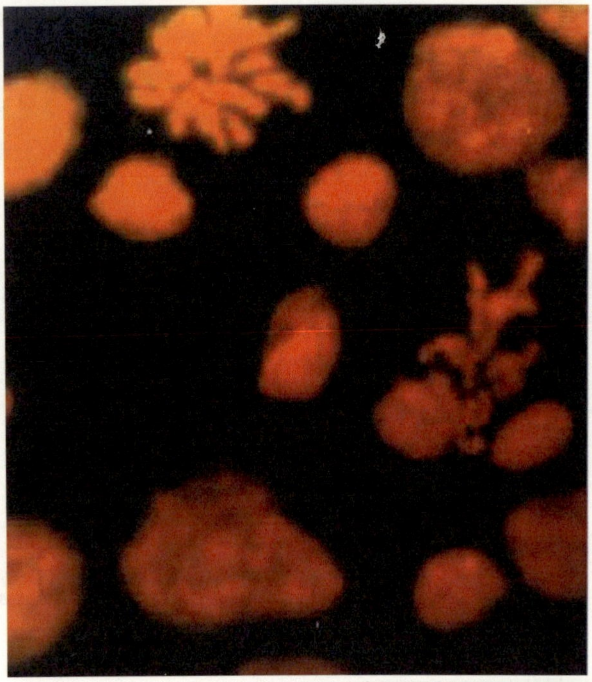

Figure 5. Propidium iodide staining of a mosaic specimen 2n = 2× – 3×. Metaphase plate showing two nuclei: diploid-triploid. 2600×.

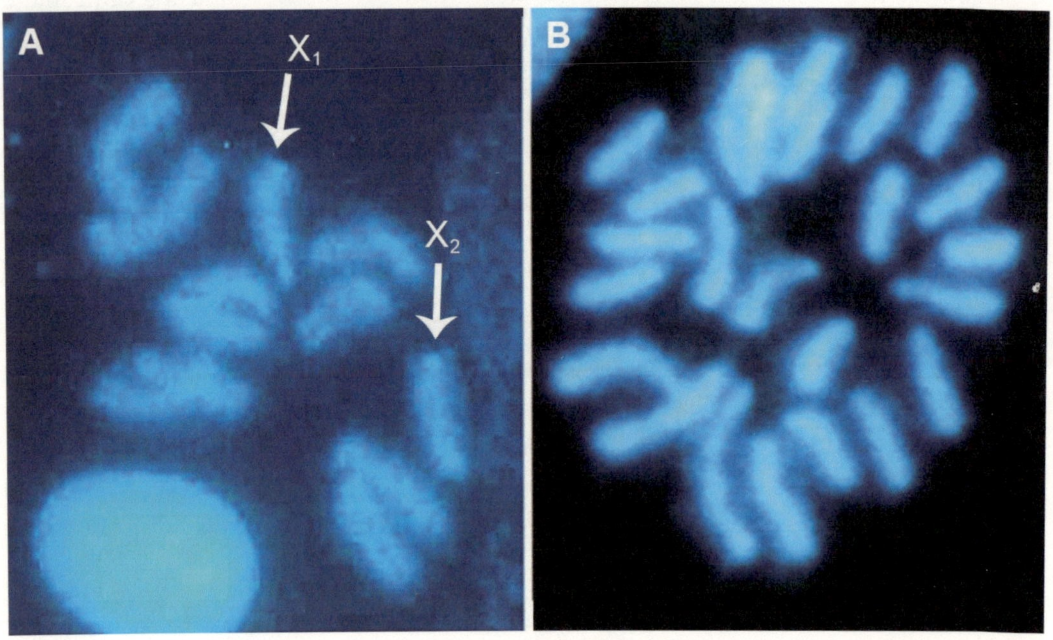

Figure 6. Hoechst staining on a mosaic specimen X_1X_2 from Brazilian stock 1220x. (A) Diploid metaphase. (B) Tetraploid metaphase. 2800×.

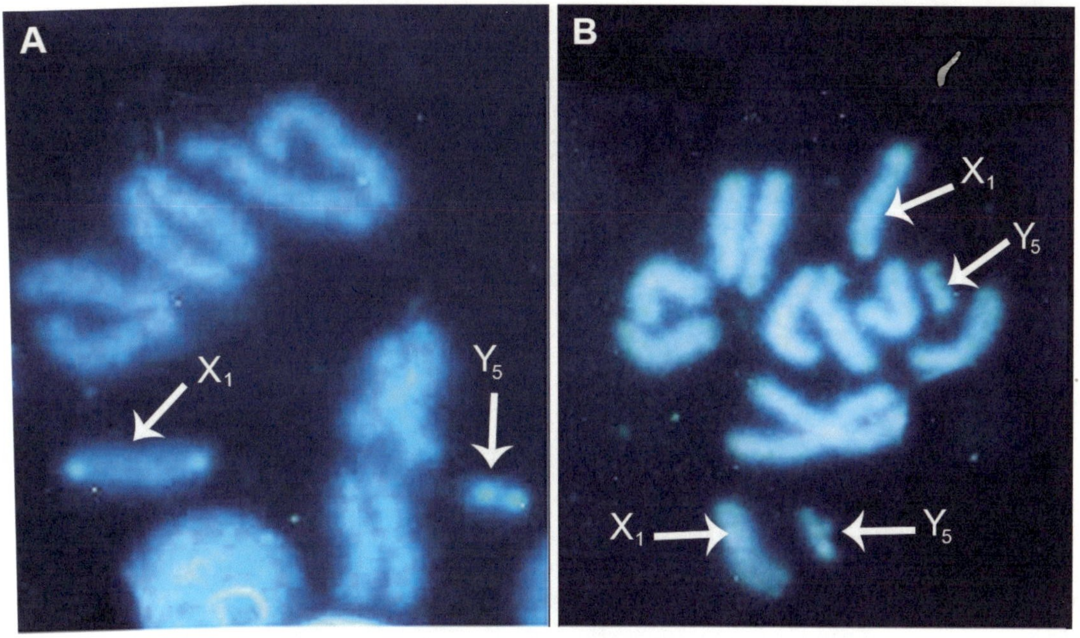

Figure 7. Hoechst staining on a X_1Y_5 mosaic individual from stock 244C. Two metaphases of the same specimen. (A) Diploid metaphase X_1Y_5. (B) Aneuploid metaphase $X_1X_1Y_5Y_5$ (sexual tetrasomic). 2600×.

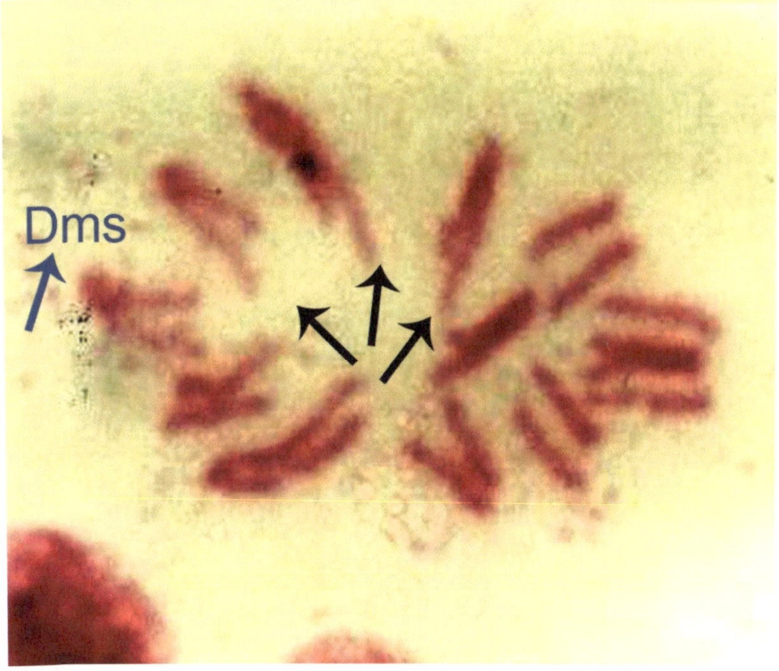

Figure 8. Metaphase showing chromosomes with unequal sister chromatids (see arrows) and double-minute chromosomes. 2800×.

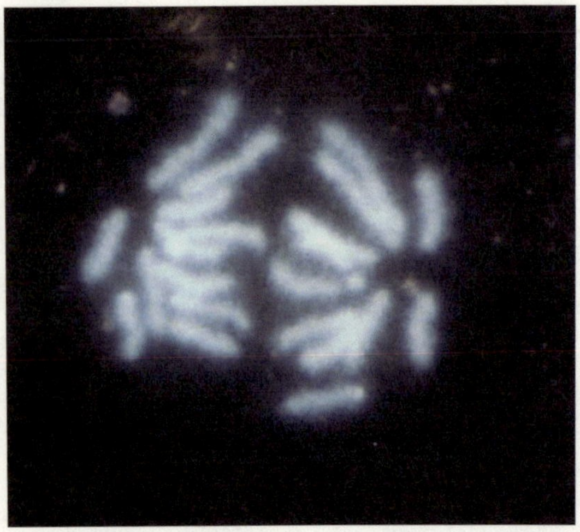

Figure 9. H-staining of a monosomic specimen 2n = 2× – 1. 2500×.

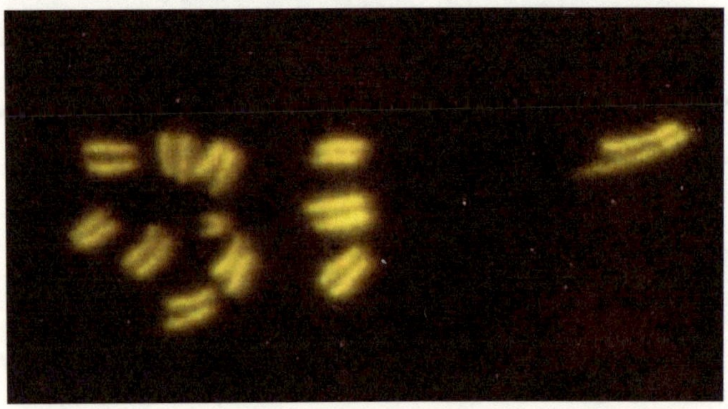

Figure 10. CMA 3 staining. Metaphase showing chromosomes with unequal chromatids.

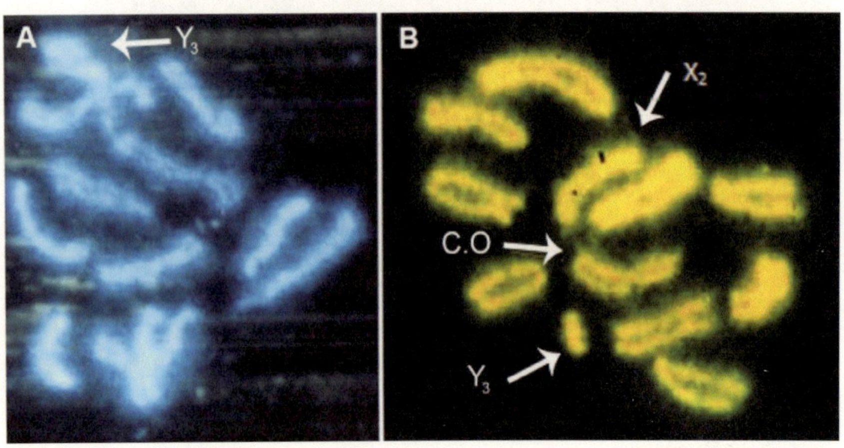

Figure 11. Stock 286. (A) Sexual aneuploid specimen 2n = 2× + 1=13, trisomic $X_1X_2Y_3$. (B) Specimen X_2Y_3 showing somatic C.O., interchange between sister chromatids.

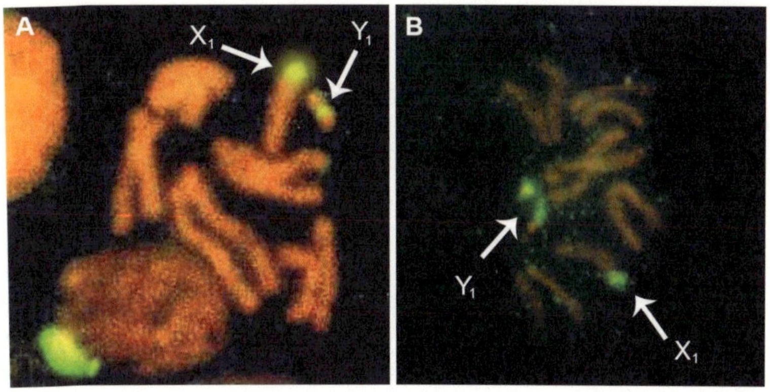

Figure 12. FISH with *C. capitata p18S* on *"f. Arg. 1."* (A and B) Different specimens from stock 215M. 2800×.

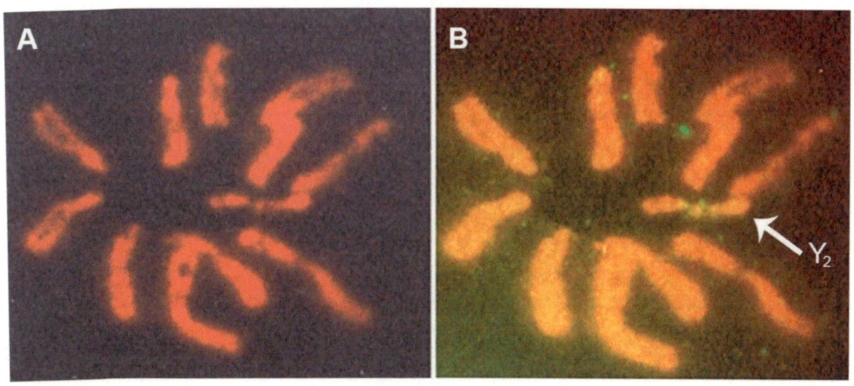

Figure 13. FISH with *C. capitata p 18S* on mitotic metaphase from stock 23M. (A) Counterstaining with propidium iodide. (B) Probe hybridizes Y_2 centromere. 2600×.

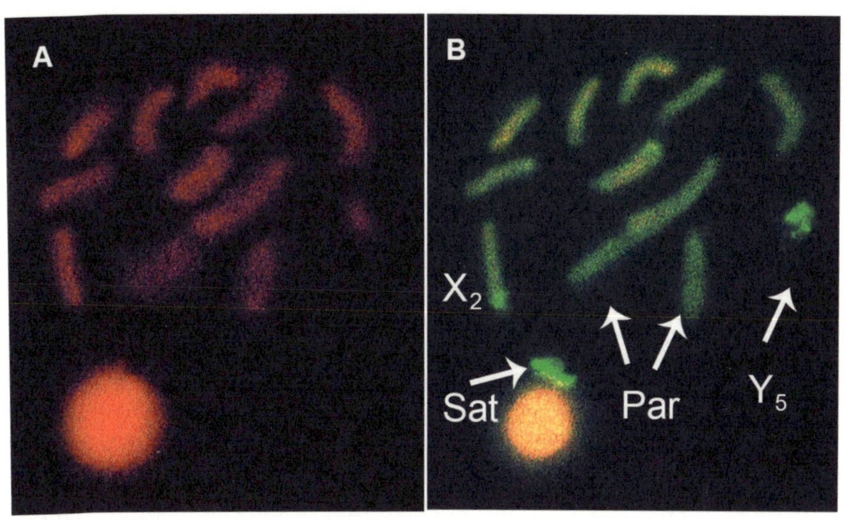

Figure 14. FISH with *C. capitata* p18S on mitotic chromosomes from a specimen X_2Y_5 of stock 1222. (A) Counterstaining with propidium iodide. (B) The probe hybridized the telomere and satellite of X_2 chromosome the whole Y_5 and an autosomal pair. 2500×.

MALES		FEMALES	
X1Y1	X1Y1+Ah	X1X1	X1X1+Ah
X2Y4	X1Y2+Ah	X1X2	X1X2+Ah
X1Y3	X1Y3+Ah	X2X2	X2X2+Ah
X2Y2	X2Y4+Ah	X2X3	X2X3+Ah
X2Y3	X2Y3+Ah	X1X3	
X2Y1	X1Y5	X1X4	X1X4+Ah
X2Y5	X2Y5+Ah	X2X4	X2X4+Ah
X1Y6	X3Y1	X4X4	X4X4+Ah
X2Y6	X3Y6		
X4Y1	X4Y5		
X4Y2	X4Y6+Ah		
X4Y4	X1Y4		
X4Y3	X3Y2		

Image 6. Karyotypes biologically compatible which were found in the studied natural populations and tested in laboratory stocks.

4. Conclusions

The normal karyotype is the most frequent karyotype known as the reference karyotype: *f Arg 1* in *A. fraterculus* and *Arg 17* in *C. capitata.*

Population cytology studies using large numbers of specimens allowed us to detect all possible combinations across generations.

The fruit fly is oviparous, its life cycle lasts around 45 days, it oviposits large numbers of eggs, has complete metamorphosis of egg and larva lives inside the fruit, pupae in the ground, and adults in the leaves of trees. Chromosomal rearrangements maintain within populations, some of them as polymorphisms similar to those of the chromosomal variants described for

Anastrepha and for *Ceratitis*. The study of the families carrying different variants proved their transmission from parents to offsprings through successive generations.

The techniques applied in our studies revealed many changes in heterochromatin and assisted in recognizing variants: N-bands are the best marker for autosome III; H-banding revealed autosomal mutations and sexual chromosomal variants such as the Y6 and double-minute chromosomes; Chromomicin A3 assisted in revealing the somatic crossing over, and FISH in recognizing rearrangements of the ribosomal cluster.

The long stretches of DNA in heterochromatin contain important sequences in health and disease that, for the most part, need to be silenced for cells to work properly.

In humans, one banding technique is applied to diagnose illnesses. It would be useful to apply different banding techniques in order to recognize new chromosomal rearrangements associated with physiological disorders. The use of several techniques on the same material should help to determine if the same mutation produces different phenotypes or behaviours when comparing different geographical populations.

Think about balanced polymorphisms such as the malaria—anemia in Eurasia, where different genotypes persist through heterozygote superiority. Could a genetic mutation that puts populations at risk for illnesses in one environmental setting expresses itself in positive ways in a different setting?

Chromosomal mutations produce variability. Variation is the key to survival and many individuals could be in the right place but in the wrong moment.

Author details

Alicia Leonor Basso Abraham

Address all correspondence to: abasso@agro.uba.ar

Cátedra de Genética, Facultad de Agronomía, Universidad de Buenos Aires, Buenos Aires, Argentina Republic

References

[1] Lerner M. The Genetic Basis of Selection. New York: John Wiley; 1958

[2] Terán H. Comportamiento alimentario y su correlación a la reproducción en hembras de *Ceratitis capitata* (Wied.) (Diptera: Trypetidae). Revista de Agronomía del Noroeste Argentino. 1977;**14**:17-34

[3] Terán H. Selección de alimentos por los machos e influencia de éstos y del espacio vital sobre el comportamiento reproductivo de hembras de Ceratitis capitata (Wied.) (Diptera: Trypetidae). Revista de Agronomía del Noroeste Argentino. 1978;**15**(2):55-66

[4] Rabossi A, Wappner P, Quesada-Allué LA. Larva to pharate adult transformation in the medfly, *Ceratitis capitata.* The Canadian Entomologist. 1992;**124**:1139-1147

[5] Manso F. Breeding technique of *Anastrepha fraterculus* (Wied.) for genetic studies. In: The South American Fruit Fly, *Anastrepha fraterculus* (Wied.); Advances in Artificial Rearing, Taxonomic Status and Biological Studies. Viena, Austria: IAEA; 1999. pp. 25-30

[6] Kerremans Ph, Gencheva E, Franz G. Genetic and cytogenetic analysis of Y-autosome translocations in the Mediterranean fruit fly *Ceratitis capitata*. Genome. 1992;**35**:264-272

[7] Willhoeft U, Franz G. Identification of the sex-determining region of the *Ceratitis capitata* Y chromosome by deletion mapping. Genetics. 1996;**144**:737-745

[8] Basso A, Lifschitz E, Manso F. Determination of intraspecific variation in heterochromatin of *Ceratitis capitata* (Wied) by C-banding. Cytobios. 1995;**83**:237-244

[9] Gatti M, Pimpinelli S, Santini G. Characterization of *Drosophila heterochromatin*. I-staining and decondensation with Hoechst 33258 and quinacrine. Chromosoma. 1976;**57**:351-375

[10] Schweizer D. Reverse fluorescence chromosome banding with Chromomicin and DAPI. Chromosoma. 1976;**58**:307-324

[11] Basso A, Sonvico A, Quesada-Allué LA, Manso F. Karyotypic and molecular identification of laboratory stocks of the South American fruit fly *Anastrepha fraterculus* (Wied.). Journal of Economic Entomology. 2003;**96**(4):1237-1244. DOI: 10.1603/0022-0493-96.4.1237

[12] Renkhawitz-Pohl R, Glaetzer K, Kuntz W. Characterization of cloned ribosomal DNA from *Drosophila hydei*. Nucleic Acids Research. 1980;**8**:4593-4611

[13] Basso A. Caraterización genética de los componentes del complejo *"Anastrepha fraterculus"* (*Anastrepha spp*. DIPTERA: Tephritidae, Trypetinae) (Wiedemann) mediante análisis de la variabilidad cromosómica [dissertation]. Argentina: Universidad de Buenos Aires; 2003. p. 234.

[14] Sonvico A, Benseñor L, Quesada-Allué LA. Caracterización del "cluster" de ADN ribosomal nuclear en poblaciones de moscas de la fruta, *Ceratitis capitata y Anastrepha fraterculus.* En: Actas Taller Internacional Sobre Programas de Control y Erradicación de Moscas de los Frutos. Buenos Aires, Argentina: SENASA; 1999

[15] Basso A, Martinez L, Manso F. The significance of genetic polymorphisms within and between founder populations of Ceratitis capitata (Wied) from Argentina. PLoS One. 2009;**4**(3):e4665. DOI: 10.1371/journal.pone.0004665

[16] Basso A, Lifschitz E. Size polymorphism of the X-chromosome due to attachment of the B-chromosome in the medfly *Ceratitis capitata* (Wied). Brazilian Journal of Genetics. 1995;**18**(2):165-171

[17] Basso A, Manso F. Are *Anastrepha fraterculus* chromosomal polymorphisms an isolation barrier? Cytobios. 1998;**93**:103-111

[18] Lifschitz E, Manso F, Basso A. Karyotype study of the South American Fruit Fly, *Anastrepha fraterculus* (Wied.) in Argentina. In: The South American Fruit Fly, *Anastrepha fraterculus* (Wied.). Advances in Artificial Rearing Taxonomic Status and Biological Studies. Viena, Austria: IAEA; 1999. pp 21-24

[19] Manso F, Basso A. Notes on the present situation of *Anastrepha fraterculus* in Argentina. In: The South American Fruit Fly, *Anastrepha fraterculus* (Wied.). Advances in Artificial Rearing Taxonomic Status and Biological Studies. Viena, Austria: IAEA; 1999. pp. 147-162

[20] Prokop A, Technau GM. The origin of postembryonic neuroblasts in the ventral nerve cord of *Drosophila melanogaster*. Development. 1991;**111**:79-88

Chromatid Abnormalities in Meiosis: A Brief Review and a Case Study in the Genus *Agave* (Asparagales, Asparagaceae)

Benjamín Rodríguez-Garay

Additional information is available at the end of the chapter

http://dx.doi.org/10.5772/intechopen.68974

Abstract

The genus *Agave* is distributed in the tropical and subtropical areas of the world and represents a large group of succulent plants, with about 200 taxa from 136 species, and its center of origin is probably limited to Mexico. It is divided into two subgenera: *Littaea* and *Agave* based on the architecture of the inflorescence; the subgenus *Littaea* has a spicate or racemose inflorescence, while plants of the subgenus *Agave* have a paniculate inflorescence with flowers in umbellate clusters on lateral branches. As the main conclusion of this study, a hypothesis rises from the described observations: *frying pan-shaped* chromosomes are formed by sister chromatid exchanges and a premature kinetochore movement in prophase II, which are meiotic aberrations that exist in these phylogenetic distant species, *Agave stricta* and *A. angustifolia* since ancient times in their evolution, and this may be due to genes that are prone to act under diverse kinds of environmental stress.

Keywords: tequila, mescal, chromatid cohesion, centromere, inversion heterorozygosity, kinetochore

1. Introduction

The genus *Agave* is distributed in the tropical and subtropical areas of the world and represents a large group of succulent plants, with about 200 taxa from 136 species, and its center of origin is probably limited to Mexico [1]. It is divided into two subgenera: *Littaea* and *Agave* based on the architecture of the inflorescence; the subgenus *Littaea* has a spicate or racemose inflorescence while plants of the subgenus *Agave* have a paniculate inflorescence with flowers in umbellate clusters on lateral branches (**Figures 1** and **2**) [1].

Agave is a young genus which originated 7.8 to 10.1 million years ago (Mya) [2]. A group of species of this genus, the subgenus *Littaea* is considered to be the most primitive of all *Agave* species as the spicate inflorescence is the most common among monocotyledons than the paniculate form of the subgenus *Agave* [1]. In this context, Eguiarte et al. [3] calculated that species of the subgenus *Littaea* group Striatae (*A. striata, A. dasyliriodes*) got separated about 8 Mya. It is important to mention that *A. stricta* also belongs to the Striatae group [1]. On the other hand, the same researchers found that *A. americana* that belongs to the subgenus *Agave* was separated about 2 Mya, thus being considered the subgenus *Agave* younger than the subgenus *Littaea*.

The groups Rigidae and Sisalanae that belong to the subgenus *Agave*, are commercially important due to their use for several purposes: (a) alcoholic beverages, such as tequila and mezcal; (b) natural long and hard fibers; and (c) steroidal and medicinal principles [2–4]. The *Agave* genus conforms a group of plant species of the Asparagaceae family (formerly Agavaceae) that belongs to the monocot class of angiosperms and because of

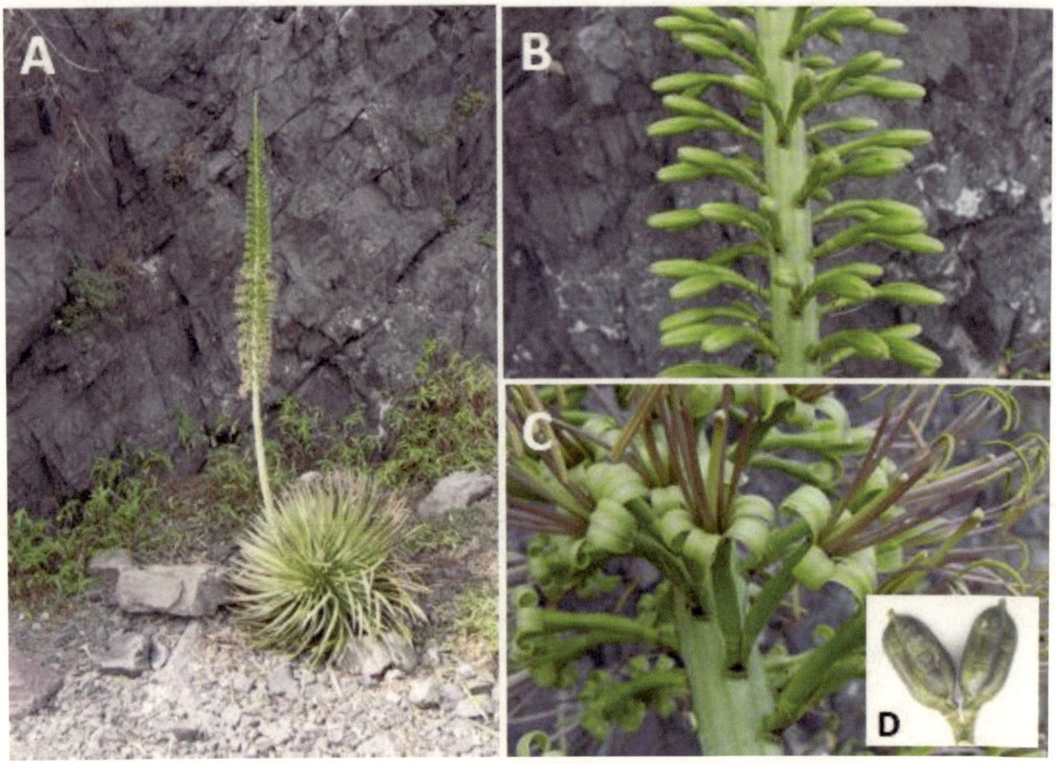

Figure 1. *Agave colimana* as an example of the subgenus *Littaea*. (A) Wild *A. colimana* plant growing in cliffs near the sea in the coast of the state of Jalisco, México. (B) Section of the spicate floral stalk showing the flower buds arranged in pairs. (C) Mature flowers arranged in pairs. (D) Immature fruits.

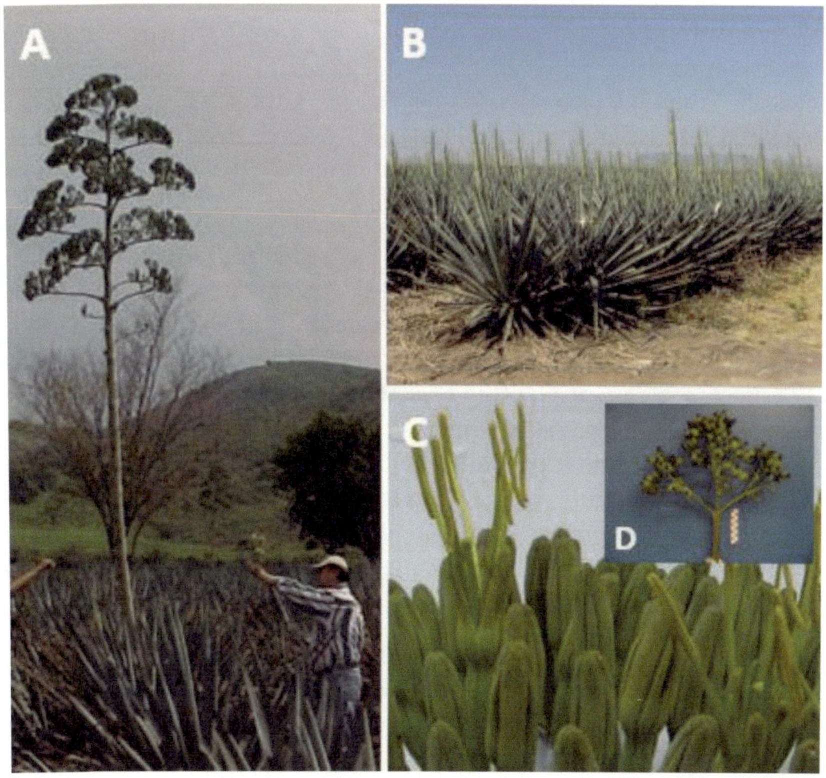

Figure 2. *Agave tequilana* as an example of the subgenus *Agave* growing near to the city of Guadalajara, Jalisco, México. (A) Mature plant of *A. tequilana* showing a paniculate inflorescence. (B) Commercial plantation with inflorescences in development ready to be cut off to allow the accumulation of sugars for the production of tequila. (C) Mature and immature flowers. (D) Immature fruits in a panicle.

its CAM metabolism and other botanical features, the genus *Agave* is gaining importance throughout the world to address the challenges that climate change is imposing with regard to food, medicine and bioenergy [4]. A good source of information about the taxonomy of the genus *Agave* is the book "Agaves of Continental North America" by Howard Scott Gentry [1].

The genus *Agave* is a semelparous perennial that produces flowers only once toward the end of its life cycle being 6–8 years for *A. tequilana* and *A. angustifolia* [5] and about 30 years for *A. Victoria-reginae* [6].

In *Agave* as in all Angiosperms, one of their main characteristics is that they possess seeds enclosed inside a fruit derived from the ovary of flowers [7]. Another important feature of angiosperms is that they have an alternation of generations in their life cycle (as in many other plants), divided in two phases: one diploid phase, which is called sporophytic, and the other haploid phase known as gametophytic phase [8–10]. The main function of the gametophytic phase is the production of haploid male and female gametes through the meiotic cell division [9, 11].

2. Meiosis (meiotic division)

The term "meiosis" (from the Greek word maiosis = μειωτικής which means reduction) was first proposed in 1905 by J. Bertland Farmer and J.E.S. Moore in reference to the nuclear division that was called "heterotype" by Walther Flemming, cell division which is responsible for the production of gametes in plants and animals [12].

Meiotic cell division is the key point process in the sexual reproduction of most of animal and plant species, through which haploid gametes are generated, and includes two successive divisions of the nucleus, where the first division is reductional and the second is equational; a failure in any or in both of these cell divisions produces chromosomal accidents which will be reflected in gamete viability or mutations that will appear in the progeny [13]. The objective of meiosis is to produce haploid gametes from original diploid cells and starts with the replication of DNA that produces four chromatids of each type of chromosome, two from the female parent and two from the male parent. These four chromatids are distributed into four final different nuclei [14]. In plants, male gametes or microgametophytes (pollen grains) are developed inside the anthers and are formed from a pollen mother cell, which undergoes a meiotic process that gives rise to a tetrad of haploid cells called microspores.

In the process of pollen development, the microspore undergoes a nonsymmetric mitotic division giving rise to a vegetative and a generative cell. The generative cell undergoes a second mitotic division producing two haploid sperms. In the meantime, the vegetative cell remains without division and produces the pollen tube, which carries the sperms, and finally reaches the ovule for the process of fertilization [15].

On the other hand, the female gametophyte develops in the ovule. One megaspore mother cell is located in the center of the ovule, which after two meiotic cell divisions gives rise to a strand of four haploid cells or megaspores. In most of angiosperms three of these megaspores degenerate, however, the cell which is the closest to the chalaza survives as the functional megaspore, this enlarges and undergoes three mitotic divisions to form the embryo sac. In general, the embryo sac follows different patterns of development in different genera and species; however, the most common pattern consists of four types of cells: three antipodal cells (at the chalazal end), one central cell containing two polar haploid nuclei (that is generally located at the center of the embryo sac), and two synergid cells flanking the egg cell, all three positioned at the micropylar end [16].

2.1. Chromosomes and chromatids in meiosis

In the meiotic process, a single round of DNA replication is followed by two rounds of chromosome segregation that generate four haploid gametes from one diploid cell [17]. To accomplish this specialized chromosome segregation, sister kinetochores (contained in the region of the chromosome called *centromere*) are attached to microtubules emanating from a spindle pole to help with the reductional segregation of homologous chromosomes (*not* sister chromatids) in the first heterotype step of the meiotic division (**Figure 3**).

Chiasmata occur between a homologous chromosome pair, and at least two of the four chromatids become unique, and different from those coming from the parents. There is the formation of bivalents in chiasmata, and this generates an adequate chromosome segregation in meiosis [21]. The chromatids that are conforming the unit called chromosome are called "sister chromatids". On the other hand, in most of organisms, homologous chromosomes have to be aligned in a precise linear manner with the help of the cytoskeleton formed by proteins that give motility to chromosomes and the intervention of the synaptonemal complex. In this manner, genetic recombination and the formation of chiasmata (stable connections between homologs formed at the sites of crossovers) take place [18]. The process of exchange of genetic material between homologous chromosomes is mediated by the action of recombination proteins and topoisomerase-like proteins that promote the breakdown of chromosomal DNA so that exchange can take place. Crossing over or recombination between sister chromatids is known as *sister chromatid exchange*. Thus, since they are identical, would not produce any new genetic variation. It has been found that chances of recombination of sister chromatids increase in meiotic cells of haploid yeast, while in mitotic cells, the chances are reduced. It is possible that several forms of ectopic recombination were favored by the lack of their genetic counterparts [19]. On the other hand, a wrong synapsis can have consequences during metaphase I, therefore, chromosomal segregation in anaphase I would occur incorrectly.

Sister chromatids are kept together by the action of the cohesin complex along the length of their arms and at their centromeres, and need to be held together in order to be segregated to opposite poles of the spindle in both mitosis and meiosis II. Sister chromatid cohesion is also involved in having homologous chromosomes together in meiosis I. Physical cohesion is dependent of the cohesin complex formed by several proteins for maintaining sister chromatids together, and the dissolution of sister-chromatid cohesion must be regulated precisely through specific control mechanisms that prevent the incorrect segregation of chromosomes [20], for example, the Spindle Assembly Checkpoint (SAC) complex that regulates the proper attachment of microtubules to kinetochores.

The cohesin complex is highly conserved in eukaryotes and is mainly composed of four conserved proteins found in yeast, animals and plants (reviewed in [21–25]). In mitosis as in meiosis, cohesins have a ring-like structure formed by SMC1, SMC2, α-kleisin (RAD21 / SCC1 in mitosis or Rec8 in meiosis) and SCC3, each element of the cohesin complex is of a key importance for proper segregation of chromosomes.

In mitosis, cell division depends on the correct separation of sister chromatids in anaphase and is accomplished by the attachment of microtubules (originated in opposite spindle poles) to sister kinetochores. Sister kinetochores are bi-oriented by being pulled to opposite poles (equational segregation) in a process of kinetochore-microtubule attachment called amphitelic. In this process that occurs in mitosis and meiosis II, sister-chromatids cohesion associated with chromatin is separated by the protease separase at the beginning of anaphase where chromosomes become bi-oriented (**Figure 3**) [26].

Kinetochores are protein complexes located at the centromeric region of the chromosome and regulate chromosome and chromatid movement, and plant kinetochores contain proteins

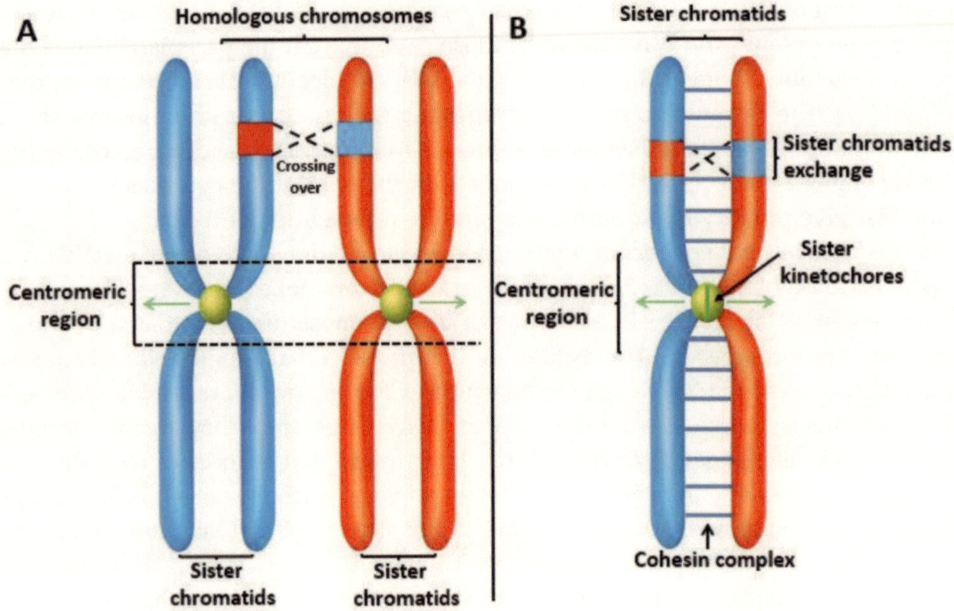

Figure 3. Schematic structure of chromosomes in meiosis. A) Homologous chromosomes showing sister chromatids, centromeric region and a crossing over. Balls represent the kinetochores and the arrows show their normal movement to opposite poles in Meiosis I. B) Metaphasic chromosome in Meiosis II showing the centromeric region which includes the kinetochores, the sister chromatids and the cohesin complex that holds together the sister chromatids. Also, an eventual sister chromatids exchange is represented. Again, the arrows show the process of normal movement of sister chromatids to opposite poles called *amphitelic bi-orientation*.

which are homologs to those found in animals and fungi kinetochores (reviewed in Ref. [27]). In this protein complex, CENH3 (a variant of histone H3) and CENPC interact internally with the centromere, while NCD80 and MIS12 interact with microtubules, and MIS12 is necessary for proper segregation of homologous chromosomes.

3. Agave cytogenetics: a case study

The genus *Agave* has been the object of cytological investigations only after 1933, since then, chromosome counts have been made on a large number of species. This genus has a bimodal complement of 10 large and 50 small chromosomes with a monoploid number of x = 30, and with varieties and species from diploid to hexaploid [5, 28–30]. Cave [31] reported regular meiosis in five diploid, two tetraploid and one hexaploid species, and irregular meiosis in two polyploids, with bridges and fragments at anaphase I. Similar cytological investigations were carried out in *Agave stricta* and *A. tequilana*, which are euploid species with the basic chromosome number of x = 30, and for which meiotic behavior heterozygous for paracentric inversions and subchromatid exchanges was described. The mentioned altered meiosis produced a number of aberrations, such as bridges and fragments at anaphase I and II [5, 32]. Also, in *A. stricta* loop chromatids were visible at prophase II, but not at metaphase II (see arrow in **Figure 4** [32]).

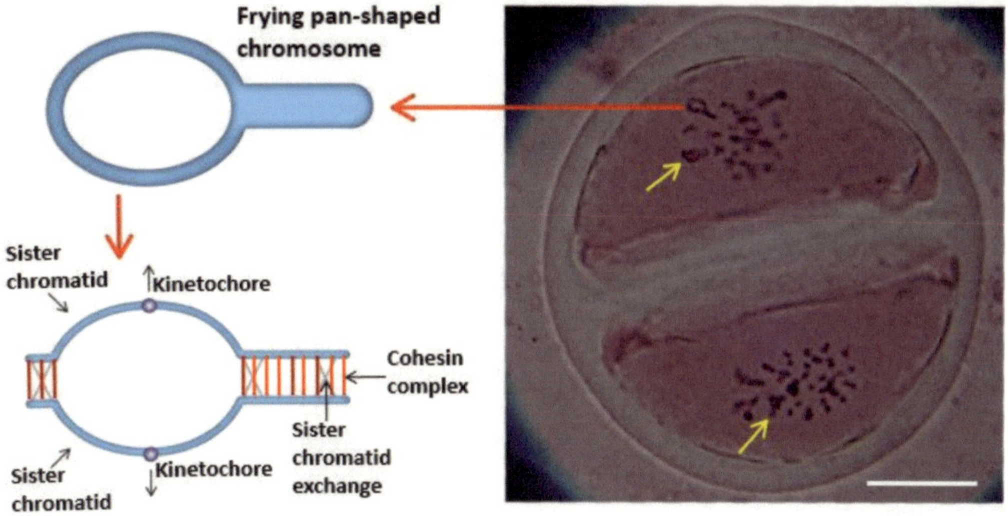

Figure 4. Schematic proposed hypothesis for the formation of *frying pan-shaped* chromosomes in prophase II of *Agave angustifolia*. White bar = 20 μm.

Agave angustifolia belongs to the subgenus *Agave* group Rigidae and is used for Mezcal production in México. The chromosome behavior in the meiosis of *Agave* species has been previously reported [5, 32–33]. Frequently, in diverse plant species, the formation of dicentric bridges and acentric fragments in Anaphase I is known as a result of inversion heterozygosity. In *A. tequilana,* the analysis of Pollen Mother Cells in anaphase I (A-I) has shown cells with normal and irregular A-I with side arm bridges (SAB), cells with one bridge and one fragment, anaphases with one or two lagging chromosomes and acentric fragments. Also, in anaphase II (A-II) some cells showed bridges, all of them leading to the production of shrunken or empty pollen grains [5].

The plant material used in this study consisted of immature anthers from the inflorescence of a plant which was an offshoot taken from a mother plant originally collected in the year 2006 in the vicinity of Sayula, Jalisco, México. This plant was called "224" as is referred in the field books and diverse files at the Plant Biotechnology Unit-CIATEJ and grown at the CIATEJ campus located in the city of Guadalajara, Jalisco, México. Fresh anthers from young buds were collected on June 2014, selected and fresh squashed in 1% acetoorceine. The best cells for meiotic chromosome analysis were photographed using an Olimpus BH2 microscope coupled with a digital Sony camera.

As the most outstanding results in this study, several aberrant meiotic divisions could be observed in the male gametogenesis. Some of the most frequent aberrations were bridges formed in anaphase I mainly due to heterozygous inversions and probably due to sister chromatid exchanges. A striking finding was a couple of *frying pan-shaped* chromosomes in each cell of several diads in prophase II before entering anaphase II (**Figure 3**),, which were highly similar to those previously reported for *Agave stricta* (see arrow in **Figure 4**) [32], a species that belongs to the subgenus *Littaea* group Striatae.

As reviewed above, the genus *Agave* is divided into two subgenera: *Littea* and *Agave*, whose most important difference is the morphology of their inflorescence, being racemose for *Littaea* and paniculate for *Agave* [1]. Also, it has been mentioned that the subgenus *Littaea* is considered to be the most primitive of the two and both separated by a span of several million years [2, 3].

On the other hand, the formation of *frying pan-shaped* configurations may be explained by putative sister chromatid exchanges, where chiasma type junctions in different points of the chromosome held the sister-chromatids and remained joined at the site of the exchange as it has been explained for regular chiasmata in a model for achiasmate homologous chromosome segregation (**Figure 5**) [34]. The phenomenon of sister-chromatid exchange may be viewed as a mechanism of double-strand break repair in plants and in general in eukaryotes. These breaks may be the product of errors caused by endogenous or exogenous kinds of stress such as reactive oxygen species (ROS), radiation [36, 37], and many other environmental kinds of stress imposed by climate change [38, 39]. Also, with regard to the cohesin complex, an example of ROS action is in the induction of loss of cohesion and chromosome errors in mammals, mainly in human females causing the phenomenon called *maternal age effect* which is produced in oocytes [40].

Furthermore, an alternative explanation for the formation of *frying pan-shaped* chromosomes is the putative aberrant loss of cohesion of arms and/or in the centromeric region of sister chromatids in meiosis II. Nowadays, it is known that the centromeric cohesin complex is protected by the

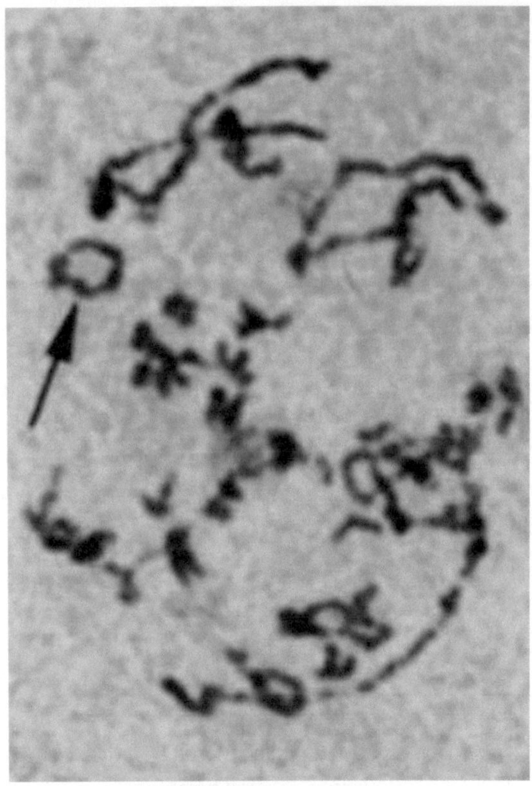

Figure 5. P II. Loop chromatid (arrow). The unaffected short arms can be seen, left. *Source:* Brandham [32]. With permission of Springer.

protein Shugoshin (Sgo1) (which means *protective deity* or *guardian* in the Japanese language). In meiosis I, sister chromatids are maintained together by the cohesin complex that contains the Rec8 subunit. At this stage, separase destroys Rec8 in the chromosome arms, while Shugoshin protects Rec8 at the centromeres. In meiosis II, the state of kinetochores of being stretched may cause Shugoshin destruction, and sister chromatid separation is facilitated by cleavage of Rec8 by separase [41]. The mechanisms of cohesion action and Shugoshin protection seem to be conserved across species such as in fission yeast and plants [23, 41, 42]. In addition, the cohesion of sister chromatids depends on an acyltransferase called Eco1/Ctf7 [43], however, this enzyme is not required for cohesin loading on DNA, but it is necessary once cohesion has been established. It has been shown that an important function of Eco1 is the acetylation of cohesin on two lysine residues that are located in the ATPase head of the SMC3 domain. Mutations of lysine residues in yeast to non-acetylated amino acid residues caused defects in cohesion [44, 45].

In this study, a putative premature loss of sister kinetochores and chromatid cohesion may be the cause of the *frying pan-shaped* chromosomes.

Finally, as a result of these meiotic errors in prophase II, aberrant anaphase II showed stretched bridges which at the end produced unbalanced meiotic end products: pollen grains (**Figures 6** and 7).

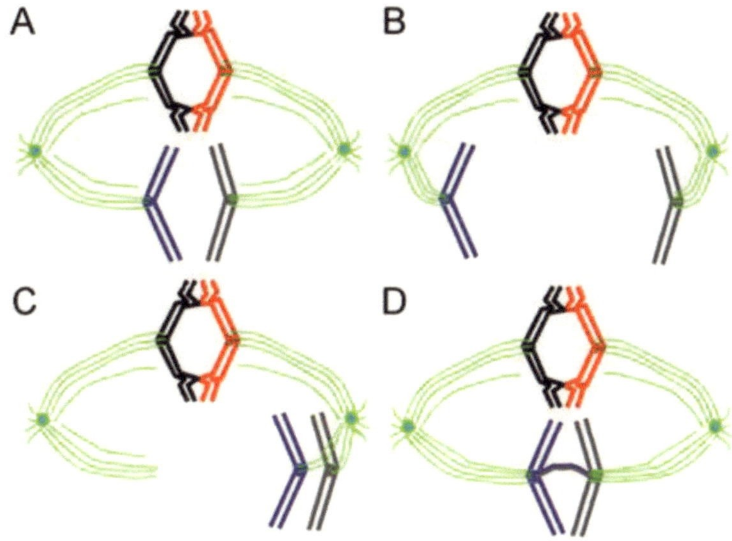

Figure 6. Model for achiasmate chromosome segregation. (A) Chiasmate homologs (red and black) are locked together by crossovers, whereas the sister chromatids are held together by cohesins (not shown). Achiasmate homologs (blue and gray) are not locked together by crossovers. Spindle (green) attachments to kinetochores (solid circles) are stabilized by tension created by pulling forces that draw chiasmate homologs to opposite poles. (B) Achiasmate chromosomes were thought not to be locked with their homologs and are able to move prematurely to one or the other spindle pole. (C) As shown by Hughes et al. [35], achiasmate homologs can be found on the same side of the metaphase plate. This is the first demonstration that this configuration can occur, and it suggests that achiasmate homologs can move in unison. (D) In addition, heterochromatic DNA threads between achiasmate homologs can be observed. These threads may provide chiasma-like function that lock homologs together and allow tension to be established between these nonexchange homologs. This tension is used by spindle forces to move achiasmate chromosomes along the spindle, orient them, make them join the mass of chiasmate chromosomes congressed at the metaphase plate, and ultimately ensures proper segregation). *Source:* Bosco [34]. With permission of Dr. Giovani Bosco.

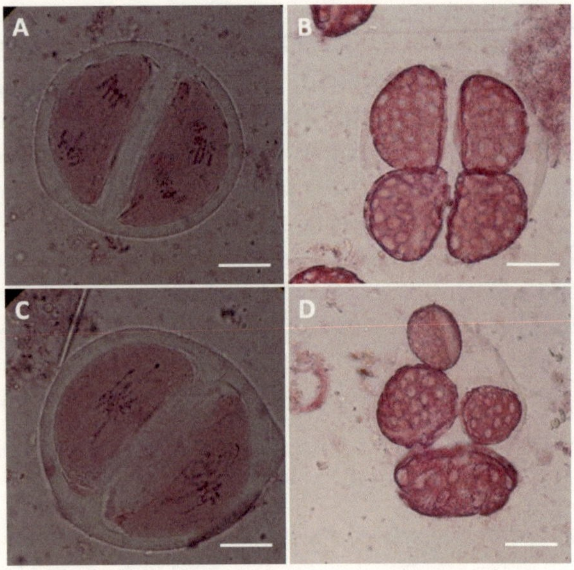

Figure 7. Consequences of normal and abnormal Meiosis II in *Agave angustifolia*. (A and B) Normal anaphase II producing normal pollen grains. (C and D) Abnormal anaphase II as a product of the abnormal sister chromatids behavior showed in **Figure 4**. Unbalanced products (pollen grains) are produced with a high and low genetic load. White bar = 20 μm.

As the main conclusion of this study, a hypothesis rises from the described observations: *frying pan-shaped* chromosomes are formed by sister chromatid exchanges and a premature kinetochore movement in prophase II, which are meiotic aberrations that exist in these phylogenetic distant species, *Agave stricta* and *A. angustifolia* since ancient times in their evolution, and this may be due to genes that are prone to act under diverse kinds of environmental stress [46].

Acknowledgements

This article was published with funds from Fideicomiso 2017 Centro de Investigación y Asistencia en Tecnología y Diseño del Estado de Jalisco (CIATEJ). The author thanks J.M. Rodríguez-Domínguez, J.R. Trinidad-Cruz, B. Tirado-Pérez, and A.M. Barranco Guzmán for reviewing the manuscript and helpful suggestions, and H. Rodríguez-Julián for the artwork of **Figures 3** and **4**.

Author details

Benjamín Rodríguez-Garay

Address all correspondence to: brodriguez@ciatej.mx

Plant Biotechnology Unit, Research Center for Assistance in Technology and Design of the State of Jalisco, El Bajío del Arenal, Zapopan, Jalisco, México

References

[1] Gentry HS. Agaves of Continental North America. Tucson, Arizona: The University of Arizona Press; 1982. p. 670

[2] Good-Avila SV, Souza V, Gaut BS, Eguiarte LE. Timing and rate of speciation in Agave (Agavaceae). Proceedings of the National Academy of Sciences of the United States of America. 2006;**103**:9124-9129. DOI: 10.1073/pnas.0603312103

[3] EguiarteLE, Souza V, Silva-Montellano A. Evolucion de la familia Agavaceae: filogenia, biología reproductiva y genetica de poblaciones. Boletín de la Sociedad Botánica de México. 2000;**66**:131-150

[4] Rodríguez-Garay B. Somatic embryogenesis in *Agave* spp. In: Loyola-Vargas VM, Ochoa-Alejo N, editors. Somatic Embryogenesis: Fundamental Aspects and Applications. Switzerland: Springer International Publishing AG; 2016.pp. 267-282. DOI: 10.1007/978- 3-319-33705-0_16

[5] Ruvalcaba-Ruiz D, Rodríguez-Garay B. Aberrant meiotic behavior in *Agave tequilana* Weber var. azul. BMC Plant Biology. 2002;**2**:10. DOI: 10.1186/1471-2229-2-10

[6] Obledo EN, Barragán-Barragán LB, Porfirio Gutiérrez-González, Ramírez-Hernández BC, Ramírez JJ, Rodríguez-Garay B. Increased photosynthetic efficiency generated by fungal symbiosis in *Agave victoria-reginae*. Plant Cell, Tissue and Organ Culture. 2003;**74**:237-241. DOI: 10.1023/A:1024046925472

[7] Li W, Ma H. Gametophyte development. Current Biology. 2002;**12**:R718-R721. DOI: http://dx.doi.org/10.1016/S0960-9822(02)01245-9

[8] Haig D. New perspectives on the angiosperm female gametophyte. Botanical Review. 1990;**56**:236-274. DOI: 10.1007/BF02858326

[9] Fan YF, Jiang L, Gong HQ, Liu CM. Sexual reproduction in higher plants I: fertilization and the initiation of zygotic program. Journal of Integrative Plant Biology. 2008;**50**:860-867. DOI: 10.1111/j.1744-7909.2008.00705.x

[10] Ma H, Sundaresan V. Development of flowering plant gametophytes. Current Topics in Developmental Biology. 2010;**91**:379-412. DOI: 10.1016/S0070-2153(10)91013-2.2010

[11] Yadegari R, Drews GN. Female gametophyte development. Plant Cell. 2004;**16**:S133–S141. DOI: http://dx.doi.org/10.1105/tpc.018192

[12] Farmer JB, Moore JES. On the meiotic phase (reduction divisions) in animals and plants. Journal of Cell Science. 1905;**s2-48**:489-558

[13] Gómez-Rodríguez VM, Rodríguez-Garay B, Barba-Gonzalez R. Meiotic restitution mechanisms involved in the formation of 2n pollen in *Agave tequilana* Weber and *Agave angustifolia* Haw. SpringerPlus. 2012;**1**:17. DOI: 10.1186/2193-1801-1-17

[14] Petronczki M, Simons MF, Nasmyth K. Un Ménage à Quatre: The molecular biology of chromosome segregation in meiosis. Cell. 2002;**112**:423-440. http://dx.doi.org/10.1016/S0092-8674(03)00083-7

[15] Mc Cormick S. Control of male gametophyte development. Plant Cell. 2004; **16**:S142–S153. http://dx.doi.org/10.1105/tpc.016659

[16] Gutiérrez-Mora A, González-Gutiérrez AG, Rodríguez-Garay B, Ascencio-Cabral A, Li-Wei L. Plant somatic embryogenesis: Some useful considerations. In: Sato K, editor. Embryogenesis. Rijeka, Croatia: InTech; 2012. pp. 229-248. DOI: 10.5772/36345

[17] Tanaka K, Watanabe Y. 2007. Sister chromatid cohesion and centromere organization in meiosis. In: Egel R, Lankenau D.-H, editors. Recombination and Meiosis. Genome Dyn Stab 2. Berlin Heidelberg: Springer-Verlag; 2007. pp. 57-79. DOI: 10.1007/7050_2007_027/ Published online: 23 June 2007

[18] Roeder GS. Meiotic chromosomes: It takes two to tango. Genes & Development. 1997;**11**: 2600-2621. DOI:10.1101/gad.11.20.2600

[19] Loidl J, Nairz K. Karyotype variability in yeast caused by nonallelic recombination in haploid meiosis. Genetics.1997;**146**:79-88

[20] Bickel SE, Orr-Weaver TL. Holding chromatids together to ensure they go their separate ways. BioEssays. 1996;**18**(4):293-300. DOI: 10.1002/bies.950180407

[21] Zamariola L, Tiang CL, De Storme N, Pawlowski W, Geelen D. Chromosome segregation in plant meiosis. Frontiers in Plant Science. 2014;**5**:279. DOI: 10.3389/fpls.2014.00279

[22] Remeseiro S, Losada A. Cohesin, a chromatin engagement ring. Current Opinion in Cell Biology. 2013;**25**(1):63-71. http://dx.doi.org/10.1016/j.ceb.2012.10.013

[23] De K, Sterle L, Krueger L, Yang X, Makaroff CA. Arabidopsis thaliana WAPL is essential for the prophase removal of cohesin during meiosis. PLoS Genetics. 2014;**10**(7):e1004497. DOI:10.1371/journal.pgen.1004497

[24] Yuan L, Yang X, Christopher A. Makaroff CA. Plant cohesins, common themes and unique roles. Current Protein & Peptide Science. 2011;**12**(2):93-104. DOI: 10.2174/138920311795684904

[25] Peters JM, Nishiyama T. Sister chromatid cohesion. Cold Spring Harbor Perspectives in Biology. 2012;**4**:a011130. DOI: 10.1101/cshperspect.a011130

[26] Yamagishi Y, Sakuno T, Goto Y, Watanabe Y. Kinetochore composition and its function: Lessons from yeasts. FEMS Microbiology Reviews. 2014;**38**:185-200. DOI: http://dx.doi.org/10.1111/1574-6976.12049

[27] Yu HG, Dawe RK, Hiatt EN, Dawe RK. The plant kinetochore. Trends in Plant Science. 2000;**5**:543-547. DOI: http://dx.doi.org/10.1016/S1360-1385(00)01789-1

[28] Pinkava DJ, Baker MA. Chromosome and hybridization studies of Agaves. Desert Plants. 1985;**7**:93-100. http://hdl.handle.net/10150/554212

[29] Moreno-Salazar SF, Esqueda M, Martínez J, Palomino G. Tamaño del genoma y cariotipo en *Agave angustifolia* y *A. rhodacantha* de Sonora, México. Revista Fitotécnia Mexicana. 2007;**30**(1):13-23. http://www.revistafitotecniamexicana.org/30-1.html

[30] Palomino G, Martínez J, Méndez I, Cepeda-Cornejo V, Barba-González R,Rodríguez-Garay B. Nuclear genome size and cytotype analysis in *Agave parviflora* Torr subsp. flexiflora Gentry & Berger (Asparagales, Asparagaceae).Caryologia. 2015;**68**(3):159-168. http://dx.doi.org/10.1080/00087114.2015.1032575

[31] Cave MS. Cytological observations on some genera of the Agavaceae. Madroño. 1964; **17**:163-170

[32] Brandham PE. Inversion heterozygosity and sub-chromatid exchanges in *Agave stricta*. Chromosoma. 1969;**26**:270-286. DOI: 10.1007/BF00326522

[33] Doughty LR. Chromosome behaviour in relation to genetics of *Agave*. I. Seven species of fibre agave. Journal of Genetics. 1936;**33**(2):198-205. DOI: 10.1007/BF02982532

[34] Bosco G. When segregation hangs by a thread. PLoS Genetics. 2009;**5**(2):e1000371. DOI:10.1371/journal.pgen.1000371

[35] Hughes SE, Gilliland WD, Cotitta JL, Takeo S, Collins KA, et al. Heterochromatic threads connect oscillating chromosomes during prometaphase I in Drosophila Oocytes. PLoS Genetics. 2009;**5**(1):e1000348. DOI:10.1371/journal.pgen.1000348

[36] Puchta H. The repair of double-strand breaks in plants: mechanisms and consequences for genome evolution. Journal of Experimental Botany. 2005;**56**:1-14. DOI:10.1093/jxb/eri025

[37] González-Barrera S, Cortés-Ledesma F, Wellinger RE, Aguilera A. Equal sister chromatid exchange is a major mechanism of Double-Strand break repair in yeast. Molecular Cell. 2003;**11**:1661-1671. DOI: http://dx.doi.org/10.1016/S1097-2765(03)00183-7

[38] Rodríguez-Garay B, Gutiérrez-Mora M,González-Gutiérrez AG. Climate change reaches the tequila country. In: Gutiérrez-Mora A, editor. Rodríguez-Garay B, Contreras-Ramos SM, Kirchmayr MR, González-Ávila M (Comps.). Sustainable and Integral Exploitation of Agave; 2014. ISBN: 978-607-96619-1-5. Published online: December 22, 2014. DOI: 10.13140/RG.2.1.2524.6882

[39] Paital B, Panda SK, Hati AK, Mohanty B, Mohapatra MK, Kanungo S, Chainy GBN. Longevity of animals under reactive oxygen species stress and disease susceptibility due to global warming. World Journal of Biological Chemistry. 2016;**7**(1):110-127. DOI: http://dx.doi.org/10.4331/wjbc.v7.i1.110

[40] Perkinsa AT, Dasa TM, Panzeraa LC, Bickela SE. Oxidative stress in oocytes during midprophase induces premature loss of cohesion and chromosome segregation errors. Proceedings of the National Academy of Sciences of the United States of America. 2016;**113**(44):E6823–E6830. DOI: 10.1073/pnas.1612047113

[41] Clift D, Marston AL. The role of shugoshin in meiotic chromosome segregation. Cytogenetic and Genome Research. 2011;**133**:234-242. DOI: 10.1159/000323793

[42] Hamant O, Golubovskaya I, Meeley R, Fiume E, Timofejeva L, Schleiffer A, Nasmyth K, Cande WZ. A REC8-dependent plant shugoshin is required for maintenance of centromeric cohesion during meiosis and has no mitotic functions. Current Biology. 2005;**15**:948-954. DOI: 10.1016/j.cub.2005.04.049

[43] Unal E, Heidinger-Pauli JM, Koshland D. DNA double-strand breaks trigger genome-wide sister-chromatid cohesion through Eco1 (Ctf7). Science. 2007;**317**:245-248. DOI: 10.1126/science.1140637

[44] Ben-Shahar TR, Heeger S, Lehane C, East P, Flynn, H, Skehel M, Uhlmann F. Eco1-dependent cohesin acetylation during establishment of sister chromatid cohesion. Science. 2008;**321**:563-566. DOI: 10.1126/science.1157774

[45] Unal E, Heidinger-Pauli J.M, Kim W, Guacci V, Onn I, Gygi SP, Koshland DE. A molecular determinant for the establishment of sister chromatid cohesion. Science. 2008;**321**:566-569. DOI: 10.1126/science.1157880

[46] Harrison CJ, Alvey E, Henderson IR. Meiosis in flowering plants and other green organisms. Journal of Experimental Botany. 2010;**61**(11):2863-2875. DOI:10.1093/jxb/erq191